PHLEBOTOMY WORKBOOK FOR THE MULTISKILLED HEALTHCARE PROFESSIONAL

D0074432

PHLEBOTOMY WORKBOOK FOR THE MULTISKILLED HEALTHCARE PROFESSIONAL

Susan King Strasinger, DA, MT(ASCP)
Director
Medical Laboratory Technician Program
Northern Virginia Community College
Annandale, Virginia

Marjorie A. Di Lorenzo, MT(ASCP)SH
Associate Faculty
Medical Assisting Program
Allan Hancock College
Santa Maria, California

Indiana University
Library
Northwest

RB
45.15
.S7
1996

Illustrations by: Mary Butters
Photography by: Frankie Harris-Lyne, CLS(NCA)
    Instructor
    Medical Laboratory Technician Program
    Northern Virginia Community College
    Annandale, Virginia

 F. A. DAVIS COMPANY • Philadelphia

WP

F. A. Davis Company
1915 Arch Street
Philadelphia, PA 19103

Copyright © 1996 by F. A. Davis Company

All rights reserved. This book is protected by copyright. No part of it may be reproduced, stored in a retrieval system, or transmitted in any form or by any means, electronic, mechanical, photocopying, recording, or otherwise, without written permission from the publisher.

Printed in the United States of America

Last digit indicates print number: 10 9 8 7 6 5 4 3 2

Publisher: Jean-François Vilain
Developmental Editor: Ralph Zickgraf
Production Editor: Marianne Fithian
Cover Designer: Steven R. Morrone

As new scientific information becomes available through basic and clinical research, recommended treatments and drug therapies undergo changes. The author(s) and publisher have done everything possible to make this book accurate, up to date, and in accord with accepted standards at the time of publication. The authors, editors, and publisher are not responsible for errors or omissions or for consequences from application of the book, and make no warranty, expressed or implied, in regard to the contents of the book. Any practice described in this book should be applied by the reader in accordance with professional standards of care used in regard to the unique circumstances that may apply in each situation. The reader is advised always to check product information (package inserts) for changes and new information regarding dose and contraindications before administering any drug. Caution is especially urged when using new or infrequently ordered drugs.

Authorization to photocopy items for internal use, or the internal or personal use of specific clients, is granted by F. A. Davis Company for users registered with the Copyright Clearance Center (CCC) Transactional Reporting Service, provided that the fee of $.10 per copy is paid directly to CCC, 222 Rosewood Drive, Danvers, MA 01923. For those organizations that have been granted a photocopy license by CCC, a separate system of payment has been arranged. The fee code for users of the Transactional Reporting Service is: 8036-8107/96 0 + $.10.

TO HARRY, MY EDITOR-IN-CHIEF
SKS

TO MY HUSBAND, SCOTT; MY SONS, MICHAEL AND CHRISTOPHER; MY PARENTS, ART AND CHARLOTTE SCHAUB; AND MY PARENTS-IN-LAW, RAY AND GLADYS DI LORENZO FOR THEIR LOVE, PATIENCE, AND CONSTANT SUPPORT IN THIS ENDEAVOR
MAD

Preface

The *Phlebotomy Workbook for the Multiskilled Healthcare Professional* and its *Instructor's Guide* are designed to meet a variety of phlebotomy training needs. These include formal phlebotomy certification programs, medical laboratory technician and medical technologist programs, medical assisting programs, and the cross-training of nurses and other allied health personnel.

The workbook format lends itself to traditional college classroom lectures, in-house training programs, and independent study for certification examinations and employee continuing education. To provide flexibility, the text is divided into three sections covering (I) general phlebotomy and healthcare information, (II) anatomy and physiology related to phlebotomy and laboratory testing, and (III) phlebotomy techniques. Chapters in Sections I and II are essentially self-contained and can be inserted into a training program at the discretion of the instructor.

The workbook integrates specific objectives, medical terminology with key terms and abbreviations, the anatomy and physiology of body systems, laboratory tests and their clinical correlations with disorders, safety and special handling procedures, phlebotomy theory and practical techniques, interpersonal skills, and quality assurance related to total quality management and continuous quality improvement.

Assessment tools, including study questions, are intended to reinforce key information. Also included are practical situation exercises and test performance evaluation forms for individual procedures. These assessment tools are printed on perforated pages, with space for written answers and notes, so that they can be torn out and handed in as homework or tests. Numerous illustrations, photographs, diagrams, charts, and tables are included to visually enhance learning.

To ease the burden on overworked instructors, the *Instructor's Guide* contains lecture outlines, answers to study questions and practical exercises, suggested audiovisual aids and their sources, additional evaluation forms, sample course schedules, individual chapter tests, and a comprehensive examination.

The *Phlebotomy Workbook for the Multiskilled Healthcare Professional* is written to comply with the guidelines established by national certifying organizations and the essentials published by the National Accrediting Agency for Clinical Laboratory Science (NAACLS). All procedures are written in accordance with the standards developed by the National Committee for Clinical Laboratory Sciences (NCCLS) and the Occupational Safety and Health Administration (OSHA), enabling this text to be used as a reference in any healthcare setting.

Acknowledgments

We are indebted to many wonderful people who aided us in our coast-to-coast endeavor to produce this workbook. First, we want to thank our families for their understanding and support, especially our husbands, for the many hours they spent at their computers and Ray Di Lorenzo for his dedication and artistic talent that provided the basis for many of the illustrations.

Without the computer and artistic expertise of Mary Butters and the photography skills of Frankie Harris-Lyne the book, as we envisioned it, would not have been possible.

The laboratory personnel at Fauquier Hospital and Prince William Hospital were most helpful in providing us with technical expertise and photographic opportunities. We are particularly grateful to Anita Sutherland, MT(ASCP), for being consistently available to provide information and to organize or participate in the photographic components.

We also appreciate the encouragement of Jean-François Vilain, Ralph Zickgraf, and Ona Kosmos from F. A. Davis and the valuable suggestions from our reviewers, including: Marilyn Barbour, MT(CLS), Indian River Community College, Fort Pierce, Florida; Suzanne W. Conner, MA, CLDir(NCA), Coop Medical Technical Program of Akron; Patricia S. Hurlbut, CMA, MT(ASCP), Waukesha County Technical Institute, Pewaukee, Wisconsin; Janice G. Lareau, MS, MT(ASCP)SH, Indiana University Northwest; and Jay W. Wilborn, MEd, MT(ASCP), Garland County Community College, Hot Springs, Arkansas.

Contents

Section I **Phlebotomy and the Healthcare Field** **1**

Chapter 1 **Introduction to Phlebotomy** **3**
Learning Objectives 3
Terminology 3
    Key Terms 3
    Abbreviations 4
Duties of the Phlebotomist 5
Desirable Personal Characteristics
    for Phlebotomists 5
Phlebotomy Education and Certification 7
Ethical and Legal Aspects of Phlebotomy 8
    Patient's Bill of Rights 8
    Legal Issues 10
Bibliography 10
Study Questions 11

Chapter 2 **Basic Medical Terminology** **15**
Learning Objectives 15
Commonly Used Prefixes 15
Commonly Used Suffixes 16
General Medical Abbreviations 17
Bibliography 18
Study Questions 19

Chapter 3 **Healthcare Delivery System** **23**
Learning Objectives 23
Terminology 23
    Roots/Combining Forms 23
    Key Terms 23
    Abbreviations 24
Hospital Organization 24

Professional Service Departments 26
    Radiology 27
    Radiation Therapy 27
    Nuclear Medicine 27
    Occupational Therapy 27
    Pharmacy 27
    Physical Therapy 27
    Respiratory Therapy 27
    Clinical Laboratory 27
Clinical Laboratory Personnel 28
    Laboratory Director (Pathologist) 28
    Laboratory Manager (Administrator) 29
    Section Supervisor 29
    Medical Technologist 30
    Medical Laboratory Technician 30
    Phlebotomist 30
Regulation of Clinical Laboratories 30
Healthcare Settings 31
Bibliography 32
Study Questions 33

Chapter 4   **Clinical Laboratory Sections** **37**
Learning Objectives 37
Hematology Section 37
    Terminology Associated with the Hematology Section 37
    Specimen Collection and Handling 38
    Tests Performed in the Hematology Section 39
    Coagulation Area of the Hematology Section 40
    Tests Performed in the Coagulation Area of
      the Hematology Section 40
Chemistry Section 42
    Terminology Associated with the Chemistry Section 42
    Specimen Collection and Handling 44
    Tests Performed in the Chemistry Section 44
Blood Bank Section 45
    Terminology Associated with the Blood Bank Section 45
    Specimen Collection and Handling 47
    Tests Performed in the Bood Bank Section 47
Serology (Immunology) Section 48
    Terminology Associated with the Serology
      (Immunology) Section 48
    Specimen Collection 49
    Tests Performed in the Serology (Immunology) Section 49

Microbiology Section 49
   Terminology Associated with the Microbiology Section 49
   Specimen Collection and Handling 51
   Tests Performed in the Microbiology Section 51
Urinalysis Section 52
   Terminology Associated with the Urinalysis Section 52
   Specimen Collection and Handling 54
   Test Performed in the Urinalysis Section 54
Bibliography 54
Study Questions 55

Chapter 5   **Safety** **61**
Learning Objectives 61
Terminology 61
   Key Terms 61
   Abbreviations 62
Biologic Hazards 62
   Handwashing 63
   Isolation Procedures 64
   Personal Protective Equipment 64
   Universal Precautions 65
Sharp Hazards 66
Chemical Hazards 67
Radioactive Hazards 68
Electrical Hazards 69
Fire/Explosive Hazards 69
Physical Hazards 70
Bibliography 70
Study Questions 71
Laboratory Safety Exercise 75

Section II   **Body Systems (Anatomy, Physiology, and Terminology)** **77**

Chapter 6   **Introduction to the Body and Integumentary System** **79**
Learning Objectives 79
Introduction to the Body 79
   Terminology 79
Directional Terms 80

Body Planes 81
Body Cavities 81
Body Systems 82
Integumentary System 83
   Terminology Associated with the
      Integumentary System 83
Function 83
Components of the Integumentary System 84
Disorders Associated with the
      Integumentary System 85
   Acne 85
   Fungal Infections 85
   Impetigo 85
   Keloid 85
   Psoriasis 85
   Skin Cancer 85
Laboratory Tests 86
Bibliography 86
Study Questions 87

Chapter 7   **Circulatory and Lymphatic Systems** **89**
Learning Objectives 89
Circulatory System 89
   Terminology Associated with the Circulatory System 89
Function 91
Blood Vessels 91
Heart 93
   Pathway of Blood Through the Heart 94
Blood 97
   Erythrocytes 97
   Leukocytes 98
      Neutrophils 99
      Lymphocytes 99
      Monocytes 99
      Eosinophils 99
      Basophils 100
   Thrombocytes 100
Coagulation 100
   Primary Hemostasis 100
   Secondary Hemostasis 100
   Fibrinolysis 100

Disorders Associated with the
   Circulatory System 101
     Blood Vessels 101
      Aneurysm 101
      Atherosclerosis 101
      Varicose Veins 101
     Heart 102
      Bacterial Endocarditis 102
      Congestive Heart Failure 102
      Myocardial Infarction 102
      Pericarditis 102
      Rheumatic Heart Disease 102
     Blood 102
      Anemia 102
      Leukemia 102
      Polycythemia 102
     Coagulation 102
      Disseminated Intravascular Coagulation 102
      Hemophilia 102
      Thrombocytopenia 102
   Laboratory Tests 103
   Lymphatic System 103
     Terminology Associated with the Lymphatic System 103
   Function 104
   Components of the Lymphatic System 104
   The Immune System 105
   Disorders Associated with the
     Lymphatic System 107
     Acquired Immunodeficiency Syndrome 107
     Hodgkin's Disease 107
     Infectious Mononucleosis 107
     Lymphoma 107
     Multiple Myeloma 107
   Laboratory Tests 107
   Bibliography 108
   Study Questions 109

Chapter 8   **Skeletal and Muscular Systems** **113**
   Learning Objectives 113
   Skeletal System 113
     Terminology Associated with the Skeletal System 113
   Function 114

Bone Composition 115
Bone Types 115
Joints 115
Disorders Associated with the Skeletal System 115
    Bone Fractures 115
    Gout 117
    Lyme Disease 117
    Osteoma 117
    Osteomalacia 117
    Osteomyelitis 117
    Osteoporosis 117
    Paget's Disease 117
    Rheumatoid Arthritis 118
    Scoliosis 118
    Spina Bifida 118
    Systemic Lupus Erythematosus 118
Laboratory Tests 118
Muscular System 118
    Terminology Associated with the Muscular System 118
Function 119
Muscle Types 119
Disorders Associated with the Muscular System 121
    Carpal Tunnel Syndrome 121
    Muscular Dystrophy 121
    Myasthenia Gravis 121
    Poliomyelitis 121
Laboratory Tests 122
Bibliography 122
Study Questions 123

Chapter 9   **Nervous and Respiratory Systems** **125**
Learning Objectives 125
Nervous System 125
    Terminology Associated with the Nervous System 125
Function 127
Structure 127
Peripheral Nervous System 127
Central Nervous System 129
Disorders Associated with the Nervous System 129
    Alzheimer's Disease 129
    Amyotrophic Lateral Sclerosis 129
    Bell's Palsy 129

Cerebral Palsy 129
Cerebrovascular Accident 130
Epilepsy 130
Meningitis 130
Multiple Neurofibromatosis 130
Multiple Sclerosis 130
Parkinson's Disease 130
Shingles 130
Laboratory Tests 130
Respiratory System 131
Terminology Associated with the Respiratory System 131
Function 132
Components of the Respiratory System 132
Disorders Associated with the
  Respiratory System 134
Asthma 134
Bronchitis 134
Chronic Obstructive Pulmonary Disease 134
Emphysema 134
Infant Respiratory Distress Syndrome 134
Lung Cancer 134
Pleurisy 135
Pneumonia 135
Pulmonary Edema 135
Strep Throat 135
Tuberculosis 135
Upper Respiratory Infection 135
Laboratory Tests 135
Bibliography 135
Study Questions 137

Chapter 10   Digestive and Urinary Systems **141**

Learning Objectives 141
Digestive System 141
Terminology Associated with the Digestive System 141
Function 143
Components of the Digestive System 143
Disorders Associated with the Digestive System 143
Appendicitis 143
Cholecystitis 144
Cirrhosis 144
Colitis 144

Crohn's Disease 145
Gastroenteritis 145
Hepatitis 145
Pancreatitis 145
Peritonitis 145
Ulcer 145
Laboratory Tests 145
Urinary System 146
Terminology Associated with the Urinary System 146
Function 146
Components of the Urinary System 147
Urine Formation 149
Disorders Associated with the Urinary System 149
Cystitis 149
Glomerulonephritis 149
Pyelonephritis 149
Renal Calculi 149
Renal Failure 150
Urinary Tract Infection 150
Laboratory Tests 150
Bibliography 150
Study Questions 151

Chapter 11   Endocrine and Reproductive Systems **155**
Learning Objectives 155
Endocrine System 155
Terminology Associated with the Endocrine System 155
Function 157
Endocrine Glands 157
Disorders Associated with the Endocrine System 159
Acromegaly 159
Addison's Disease 159
Cushing's Disease 159
Diabetes Insipidus 160
Diabetes Mellitus 160
Dwarfism 161
Gigantism 161
Graves' Disease 161
Hyperinsulinism 161
Hypoglycemia 161
Myxedema 161
Laboratory Tests 161

Reproductive System 161
   Terminology Associated with the Reproductive System 161
Function 163
Components of the Reproductive System 163
Disorders Associated with the
   Reproductive System 165
   Carcinoma 165
   Endometriosis 165
   Fibroids 165
   Pelvic Inflammatory Disease 165
   Premenstrual Syndrome 166
   Sexually Transmitted Diseases 166
   Toxic Shock Syndrome 166
Laboratory Tests 166
Bibliography 166
Study Questions 167

Section III   Phlebotomy Techniques 171

Chapter 12   Venipuncture Equipment 173
Learning Objectives 173
Terminology 173
   Key Terms 173
   Abbreviations 173
Organization of Equipment 174
Needles 175
Needle Disposal Systems 176
Needle Adapters 176
Collection Tubes 178
   Principles of Color-Coded Tubes 179
   Order of Draw 182
Syringes 185
Winged Infusion Sets 185
Tourniquets 185
Puncture Site Protection Supplies 187
Additional Supplies 187
Bibliography 187
Study Questions 189
Venipuncture Equipment Selection Exercise 193
Evaluation of Equipment Selection and Assembly 195

Chapter 13 Routine Venipuncture **197**

Learning Objectives 197
Terminology 197
    Key Terms 197
Requisitions 198
Greeting the Patient 199
Patient Identification 200
Patient Preparation and Positioning 201
Equipment Assembly 202
Tourniquet Application 202
Site Selection 203
Cleansing the Site 206
Examination of Puncture Equipment 207
Performing the Venipuncture 207
Removal of the Needle 210
Disposal of the Needle 211
Labeling the Tubes 211
Bandaging the Patient's Arm 212
Leaving the Patient 212
Completing the Venipuncture Procedure 212
Summary of Venipuncture Technique with a
    Vacuum Tube 213
Bibliography 213
Study Questions 215
Evaluation of Tourniquet Application and
    Vein Selection 219
Evaluation of Venipuncture Technique Using an
    Evacuated Tube 221

Chapter 14 Venipuncture Complications **223**

Learning Objectives 223
Terminology 223
    Key Terms 223
    Abbreviation 224
Requisitions 224
Greeting the Patient 224
Patient Identification 225
Patient Preparation 225
Equipment Assembly 226

Tourniquet Application 226
Site Selection 227
   Areas to Be Avoided 227
   Using Central Venous Catheters 228
Cleansing the Site 229
Examination of Puncture Equipment 229
Performing the Venipuncture 229
   Using a Syringe 229
   Using a Butterfly 230
   Complications 230
   Hemolyzed Specimens 232
Removal of the Needle 233
Disposal of the Needle 233
Labeling the Tubes 233
Bandaging the Patient's Arm 234
Leaving the Patient 234
Completing the Venipuncture Procedure 234
Bibliography 234
Study Questions 235
Venipuncture Complications Exercise 239
Evaluation of Venipuncture Technique
   Using a Syringe 243
Evaluation of Venipuncture Technique
   Using a Butterfly 245

Chapter 15   **Special Venipuncture Collection** **247**
Learning Objectives 247
Terminology 247
   Key Terms 247
   Abbreviations 248
Fasting Specimens 248
Timed Specimens 248
   Two-Hour Postprandial Glucose 249
   Glucose Tolerance Test 249
   Diurnal Variation 250
   Therapeutic Drug Monitoring 250
Blood Cultures 250
Special Specimen Handling Procedures 252
   Cold Agglutinins 252
   Chilled Specimens 252

Specimens Sensitive to Light 252
Legal (Forensic) Specimens 252
Bibliography 254
Study Questions 255
Special Venipuncture Collection Exercise 257
Evaluation of Blood Culture Collection Technique 259

Chapter 16   Dermal Puncture **261**

Learning Objectives 261
Terminology 261
Key Terms 261
Composition of Capillary Blood 262
Dermal Puncture Equipment 262
Skin Puncture Devices 263
Microspecimen Containers 264
Capillary Tubes 264
Micropipets 265
Microcollection Tubes 265
Micropipet and Dilution System 265
Additional Dermal Puncture Supplies 266
Dermal Puncture Procedure 267
Phlebotomist Preparation 267
Patient Identification and Preparation 267
Site Selection 267
Heel Puncture Sites 268
Finger Puncture Sites 268
Summary of Dermal Puncture Site Selection 269
Cleansing the Site 269
Performing the Puncture 270
Specimen Collection 270
Order of Draw 271
Labeling the Specimen 272
Completion of the Procedure 272
Summary of Dermal Puncture Technique 272
Bibliography 273
Study Questions 275
Dermal Puncture Exercise 279
Evaluation of a Microtainer Collection
by Heel Stick 281
Evaluation of Finger Stick on an Adult Patient 283
Evaluation of Unopette Collection on a
2-Year-Old Child 285

Chapter 17 Special Dermal Puncture **287**

Learning Objectives 287
Terminology 287
   Key Terms 287
   Abbreviations 287
Collection of Neonatal Bilirubins 288
Preparation of Blood Smears 289
Blood Smears for Malaria 290
Bleeding Time 292
Neonatal Screening 294
Ancillary (Bedside) Blood Glucose Test 296
Bibliography 296
Study Questions 297
Special Dermal Puncture Exercise 301
Evaluation of Blood Smear Preparation 303
Evaluation of Bleeding Time Technique 305
Evaluation of Neonatal Filter Paper Collection 307
Evaluation of Bedside Glucose Testing 309

Chapter 18 Arterial Blood Collection **311**

Learning Objectives 311
Terminology 311
   Key Terms 311
   Abbreviations 312
Arterial Blood Gases 312
Arterial Puncture Equipment 313
Arterial Puncture Procedure 314
   Phlebotomist Preparation 314
   Patient Preparation 315
   Site Selection 315
   Modified Allen Test 315
   Preparing the Site 316
   Performing the Puncture 316
   Completion of the Procedure 317
   Summary of Steps in the Arterial Puncture 318
Specimen Handling 318
Arterial Puncture Complications 319
Capillary Blood Gases 320
Bibliography 320
Study Questions 321

Arterial Puncture Exercise 325
Evaluation of Modified Allen Test Performance 327
Evaluation of Arterial Puncture Technique 329
Evaluation of Capillary Blood Gas Collection 331

Chapter 19 Additional Duties of the Phlebotomist **333**
Learning Objectives 333
Terminology 333
    Key Terms 333
    Abbreviations 334
Patient Instruction 334
    Urine Specimen Collection 335
    Fecal Specimen Collection 336
    Semen Specimen Collection 336
Collection of Throat Cultures 337
Blood Donor Collection 337
    Donor Selection 337
    Donor Collection 338
Collection of Sweat Electrolytes 339
Receiving and Transporting Specimens 340
Specimen Processing, Accessioning,
    and Shipping 341
Use of the Laboratory Computer 343
Bibliography 345
Study Questions 347

Chapter 20 Quality Phlebotomy **353**
Learning Objectives 353
Terminology 353
    Key Terms 353
    Abbreviations 354
Quality Assurance 354
    Procedure Manual 355
    Variables/Indicators 355
    Ordering of Tests 355
Specimen Collection 357
    Patient Identification 357
    Phlebotomy Equipment 357
    Patient Preparation 359
    Tourniquet Application 361
    Site Selection 361
    Cleansing the Site 361

Performing the Puncture 362
Disposal of Puncture Equipment 362
Transportation of Specimens 362
Specimen Processing 363
Total Quality Management 364
Bibliography 365
Study Questions 367

Index **373**

SECTION I   Phlebotomy and the Healthcare Field

CHAPTER 1

Introduction to Phlebotomy

Learning Objectives

Upon completion of this chapter, the reader will be able to:

1 Define the terms and abbreviations in this chapter.
2 State the duties of a phlebotomist.
3 Describe the importance of a professional public image for the phlebotomist.
4 Describe personal characteristics that are important in a phlebotomist.
5 Discuss the importance of communication and interpersonal skills for the phlebotomist within the laboratory, with patients, and with personnel in other departments of the hospital.
6 Discuss the purpose of formal phlebotomy education programs.
7 List the professional agencies that provide phlebotomy certification.
8 Explain how the Patient's Bill of Rights involves the phlebotomist.
9 Define ethics as applied to the laboratory profession.
10 Define medical law and state how it differs from ethics.
11 Discuss why medical ethics and medical law are necessary in the practice of medicine.
12 Give examples of how phlebotomists could be involved in medical malpractice actions.

Terminology

Key Terms	Definition
Accreditation	Process by which a program or institution documents meeting established guidelines
Assault	Attempt or threat to touch or injure another person
Battery	Unauthorized physical contact
Certification	Documentation assuring that an individual has met certain professional standards
Civil law suit	Court action between individuals, corporations, government bodies, or other organizations (compensation is monetary)
Confidentiality	Maintaining the privacy of information
Criminal law suit	Court action brought by the state for committing a crime against public welfare (punishment is imprisonment and/or a fine)
Ethics	Principles of personal and professional conduct
Informed consent	Patient's right to know the method and risks before agreeing to treatment
Invasion of privacy	Unauthorized release of information

Terminology
Continued

Key Terms	Definition
Litigation	Law suit
Malpractice	Medical care that does not meet a reasonable standard and results in harm
Negligence	Failure to perform duties according to accepted standards
Patient's Bill of Rights	Document written by the American Hospital Association stating the patient's rights during treatment
Phlebotomy	Puncture or incision into a vein to obtain blood
Professionalism	Conduct and qualities that portray a professional
Tort	Wrongful act committed by one person against another person or property

Abbreviations	Definition
AMT	American Medical Technologists
ASCLS	American Society for Clinical Laboratory Science
ASCP	American Society of Clinical Pathologists
ASPT	American Society of Phlebotomy Technicians
CEU	Continuing Education Unit
CLPlb	Certified Laboratory Phlebotomist
CPT	Certified Phlebotomy Technician
NCA	National Certification Agency for Medical Laboratory Personnel
NPA	National Phlebotomy Association
PBT	Phlebotomy Technician
RPT	Registered Phlebotomy Technician

Defined as "an incision into a vein," **phlebotomy** is one of the oldest medical procedures, dating back to the early Egyptians. The practice of "bloodletting" was used to cure disease and maintain the body in a state of well-being. Hippocrates believed that disease was caused by an excess of body fluids, including blood, bile, and phlegm and that removal of the excess would cause the body to return to or maintain a healthy state. Techniques for bloodletting included suction cup devices with lancets that pulled blood from the incision; the application of blood-sucking worms, called "leeches," to an incision; and barber surgery, in which blood from the incision produced by the barber's razor was collected in a bleeding bowl. The familiar red and white striped barber pole symbolizes this last technique and represents red blood and white bandages. Bloodletting is now called "therapeutic phlebotomy" and is used as a treatment for only a small number of blood disorders.

Currently a much more important role for phlebotomy is the collection of blood specimens for laboratory analysis to diagnose and monitor medical conditions. The use of equipment designed to minimize patient discomfort and the use of aseptic techniques have replaced the earlier practices.

Due to the increase in the number and complexity of laboratory tests and the need to increase the efficiency and cost-effectiveness of health care, phlebotomy has become a specialized area of clinical laboratory practice and has resulted in the creation of the job title "phlebotomist." This development supplements, but does not replace, the previous practice, in which the same laboratory employees collected and analyzed the specimens. Therefore, phlebotomy remains a part of laboratory training programs for analytical personnel because phlebotomists are not available at all times and in all situations.

The specialization of phlebotomy has expanded rapidly and with it the role of the phlebotomist. These changes have resulted in the need to replace on-the-job training with structured phlebotomy training programs leading to certification in phlebotomy. Phlebotomists are no longer just "taking blood" but are recognized as key players on the healthcare team.

In this expanded role the phlebotomist must have knowledge of the healthcare system, the anatomy and physiology related to laboratory testing and phlebotomy, the collection and transport requirements for tests performed in all sections of the laboratory, documentation and patient records, and the interpersonal skills needed to provide quality patient care. The phlebotomist is often the only personal contact a patient has with the laboratory and can leave a lasting impression of the quality of not only the laboratory but the entire healthcare setting.

DUTIES OF THE PHLEBOTOMIST

A phlebotomist is a person trained to obtain blood specimens by venipuncture and microtechniques. In addition to technical, clerical, and interpersonal skills, the phlebotomist must develop strong organizational skills to efficiently handle a heavy workload and maintain accuracy, often under stressful conditions.

Major duties and responsibilities of the phlebotomist include:

1   Correct identification of the patient prior to sample collection
2   Collection of the appropriate amount of blood by venipuncture or dermal puncture for the specified tests
3   Selection of the appropriate specimen containers for the specified tests
4   Correct labeling of all specimens with the required information
5   Appropriate transportation of specimens back to the laboratory in a timely manner
6   Effective interaction with patients and hospital personnel
7   Processing of specimens for delivery to the appropriate laboratory departments
8   Performance of computer operations and record keeping pertaining to phlebotomy
9   Observation of all safety regulations
10 Attendance at continuing education programs

DESIRABLE PERSONAL CHARACTERISTICS FOR PHLEBOTOMISTS

Phlebotomists are part of a service-oriented industry, and specific personal characteristics are necessary to be successful in this area.

DEPENDABILITY   Laboratory testing begins with specimen collection and relies on the phlebotomist to report to work whenever scheduled and on time.

COMPASSION   Phlebotomists deal with sick, anxious, and frightened patients every day. They must be sensitive to their needs, understand a patient's concern about a possible diagnosis or just the fear of a needle, and take the time to reassure each patient. A smile and a cheerful tone of voice are simple techniques that can put a patient more at ease.

HONESTY   The phlebotomist should never hesitate to admit a mistake, as a misidentified patient or mislabeled specimen can be critical to patient safety.

INTEGRITY   Patient **confidentiality** must be protected and patient information is never discussed with anyone who does not have a professional need to know it.

APPEARANCE   Each organization specifies the dress code it considers most appropriate, but common to all is a neat and clean appearance that portrays a professional attitude to the patient. Laboratory coats should be clean and pressed, and completely buttoned; shoes should be polished. Excessive jewelry, makeup, and perfume should not be worn, and long hair must be neatly pulled back. Personal hygiene is extremely important because of the close patient contact, and close attention should be paid to bathing, deodorants, and mouthwashes. In general, a sloppy appearance indicates a tendency toward sloppy performance.

COMMUNICATION SKILLS   Good communication skills are needed for the phlebotomist to function as the liaison between the laboratory and the patients, their family and visitors, and other healthcare personnel. The three components of communication — verbal skills, listening skills, and nonverbal skills or body language — all contribute to effective communication by the phlebotomist.

1   *Verbal skills* enable phlebotomists to introduce themselves, explain the procedure, reassure the patient, and help to assure the patient that the procedure is being competently performed. Barriers to verbal communication that must be considered include physical handicaps such as deafness, patient emotions, the level of patient education, age, and language proficiency. By recognizing these barriers the phlebotomist can be better equipped to communicate with the patient. When talking to a hearing-impaired patient it is important to speak loudly and clearly and to look directly at the patient to facilitate lip reading. Using a calm tone of voice may alleviate the fears of an emotional patient. To help the patient understand the procedure, the phlebotomist must speak to the age and educational level of the patient. Use age-appropriate phrases and avoid medical jargon by using terminology appropriate for lay persons. Every attempt should be made to locate someone who can translate for patients who do not speak the English language. Most hospitals maintain a list of interpreters.

2   *Listening skills* are a key component of communication. Allow the patient to express feelings and anxieties. Actively interact by providing appropriate feedback to let the patient know that you understand and care. Active listening involves looking directly at the patient with complete attention.

3   *Nonverbal skills* or body language include facial expressions, posture, and eye contact. Positive body language is demonstrated by a phlebotomist who walks briskly into the room, displays a smile, and looks directly at the patient while talking. This makes patients feel that they are important and you care about them and your work. Notice the phlebotomist and patient in Figure 1 – 1. Conversely, shuffling into the room, avoiding eye contact, and gazing out the window while talking are examples of negative body language and indicate boredom and disinterest in the patients and their tests.

4   *Telephone skills* are essential for phlebotomists. The phlebotomy department frequently acts as a type of switchboard for the rest of the laboratory because of its location in the central processing area of the laboratory. This is a prime example of the phlebotomist's role as a liaison for the laboratory, and poor telephone skills will affect the image of the laboratory. Phlebotomists should have a

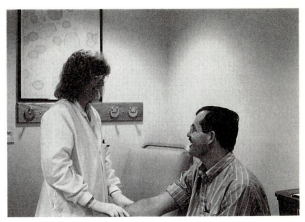

FIGURE 1–1. Phlebotomist communicating with a patient.

thorough understanding of the telephone system with regard to transferring calls, placing calls on hold, and paging personnel.

To observe the rules of proper telephone etiquette:

- Answer the phone promptly and politely, stating the name of the department and your name.
- Always check for an emergency before putting someone on hold, and return to calls that are on hold as soon as possible. This may require returning the current call after you have collected the required information.
- Keep writing materials beside the phone for recording information such as the location of emergency blood collections, requests for test results, and numbers for returning calls.
- Make every attempt to help the callers, and if you cannot help, transfer them to another person or department that can. It is also helpful to give callers the number to which you are transferring them.
- Provide accurate and consistent information by keeping current with laboratory policies, looking up information published in department manuals or asking a supervisor.
- Speak clearly and make sure you understand what the caller is asking and that the caller understands the information you are providing.

PHLEBOTOMY EDUCATION AND CERTIFICATION

Structured phlebotomy education programs have recently been developed by hospitals, community colleges, and technical institutions and have always been a part of medical laboratory technician and medical technologist programs. The length and format of these programs vary considerably; however, the goal of providing the healthcare field with phlebotomists that are knowledgeable in all aspects of phlebotomy is universal. The training programs are designed to incorporate a combination of classroom instruction and clinical practice. Most programs follow guidelines developed by national phlebotomy organizations to ensure the quality of the program, to meet national **accreditation** requirements, and to prepare graduates to sit for a national certifying examination.

Obtaining **certification** from a nationally recognized professional organization should be a goal of all phlebotomists, as it serves to enhance their position within

TABLE 1–1. **PHLEBOTOMIST CERTIFICATIONS**

Certifying Organization	Phlebotomist Designation
American Medical Technologists (**AMT**)	Registered Phlebotomy Technician, **RPT** (AMT)
American Society of Clinical Pathologists (**ASCP**)	Phlebotomy Technician, **PBT** (ASCP)
American Society of Phlebotomy Technicians (**ASPT**)	Certified Phlebotomy Technician, **CPT** (ASPT)
National Certification Agency for Medical Laboratory Personnel (**NCA**)	Clinical Laboratory Phlebotomist, **CLPlb** (NCA)
National Phlebotomy Association (**NPA**)	Certified Phlebotomy Technician, **CPT** (NPA)

the healthcare field and documents the quality of their skills and knowledge. Certification examinations can be taken by phlebotomists upon completion of a structured educational program that meets the standards of the certifying organization, or by documentation of experience that meets specified standards. Certification examinations are offered by the organizations listed in Table 1–1. After attaining a satisfactory score, phlebotomists can indicate this achievement by placing the initials of the certifying agency behind their names.

Membership in a professional organization enhances the **professionalism** of a phlebotomist by providing increased opportunities for continuing education. Professional organizations present seminars and workshops, publish journals containing information on new developments in the field, and represent the profession at state and national levels to influence regulations affecting the profession.

All healthcare professionals are expected to participate in continuing education activities. Attendance at many workshops and seminars is documented by the issuing of certificates containing continuing education units (**CEUs**). Equally important is attending staff meetings, reading pertinent memoranda, and observing notices placed on bulletin boards or in newsletters.

ETHICAL AND LEGAL ASPECTS OF PHLEBOTOMY

Principles of right and wrong called the "code of ethics" provide the personal and professional rules of performance and moral behavior as set by members of a profession. Medical **ethics** focus on the patient to assure that all members of a healthcare team possess and exhibit the skill, knowledge, training, and professionalism necessary to serve the patient. Phlebotomists are expected to follow this code by performing the duties specified in their job description, adhering to established standards of performance, and continuing to improve their knowledge and skills.

Patient's Bill of Rights

A document published by the American Hospital Association called the **Patient's Bill of Rights** specifies what the patient has a right to expect during medical treatment. A patient's rights and dignity must be protected in the process of providing quality care. The document addresses the following 12 areas:

1   Patients have the right to considerate and respectful care.
2   Patients have the right to obtain from their physician complete current information about their diagnosis, treatment, and prognosis in terms patients can be reasonably expected to understand.
3   Patients have the right to receive from a physician information necessary to

give **informed consent** prior to a procedure. The information should include knowledge of the proposed procedure, with risks and probable duration of incapacitation. In addition, the patient has a right to information about medically significant alternatives.

4   Patients have the right to refuse treatment to the extent permitted by law and to be informed of the medical consequences of their action.

5   Patients have the right to privacy in their medical care. Case discussion, consultation, examination, and treatment should be conducted discreetly. Those not directly involved with a patient's care must have the patient's permission to be present.

6   Patients have the right to expect that all communication and records pertaining to their care be treated as confidential.

7   Patients have the right to expect the hospital to make a reasonable response to their request for services and to provide evaluation, service, and referral as indicated.

8   Patients have the right to obtain information as to any relationship of their hospital with other healthcare and educational institutions, insofar as their care is concerned, and to the professional relationship among individuals who are treating them.

9   Patients have the right to be advised if the hospital proposes to engage in or perform human experimentation affecting their care or treatment. Patients have the right to refuse to participate in research projects.

10 Patients have the right to expect continuity of care, including future appointments and instructions on continuing healthcare requirements after discharge.

11 Patients have the right to examine and receive an explanation of their bill, regardless of the source of payment.

12 Patients have the right to know what hospital rules and regulations apply to their conduct as a patient.

The phlebotomist is directly involved with several sections of the Patient's Bill of Rights including:

1   Patients may be difficult to deal with because they are afraid to be in the hospital or are angry because they have just received an unfavorable diagnosis; however, the phlebotomist must still treat them with respect and consideration.

2   Notice that it is the physician not the phlebotomist that must provide information concerning the purpose of test procedures. When questioned, phlebotomists should refer the patient to their physician. Also laboratory test results are reported only to physicians or their designated representatives and are never given to patients or their family members.

4   The patient has the right to refuse to have blood drawn. If, after you have explained the procedure and explained that it was requested by the physician to provide treatment, the patient still refuses, do not forcibly obtain the sample. Notify the nursing staff or the physician of the patient's refusal and note this information on the requisition form.

5   The patient's condition and laboratory test results are confidential and must not be discussed with anyone who is not directly involved with the patient's care or testing. Do not discuss patient information in elevators or in the cafeteria where it may be overheard by bystanders.

Legal Issues

Failure to respect patients' rights can result in legal action initiated by the patient or the patient's family. Medical law regulates the conduct of members of the healthcare professions. It differs from ethics, which are recommended standards, by being legally required conduct. **Litigation** initiated as a result of illegal actions can be at the local, state, or national level and can result in criminal or civil prosecution. Penalties may include revocation of professional licenses, monetary fines, or imprisonment.

A **criminal law suit** is an action initiated by the state for committing an illegal act against the public welfare and can be punishable by imprisonment. A **civil law suit** is a court action between parties seeking monetary compensation for an offense. A wrongful act committed by one person against another is called a **tort**. The threat to touch another person without their consent is termed **assault** and the actual touching is **battery**. These are charges that could be initiated against a phlebotomist who forcibly tries to collect a sample from a patient who refuses to have blood drawn. Release of confidential information is considered an **invasion of privacy**.

Medical **malpractice** is misconduct or lack of skill by a healthcare professional that results in injury to the patient. **Negligence**, which is defined as failure to give reasonable care by the healthcare provider, must be proven. Examples of medical malpractice that could involve the phlebotomist include failure to raise a bedrail that has been lowered during the phlebotomy procedure, resulting in the patient falling out of bed; performing an unauthorized arterial puncture, producing an arteriospasm or excessive bleeding; or a misidentification of a patient or specimen, resulting in inappropriate treatment or death.

All healthcare workers should carry malpractice insurance. Most institutions have policies covering all workers, and the phlebotomist should confirm this coverage at the time of employment.

BIBLIOGRAPHY

Clerc, JM: An Introduction to Clinical Laboratory Science. CV Mosby, St. Louis, 1992.

Lewis, MA, and Tamparo, CD: Medical Law, Ethics, and Bioethics in the Medical Office, ed. 3. FA Davis, Philadelphia, 1993.

Marshall, JR: Fundamental Skills for the Clinical Laboratory Professional. Delmar Publishing, Albany, NY, 1993.

Study Questions

1. Number (1 to 5) the following developments in the history of phlebotomy in chronological order.

    a. _____ Development of structured phlebotomy training programs

    b. _____ Hippocrates' theory on the relationship between excess body fluids and disease

    c. _____ Collection of blood for diagnostic testing

    d. _____ Certification of phlebotomists

    e. _____ Appearance of the barber pole symbol

2. State a way that failure of the phlebotomist to demonstrate the following characteristics could affect the quality of patient care.

    a. Dependability _____

    _____

    _____

    b. Compassion _____

    _____

    _____

    c. Honesty _____

    _____

    _____

    d. Integrity _____

    _____

    _____

3. Why is the appearance and personal hygiene of the phlebotomist important to the patient?

    _____

    _____

    _____

4. List four barriers to effective verbal communication and state a means to overcome each.

    a. _____

    _____

    _____

    b. _____

    _____

    _____

   c. _____

     _____

     _____

   d. _____

     _____

     _____

5. State two behaviors that represent negative body language.

   a. _____

   b. _____

6. How can a phlebotomist demonstrate good telephone communication skills in the following situations?

   a. Placing a call on hold _____

     _____

     _____

   b. Providing instructions to a patient _____

     _____

     _____

   c. Receiving a request for information about a radiology procedure _____

     _____

     _____

7. Provide the name of the organization for each abbreviation and the initials used to identify phlebotomists certified by each agency.

Organization		**Initials**
a. ASCP _____		_____
b. NPA _____		_____
c. NCA _____		_____
d. ASPT _____		_____
e. AMT _____		_____

8. State an action by a phlebotomist that would violate sections 1, 2, 4, and 5 of the Patient's Bill of Rights.

   a. Section 1 _____

     _____

     _____

b. Section 2 _____

_____

_____

c. Section 4 _____

_____

_____

d. Section 5 _____

_____

_____

9. List two patient's rights that could result in a lawsuit if the phlebotomist did not observe them.

a. _____

b. _____

10. The principles of right and wrong are called _____.

11. Differentiate between a criminal and a civil law suit.

_____

_____

12. Describe two incidents that could cause a phlebotomist to be charged with negligence.

a. _____

_____

b. _____

_____

13. A phlebotomist is asked to go to the intensive care unit (ICU) to draw blood from a patient diagnosed with AIDS. The phlebotomist is very rude and abrupt with the patient. Is this an example of ethical or legal misconduct?

_____

14. A requisition for a type and crossmatch for 2 units of blood on a preoperative patient was delivered to the laboratory. The phlebotomist noted that the patient was in Room 410, Bed 1. When the phlebotomist went to Room 410, there was only one patient in the room and the phlebotomist drew blood from that patient. The Blood Bank processed the specimen and prepared Group B blood for the patient. During surgery the patient

developed symptoms consistent with a transfusion reaction after receiving 1 unit of blood. The patient's blood was retyped as Group A. What could have happened in this case? Is the phlebotomist legally responsible?

_____

_____

_____

_____

15. A hometown professional football player was admitted to the hospital for blood work. Tests to rule out cancer of the prostate were ordered. The phlebotomist obtained the blood specimens and delivered them to the lab. After work he/she excitedly told his/her friends of the famous person and the sad reason he was in the hospital. Is there anything ethically or legally wrong with this scenario? Explain your answer.

_____

_____

_____

_____

16. Informed consent is a right of the patient. Explain the role the phlebotomist has in ensuring this right.

_____

_____

_____

_____

CHAPTER 2 # Basic Medical Terminology

Learning Objectives

Upon completion of this chapter, the reader will be able to:

1 Define and state the purpose of prefixes, roots, suffixes, and combining forms.
2 Correctly form medical terms using prefixes, roots, suffixes, and combining forms.
3 State the meaning of the commonly used prefixes and suffixes and define the general medical abbreviations in this chapter.

Medical terminology is derived primarily from the classic Greek and Latin languages. However, it is not necessary to master either of these languages to obtain a solid background in basic medical terminology. Medical terms consist of combinations of three major word parts: prefixes, roots, and suffixes. The same prefixes and suffixes are frequently used with different roots; therefore, knowledge of a small number of commonly used prefixes, roots, and suffixes can provide the phlebotomist with an extensive medical vocabulary, and will provide the phlebotomist with the medical communication skills necessary for successful job performance.

Prefixes are letters or syllables added to the beginning of a root to alter its meaning. Likewise, suffixes are letters or syllables added to the end of a root to alter its meaning. In medical terminology suffixes often indicate a condition or a type of procedure.

The most commonly used prefixes and suffixes are presented in this chapter. Roots and combining forms and specific suffixes will be introduced as they pertain to the material being discussed. It will be necessary to memorize these common prefixes and suffixes. This will be easier if you relate them to terms that are already familiar to you.

Example: In medical terminology, the prefix "post-" means "after" just as it does in the term "postgraduate."

The suffix "-ectomy" means "surgical removal," and the term "tonsillectomy" is a familiar word to most people.

COMMONLY USED PREFIXES

Prefixes	Meaning
a-, an-	no, not, without
ab-	away from
ad-	toward
anti-, contra-	against

COMMONLY USED PREFIXES
Continued

Prefixes	Meaning
bi-	two
circum-, peri-	around
co-, con-	together, with
dys-	difficult, painful
ecto-, exo-, extra-	outside
endo-, intra-	inside, within
epi-	on, over
hetero-	different
homo-	same
hydro-	water
hyper-	increased
hypo-	decreased
inter-	between
iso-	equal
macro-	large
mal-	bad, ill
meta-	beyond
micro-	small
mono-, uni-	one
multi-, poly-	many
neo-	new
pan-	all
post-, retro-	after
pre-, ante-	before, in front
pseudo-	false
sub-	below
supra-, super-	above
trans-	across

COMMONLY USED SUFFIXES

Suffixes	Meaning
-algia	pain
-centesis	surgical puncture
-ectomy	surgical removal
-gram	written record
-graphy	method of recording
-ic	pertaining to
-itis	inflammation
-logist	one who studies
-logy	study of
-megaly	enlargement
-oid	like, similar to
-oma	tumor
-osis, iasis	abnormal condition
-ostomy	surgical opening

COMMONLY USED SUFFIXES
Continued

Suffixes	Meaning
-pathy	disease
-phobia	fear
-plasty	surgical repair
-scope	instrument for viewing
-scopy	visual examination
-stasis	controlling, standing still
-tome	instrument for cutting
-tomy	incision
-toxic	poison

Roots are the main part of a word and may be combined with prefixes, suffixes, or other roots. They frequently refer to body components. The combining form of a root contains a vowel, usually an "o," which is used to facilitate pronunciation when the root is combined with a word part that does not begin with a vowel.

> *Example:* The root word for "heart" is "cardi"
> The combining form is "cardi/o"
> The study of the heart is "cardiology"

Specific root words and combining forms will be listed in later chapters.

Abbreviations are used to shorten words, names, or phrases. Numerous abbreviations are used in the medical field to represent terms, names of organizations, or common medical phrases. Laboratory tests are frequently abbreviated, and phlebotomists must become familiar with these abbreviations.

General medical abbreviations are listed in this chapter, and those relating to particular hospital and laboratory areas, body systems, tests, and phlebotomy techniques are included with the appropriate chapters.

GENERAL MEDICAL ABBREVIATIONS

Abbreviations	Definition
ASAP	As soon as possible
cc, cm³	Cubic centimeter
cm	Centimeter
CPR	Cardiopulmonary resuscitation
DOA	Dead on arrival
DOB	Date of birth
Dx	Diagnosis
g, gm	Gram
Hx	History
IM	Intramuscular
IV	Intravenous
kg	Kilogram
mg	Milligram
mL	Milliliter
mm	Millimeter

GENERAL MEDICAL ABBREVIATIONS
Continued

Abbreviations	Definition
NB	Newborn
NPO	Nothing by mouth
post-op	After surgery
pre-op	Before surgery
PRN	Allowable as needed
q	Every
qh	Every hour
qid	Four times a day
QNS	Quantity nonsufficient
R/O	Rule out
Rx	Prescription/treatment
STAT	Immediately
μL	Microliter

BIBLIOGRAPHY

Gylys, BA: Medical Terminology Simplified: A Programmed Learning Approach by Body Systems. FA Davis, Philadelphia, 1993.

Gylys, BA, and Wedding, ME: Medical Terminology: A Systems Approach, ed. 3. FA Davis, 1995, Philadelphia.

Leonard, PC: Building a Medical Vocabulary. WB Saunders, Philadelphia, 1993.

Study Questions   1. To each of the commonly used prefixes add a root to form a word with which you are familiar. It does not have to be medical terminology but should represent the meaning of the prefix. See example.

a <u>TYPICAL</u>	exo _____	multi _____
ab _____	extra _____	neo _____
ad _____	hetero _____	pan _____
an _____	homo _____	peri _____
ante _____	hydro _____	poly _____
anti _____	hyper _____	post _____
bi _____	hypo _____	pre _____
circum _____	inter _____	pseudo _____
co _____	intra _____	retro _____
con _____	iso _____	sub _____
contra _____	macro _____	super _____
dys _____	mal _____	supra _____
ecto _____	meta _____	trans _____
endo _____	micro _____	uni _____
epi _____	mono _____	

2. Find 10 commonly used suffixes that you can add to a root or a combining form and create a word that is familiar to you.

a. _____

b. _____

c. _____

d. _____

e. _____

f. _____

g. _____

h. _____

i. _____

j. _____

3. Translate the following statements.

a. A **pre-op** patient must be **NPO**.

_____

_____

b. The **STAT** specimen drawn by the phlebotomist was **QNS** to **R/O** a **Dx** of heart disease.

_____

_____

_____

c. A **post-op** patient receives 25 **mg** of **IV** pain medication, **PRN**.

_____

_____

_____

4. Find a suffix

For each of the following definitions, find the suffix in the word puzzle and circle it. Suffixes may be horizontal, vertical, or diagonal, and may be spelled backward.

like _____ oid _____   surgical puncture _____

study of _____   surgical removal _____

disease _____   written record _____

pain _____   method of recording _____

poison _____   surgical repair _____

controlling _____   instrument for cutting _____

enlargement _____   surgical opening _____

tumor _____   instrument for viewing _____

inflammation _____

C	F	B	I	A	D	X	E	T	M
E	Y	W	Y	L	O	G	Y	S	A
N	T	Q	H	G	P	G	I	T	R
T	S	I	T	I	R	S	X	O	G
E	A	N	A	A	A	Y	A	X	E
S	L	A	P	T	J	M	M	I	C
I	P	H	S	I	H	O	O	C	T
S	Y	M	E	M	O	T	I	U	O
S	C	O	P	E	K	S	I	D	M
Y	L	A	G	E	M	O	H	S	Y

5. Find a definition or abbreviation
   Identify the following abbreviations or definitions and then find the answer in the word puzzle and circle it. Answers may be horizontal, vertical, or diagonal, and may be spelled backward.

   cm _____Centimeter_____   As soon as possible _____

   Dx _____   Intravenous _____

   NB _____   Four times a day _____

   mg _____   Allowable as needed _____

   R/O _____   Date of birth _____

   Immediately _____   Quantity nonsufficient _____

   Prescription _____   Nothing by mouth _____

   Before surgery _____   Cardiopulmonary resuscitation ___

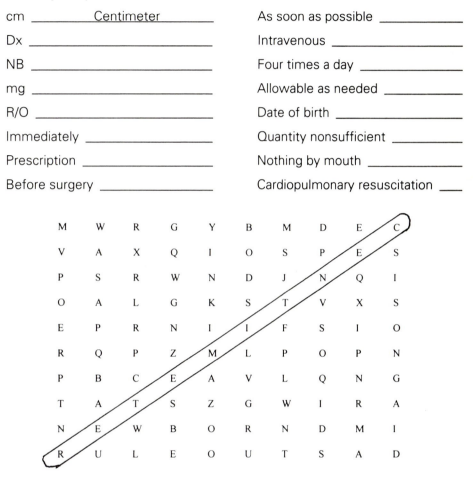

M	W	R	G	Y	B	M	D	E	C
V	A	X	Q	I	O	S	P	E	S
P	S	R	W	N	D	J	N	Q	I
O	A	L	G	K	S	T	V	X	S
E	P	R	N	I	I	F	S	I	O
R	Q	P	Z	M	L	P	O	P	N
P	B	C	E	A	V	L	Q	N	G
T	A	T	S	Z	G	W	I	R	A
N	E	W	B	O	R	N	D	M	I
R	U	L	E	O	U	T	S	A	D

CHAPTER 3 Healthcare Delivery System

Learning Objectives

Upon completion of this chapter, the reader will be able to:

1 State the meaning of the roots and define the terms and abbreviations associated with the healthcare delivery system.
2 List the various hospital services.
3 Describe the major functions of the hospital departments.
4 Describe the organizational structure of the clinical laboratory.
5 State the qualifications for laboratory personnel.
6 Discuss the role of JCAHO, CAP, NCCLS, and CLIA '88 in the regulation and accreditation of laboratories.
7 Identify the different types of laboratory settings in which a phlebotomist may be employed.

Terminology

Roots/Combining Forms	Meaning
path/o	disease
ped/i	children
pharmac/o	drug
phleb/o	vein
radi/o	x-ray, radiant energy

Key Terms	Definition
Electrocardiography	Recording of variations in the electrical activity of the heart muscle
Electroencephalog- raphy	Recording of electrical changes in various areas of the brain
Neonatal	Pertaining to the first 4 weeks after birth
Oncology	Branch of medicine specializing in tumors
Pathology	Branch of medicine specializing in the study of disease
Pediatric	Pertaining to the treatment of children
Pharmacology	The study of drugs
Phlebotomist	Specialist in the incision into a vein
Radiologist	Physician specializing in radiant energy interpretation

Terminology
Continued

Abbreviations	Definition
CAP	College of American Pathologists
CCU	Cardiac care unit
CLIA '88	Clinical Laboratory Improvement Act of 1988
CLS	Clinical laboratory scientist (MT)
CLT	Clinical laboratory technician (MLT)
CNA	Certified nursing assistant
CT	Cytotechnologist
DO	Doctor of Osteopathy
DRG	Diagnostic related group
ER	Emergency room
GYN	Gynecology
HMO	Health maintenance organization
ICU	Intensive care unit
JCAHO	Joint Commission on Accreditation of Healthcare Organizations
L & D	Labor and delivery
LPN	Licensed practical nurse
MD	Doctor of Medicine
MLT	Medical laboratory technician (CLT)
MRI	Magnetic resonance imaging
MT	Medical technologist (CLS)
NCCLS	National Committee for Clinical Laboratory Standards
OB	Obstetrics
OP	Outpatient
OR	Operating room
OT	Occupational therapy
PA	Physician's assistant
POL	Physician office laboratory
PPO	Preferred provider organization
PT	Physical therapy
RN	Registered nurse

As members of the healthcare delivery system, **phlebotomists** should have a basic knowledge of the various healthcare settings in which they may be employed. This chapter covers the organization of hospitals, functions of hospital departments, clinical laboratory organization and personnel, accreditation policies, and alternative healthcare settings.

HOSPITAL ORGANIZATION

A typical hospital consists of a Board of Trustees, a Chief of Staff, a hospital administrator and assistant administrators for service areas. The hospital is governed by the Board of Trustees, who are private citizens. The board is ultimately responsible for the hospital operations and the medical staff. The Chief of Staff is the head of the medical team and acts as the liaison between the physicians, the Board of Trustees, and the hospital administrator. The Board of Trustees hires the hospital administrator to manage the hospital operations. This person may be assisted by assistant administrators who head each of the four main services of the hospital. The four services of a hospital are the professional service, nursing service, support service, and fiscal service.

PROFESSIONAL SERVICES   The service consisting of the departments of the hospital that assist the physician in the diagnosis and treatment of disease. Radiology, radiation therapy, nuclear medicine, occupational therapy, pharmacy, physical therapy, respiratory therapy, and the clinical laboratory are the main departments in this service. Other branches of professional services include **electrocardiography** and **electroencephalography**. The phlebotomist belongs to this group as part of the clinical laboratory staff.

NURSING SERVICES   The service dealing directly with patient care. It consists of the cardiac care unit (**CCU**), central supply, emergency room (**ER**), epidemiology, hospital units, infection control, intensive care unit (**ICU**), nursery, and operating room (**OR**). Healthcare team members associated with this service are registered nurses (**RN**), licensed practical nurses (**LPN**), certified nursing assistants (**CNA**), and the unit secretary or ward clerk. Phlebotomists interact most often with this service.

SUPPORT SERVICES   The service maintaining the hospital. Food service, grounds care, housekeeping, human resources, laundry, maintenance, purchasing, and security belong to this service.

FISCAL SERVICES   The service managing the business aspect of a hospital. Included in this service are accounting, admitting, the business office, credit and collection, data processing, and medical records (health information technology).

A hospital organizational chart is shown in Figure 3–1. Organizational charts are designed to define the position of each employee with regard to authority, responsibility, and accountability. Hospital organizational charts are further broken down into department organizational charts. Job descriptions and evaluations are based on organizational structure.

Hospital clinical laboratories employ the most phlebotomists. The need for phlebotomists depends on the size of the hospital.

A small hospital consists of less than 75 beds and performs primary care and general laboratory testing, as opposed to the specialized services found in larger hospitals. Phlebotomists may only be required on the day shift.

A medium-sized hospital of up to 300 beds requires a laboratory to function 24 hours per day, 7 days a week. The laboratory is departmentalized and may require phlebotomy coverage for the day and evening shifts.

A large hospital with more than 300 beds requires phlebotomy coverage for all three shifts, and the laboratory provides more specialized services. Many factors, such as a busy ER and the inclusion of certain specialties (e.g., a cardiac unit for open heart surgery, **oncology** units, pediatrics, obstetrics [**OB**], neonatology, ICU, CCU, **neonatal** ICU, burn centers, or dialysis units) increase phlebotomy staffing requirements of hospitals. Teaching hospitals with residents, interns, and allied health programs have significantly higher workloads. Large hospitals with specialized clinics such as cancer clinics, **pediatric** clinics, or industrial clinics have high outpatient (**OP**) workloads and demand larger phlebotomy staffs.

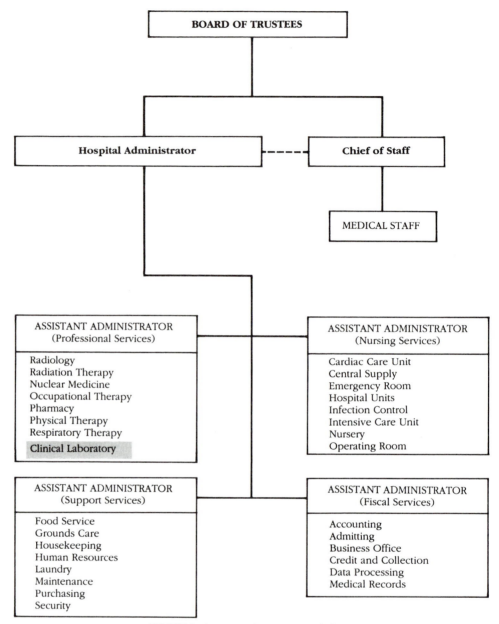

FIGURE 3–1. Hospital organizational chart.

PROFESSIONAL SERVICE DEPARTMENTS

The patient is often transported to different areas of the hospital; therefore, the phlebotomist must be familiar with the location of each department, the nature of the procedures performed in the department, and the safety precautions pertaining to that department. In addition the phlebotomist must interact with all hospital professionals in each department. The professional image of the laboratory is projected by the phlebotomist to the rest of the hospital staff and the patients.

Radiology

The radiology department utilizes various forms of radiant energy to diagnose and treat disease. Some of the techniques include x-rays of teeth and bones, computerized axial tomography (CAT or CT scan), contrast studies using barium sulfate, cardiac catheterization, fluoroscopy, ultrasound, and magnetic resonance imaging (**MRI**). A **radiologist**, who is a physician, administers diagnostic procedures and interprets x-rays. The allied healthcare professional in this department is a radiographer.

Radiation Therapy

The radiation therapy department utilizes high-energy x-rays or ionizing radiation to stop the growth of cancer cells. Radiation therapy technologists perform these procedures. Because radiation therapy may affect the bone marrow, blood tests are often performed by the laboratory to monitor the patients.

Nuclear Medicine

The nuclear medicine department studies the characteristics of radioactive substances in the diagnosis and treatment of disease. Radioactive materials, called radioisotopes, emit rays as they disintegrate and the rays are measured on specialized instruments. Two types of tests are used. In vitro tests analyze blood and urine specimens using radioactive materials to detect levels of hormones, drugs, and other substances. In vivo tests involve administering radioactive material to the patient by intravenous injection and measuring the emitted rays to examine organs and evaluate their function. Examples of these procedures are bone, brain, liver, and thyroid scans. Therapeutic doses of radioactive material also can be given to a patient to treat diseases. Nuclear medicine technologists perform these procedures under the supervision of a physician.

Occupational Therapy

The occupational therapy (**OT**) department teaches techniques that enable patients with physical, mental, or emotional disabilities to function within their limitations in daily living. Occupational therapists provide this instruction.

Pharmacy

The pharmacy department dispenses the medications prescribed by physicians. The phlebotomist is often responsible for the collection of specifically timed specimens used to monitor the blood level of certain medications. Persons trained to dispense medications are called pharmacists.

Physical Therapy

The physical therapy (**PT**) department provides treatment to patients that have been disabled due to illness or injury by using procedures involving water, heat, massage, ultrasound, and exercise. Physical therapists are the professionals trained to provide this therapy.

Respiratory Therapy

Respiratory therapists provide treatment in breathing disorders and often perform the arterial punctures used to evaluate arterial blood gases that are discussed in Chapter 18.

Clinical Laboratory

The clinical laboratory provides data to the healthcare team to aid in determining the diagnosis, treatment, and prognosis of a patient.

The laboratory is divided into two areas, anatomical and clinical. The anatomical area is divided into the cytology and histology sections and may include a cytogenetics section. Surgical specimens, frozen sections, surgical biopsies, cytologic specimens, and autopsies are analyzed here.

In the cytology section, cytotechnologists (**CT**) process and examine tissue and body fluids for abnormal cells such as cancer cells. A Pap smear is one of the most common tests.

In the histology section, histologists process and stain tissue obtained during autopsy or surgery for examination by the pathologist.

Cytogenetics is the section where chromosome studies are performed to detect genetic disease. Blood, amniotic fluid, tissue, and bone marrow specimens can be analyzed.

The clinical area is divided into specialized sections: hematology/coagulation, chemistry, blood bank, serology (immunology), microbiology, urinalysis, and phlebotomy. In the clinical laboratory, blood, bone marrow, microbiology specimens, urine, and other body fluids are analyzed. See Figure 3–2 for an organizational chart of the clinical laboratory.

CLINICAL LABORATORY PERSONNEL

The laboratory employs a large number of personnel, whose qualifications vary with their job description. Most personnel are required to be certified by a national organization. Some states require an additional state licensure, and the number of these is currently increasing. See Figure 3–3 for an organizational chart of clinical laboratory personnel.

Laboratory Director (Pathologist)

The director of the laboratory is usually a pathologist, a physician who has completed a 4- to 5-year pathology residency. A pathologist is a specialist in the study of disease and may specialize in clinical **pathology**, anatomic pathology, or both. Clinical pathology is the interpretation of clinical laboratory test results to diagnose disease. Anatomic pathology is the study of tissue, including surgical and autopsy specimens.

The pathologist is the liaison between the medical staff and the laboratory staff, and acts as a consultant to physicians regarding a patient's diagnosis and treatment.

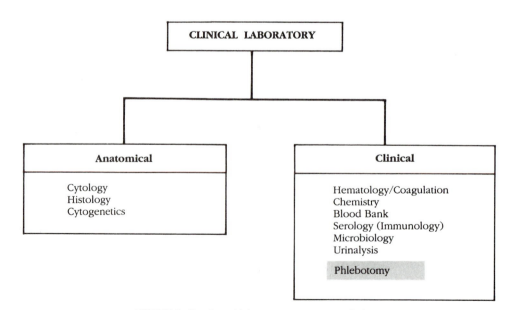

FIGURE 3–2. Clinical laboratory organizational chart.

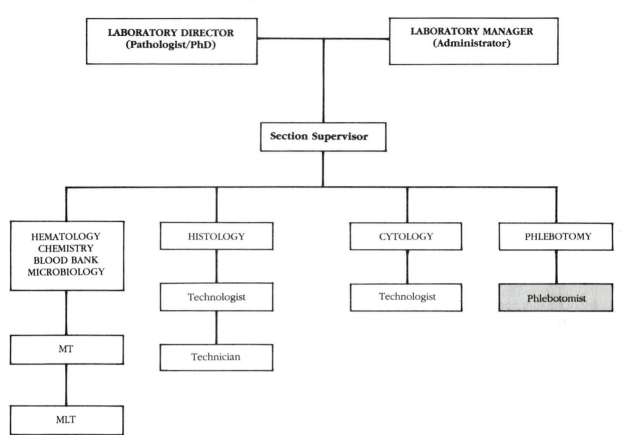

FIGURE 3–3. Clinical laboratory personnel organizational chart.

Direct responsibility lies with the pathologist for the anatomic and clinical areas of the laboratory. Responsibilities include establishing laboratory policies, interpreting test results, performing bone marrow biopsies and autopsies, and diagnosing disease from tissue specimens or cell preparations. Often the laboratory director has one or more associate pathologists to assist with the laboratory responsibilities. The laboratory director may also be a laboratory specialist who possesses a doctorate degree.

Laboratory Manager (Administrator)

The laboratory manager is responsible for overall technical and administrative management of the laboratory, including personnel and budgets. The laboratory manager is usually a medical technologist with a master's degree and 5 or more years of laboratory experience. The additional education is often in either administration or business. The laboratory manager acts as a liaison between the laboratory staff, the administrator of professional services, and the laboratory director.

Section Supervisor

The section supervisor is a medical technologist with experience and expertise related to the particular laboratory section. Many section supervisors have a specialty certification in hematology, chemistry, blood banking, immunology, or microbiology. The section supervisor is accountable to the laboratory manager. Responsibilities of the section supervisor include reviewing all laboratory test results; consulting with the pathologist on the abnormal test results; scheduling personnel; maintaining automated instruments by implementing preventive maintenance procedures and quality control measures; preparing budgets; maintaining reagents and supplies; orienting, evaluating, and teaching personnel; and providing research and development protocols for new test procedures.

Medical Technologist

The medical technologist (**MT**) or clinical laboratory scientist (**CLS**) has a bachelor's degree in medical technology or in a biologic science and 1 year of training in an accredited medical technology program. The technologist reports to the section supervisor or laboratory director. A medical technologist performs laboratory procedures that require independent judgment and responsibility with minimal technical supervision; maintains equipment and records; performs quality assurance and preventive maintenance activities related to test performance; and may function as a supervisor, educator, manager, or researcher within a medical laboratory setting. Some of the medical technologist's duties are to evaluate and solve problems related to the collection of specimens, perform complex laboratory procedures, perform and analyze quality control data, report and answer inquiries regarding test results, troubleshoot equipment, participate in the evaluation of new test procedures, and provide education to new employees and students.

Medical Laboratory Technician

A medical laboratory technician (**MLT**) or clinical laboratory technician (**CLT**) usually has a 2-year associate degree from an accredited college medical laboratory program. A medical laboratory technician performs routine laboratory procedures according to established protocol under the supervision of a technologist, supervisor, or laboratory director. The duties of the MLT include collecting and processing biologic specimens for analysis, performing routine analytic tests, recognizing factors that affect test results, recognizing abnormal results and reporting them to a supervisor, recognizing equipment malfunctions and reporting them to a supervisor, performing quality control and preventive maintenance procedures, maintaining accurate records, and demonstrating laboratory technical skills to new employees and students.

Phlebotomist

The phlebotomist collects blood from patients for the purpose of laboratory analysis. The phlebotomist must have a high school diploma and usually has completed a structured phlebotomy training program. Certified phlebotomy technicians have passed a national certifying examination. The phlebotomist is trained to properly identify the patient; obtain the correct amount of blood by venipuncture or microtechnique, utilizing the correct equipment and collection tubes; properly label and transport specimens to the laboratory; prepare specimens to be delivered to the laboratory sections; and observe all safety and quality control policies. Test collection requirements vary with each department; therefore, the phlebotomist must interact with and have knowledge of all the sections in the laboratory.

REGULATION OF CLINICAL LABORATORIES

Hospital laboratories are governed by regulations that provide guidelines and rules for quality patient care. Accrediting agencies, such as the Joint Commission on Accreditation of Healthcare Organizations (**JCAHO**) and the College of American Pathologists (**CAP**), exist to assure a high standard of care for patients.

The preferred accrediting agency for hospitals is JCAHO. Every 3 years hospitals are accredited; compliance with the regulations is ensured by an on-site visit to the facility by an inspection team. If deficiencies are present, the hospital must correct them within a specified time frame and may be reinspected.

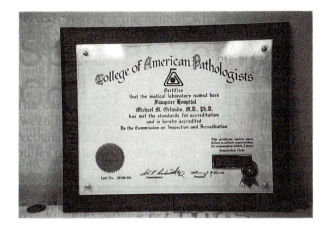

FIGURE 3–4. Accreditation certificate from the College of American Pathologists (CAP).

Accredited laboratories are inspected by CAP (Fig. 3–4), which provides laboratory inspection and proficiency testing. Samples for proficiency testing are sent to each section and specified test procedures are performed. The results of these procedures are compared with the range of results of all participating laboratories throughout the country. Incorrect values indicate a problem with a procedure. Such problems must be corrected, and the corrective action must be documented. Inspection teams comprised of pathologists and medical technologists visit the laboratory every 2 years to review procedures, personnel qualifications, and record documentation.

Usually a laboratory that is accredited by CAP is recognized by JCAHO and does not undergo two inspections. In order to receive reimbursement for Medicare or Medicaid, the laboratory must be accredited by an approved accrediting agency.

National standards and guidelines are set for laboratories by the National Committee for Clinical Laboratory Standards (**NCCLS**), a national nonprofit organization that provides recommendations for laboratory procedures and evaluations.

In 1988, a bill was introduced into Congress called the Clinical Laboratory Improvement Act of 1988 (**CLIA '88**) that mandated regulation of all laboratories, with the same standards for laboratory testing in physician office laboratories, nursing home facilities, clinics, hospital laboratories, government laboratories, health maintenance organizations, or independent laboratories. The classification of laboratories is based on the complexity of testing performed, and personnel qualifications are specified for various levels of test complexity. Implementation of CLIA has not yet been fully accomplished and regulations continue to change.

HEALTHCARE SETTINGS

Phlebotomists may be employed in other medical facilities such as physician office laboratories, health maintenance organizations, reference laboratories, urgent care centers, nursing home facilities, and clinics.

Physician office laboratories (**POLs**) can range from single practitioners doing simple screening tests to large group medical practices requiring specialized testing. A central on-site laboratory provides convenience to the patient.

Health maintenance organizations (**HMOs**) are group practice centers that provide all medical services in one location. Physicians offices, radiology, laboratory, electrocardiography services, and outpatient surgery can be performed in the center. One prepaid fee is paid by a member for all services instead of the patient being billed for each service.

Preferred provider organizations (**PPOs**) provide medical care to an established group of patients. A business agreement between the physician and an insurer predetermines fees for specific services. Specific providers must be used to receive the preset discounted rate.

Large independent reference laboratories perform routine and highly specialized tests that cannot feasibly be done in smaller laboratories. Phlebotomists may perform both on-site and off-site collections.

Due to changes in the healthcare system and efforts to cut costs, the length of stay for a patient in the hospital is decreasing and more tests are being performed on an outpatient basis and in different types of settings. The implementation of diagnostic related groups (**DRGs**) by the federal government in an effort to limit the number of diagnostic procedures performed and the length of hospital stays has had an impact on the clinical laboratory. The DRG system classifies patients into diagnostic categories related to body systems and the illnesses associated with them. A total of 467 illness categories have been developed and classification of patients is based on primary and secondary diagnoses, age, treatment performed, and status on discharge. This system determines the amount of money the government will pay for a patient's care, regardless of the number of tests performed. Therefore, laboratory tests and other procedures must be kept within the specified DRG guidelines or the additional cost must be absorbed by the healthcare institution. Emphasis is also being placed on preventive medicine, which has increased the number of wellness clinics for health screening. The need for providers of home health care will continue to increase. The role of phlebotomists will certainly be affected by these changes.

BIBLIOGRAPHY

Clerc, JM: An Introduction to Clinical Laboratory Science. CV Mosby, St. Louis, 1992.
Sazama, JD: Licensure of laboratory personnel. Laboratory Medicine, ASCP, April, 1993.

Study Questions

1. Using the basic terminology and the terminology in this chapter, define the following:

   a. Pathologist   _____

   b. Radiologist   _____

   c. Phlebotomy   _____

   d. Cytology   _____

   e. Encephalography _____

2. Describe the following situations by defining the underlined words:

   a. The patient in the ER was DOA.

   _____

   _____

   b. An OP was taken to Radiology at the HMO.

   _____

   _____

   _____

   c. A request was made for a STAT phlebotomy in the ICU.

   _____

   _____

   _____

   d. The RN in L & D requested 10 mL of blood be drawn from an OB patient ASAP.

   _____

   _____

   _____

   _____

   _____

   e. The MT performed the tests requested by the pathologist on samples drawn by the CPT.

   _____

   _____

   _____

3. Name the four services in a hospital and a department of each.

Service   **Department**

a. _____   _____

b. _____   _____

c. _____   _____

d. _____   _____

4. Describe the qualifications of a pathologist.

_____

_____

_____

5. Differentiate between the two divisions of the hospital laboratory. Indicate the sections in each.

Division   **Sections**

a. _____   _____

                            _____

b. _____   _____

                            _____

                            _____

6. State three different settings where phlebotomists may be employed other than the hospital.

a. _____

b. _____

c. _____

7. Discuss possible differences in phlebotomy staffing among small, medium-sized, and large hospitals.

_____

_____

_____

8. List two similarities and two differences between a medical laboratory technician and a medical technologist.

Similarity   **Difference**

a. _____   _____

b. _____   _____

9. Using the laboratory organizational chart, answer the following questions:

   a. To whom would the phlebotomist report the failure to obtain a blood specimen? _____

   b. Would a medical technologist report to a medical laboratory technician or a section supervisor? _____

10. Name two accrediting agencies for laboratories.

   a. _____

   b. _____

CHAPTER 4 Clinical Laboratory Sections

Learning Objectives

Upon completion of this chapter, the reader will be able to:

1   State the meaning of the roots and suffixes and define the terms and abbreviations associated with the sections of the clinical laboratory.
2   Discuss the basic organization of the hematology, chemistry, blood bank, serology/immunology, microbiology, and urinalysis sections.
3   Describe the appropriate collection and handling of specimens analyzed in the individual clinical laboratory sections.
4   Identify the most common tests performed in the individual clinical laboratory sections and state their function.

HEMATOLOGY SECTION

Terminology Associated with the Hematology Section

Roots/Combining Forms	Meaning
bas/o	alkaline blue dye
coagul/o	clotting
eosin/o	acidic red dye
hem/o, hemat/o	blood
morph/o	form

Suffixes	Meaning
-blast	immature cell
-cyte	cell
-globin	protein
-penia	decrease in cell numbers
-philia	increase in cell numbers

Key Terms	Definition
Anemia	Deficiency of red blood cells
Anticoagulant	Substance that prevents blood from clotting
Clot	Blood that has coagulated
Granulocyte	White blood cell with granules
Hemolysis	Destruction of red blood cells
Hemostasis	Stoppage of blood flow from a damaged blood vessel
Leukemia	Malignant overproduction of white blood cells
Morphology	The study of structures

37

Terminology Associated with the Hematology Section
Continued

Abbreviations	Definition
APTT (PTT)	Activated partial thromboplastin time
BT	Bleeding time
CBC	Complete blood count
Diff	White blood cell differential
ESR (Sed rate)	Erythrocyte sedimentation rate
FDP	Fibrin degradation products
Hct	Hematocrit
Hgb, Hb	Hemoglobin
LE	Lupus erythematosus
MCH	Mean corpuscular hemoglobin
MCHC	Mean corpuscular hemoglobin concentration
MCV	Mean corpuscular volume
Plt	Platelet
PT	Prothrombin time
RBC	Red blood cell
RDW	Red cell distribution width
Retic	Reticulocyte
TT	Thrombin time
WBC	White blood cell

Hematology is the study of the formed (cellular) elements of the blood. In this section the cellular elements, red blood cells (**RBC**s), white blood cells (**WBC**s), and platelets (**Plt**s) are enumerated and classified in all body fluids and in the bone marrow. These cells, which are formed and mature in the bone marrow, are released into the blood stream as needed to carry oxygen, provide immunity against infection, and aid in blood clotting.

By examining the cells in a blood specimen, disorders such as **leukemia**, **anemia**, other blood diseases, and infection can be detected and the treatment monitored (Fig. 4–1).

Specimen Collection and Handling

The most common body fluid analyzed in the hematology section is whole blood (a mixture of cells and plasma). A whole blood specimen is obtained by using a collection tube with an **anticoagulant** to prevent clotting of the specimen. Most tests performed in the hematology section require blood that has been collected in lavender top tubes containing the anticoagulant, ethylenediaminetetraacetic acid (EDTA) (see Chapter 12). Immediate inversion of this tube eight times is critical to prevent clotting and ensure accurate blood counts.

Blood is analyzed either whole, as plasma, or as serum. The liquid portion of blood is called plasma if it is obtained from a specimen that has not been allowed to **clot**. Clotting is prevented by collecting the specimen in a tube containing an anticoagulant. If the specimen is allowed to clot, the liquid portion is called serum. The major difference between plasma and serum is that plasma contains the protein fibrinogen and serum does not. Refer to Figure 7–7 to see the role of fibrinogen in the clotting process. Figure 4–2 illustrates the differences between plasma and serum. It is important to differentiate between plasma and serum, as many laboratory tests are designed to be performed specifically on either plasma or serum.

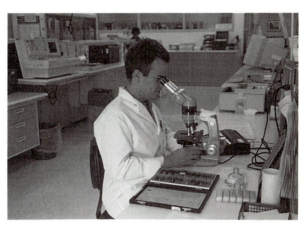

FIGURE 4–1. A technician examining blood cells in the hematology section.

Tests Performed in the Hematology Section

A complete blood count (**CBC**) is the primary analysis performed in the hematology section and is usually performed on automated instruments using whole blood (Fig. 4–3). Very often it is ordered on a STAT basis. The tests in Table 4–1 are a part of a CBC or they may be ordered separately.

Other tests performed in the hematology section include:

Body fluid analysis	Determines the number and type of cells in various body fluids
Bone marrow	Determines the number and type of cells in the bone marrow
Eosinophil count	Determines the number of eosinophils in blood or nasal secretions (elevated in allergies or parasitic infection)
Erythrocyte sedimentation rate (**ESR**)	Determines the rate of red blood cell sedimentation (nonspecific test for inflammatory disorders)
Lupus erythematosus (**LE**) prep	Test for systemic lupus erythematosus
Osmotic fragility	Determines the ability of red blood cells to absorb liquid without lysing
Plasma hemoglobin	Detects intravascular **hemolysis**
Reticulocyte (**Retic**) count	Evaluates bone marrow production of red blood cells
Sickle cell	Screening test for Hgb S (sickle cell anemia)
Special stains	Determine the type of leukemia (phlebotomists must often obtain blood smears)

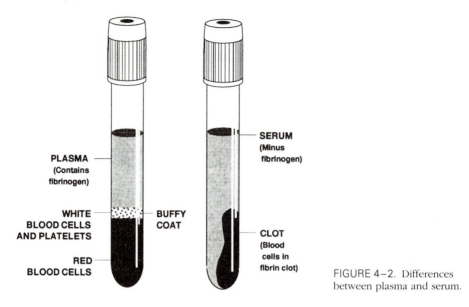

FIGURE 4–2. Differences between plasma and serum.

Coagulation Area of the Hematology Section

The coagulation laboratory is usually a part of the hematology section, but may be a separate section in larger laboratories. In this area the overall process of **hemostasis** is evaluated; this includes platelets, blood vessels, coagulation factors, fibrinolysis, inhibitors, and anticoagulant therapy (heparin and coumadin). Plasma from a specimen drawn in a light-blue top tube with the anticoagulant, sodium citrate, is the specimen most frequently analyzed. The blood specimen must be returned to the laboratory for analysis within 30 minutes.

Tests Performed in the Coagulation Area of the Hematology Section

The tests most frequently performed in the coagulation area of the hematology section and their function are presented in Table 4–2.

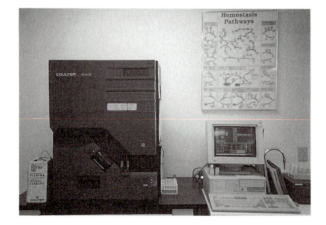

FIGURE 4–3. An automated hematology analyzer.

TABLE 4–1. **COMPLETE BLOOD COUNT**

Test	Function
Differential (**Diff**)	Determines the percentage of the different types of white blood cells and evaluates red blood cell and platelet **morphology** (may be examined microscopically on a peripheral blood smear stained with Wright's stain)
Hematocrit (**Hct**)	Determines the volume of red blood cells packed by centrifugation (expressed as a percent)
Hemoglobin (**Hgb**)	Determines the oxygen-carrying capacity of red blood cells
Indices	Calculations to determine the size of red blood cells and the amount of hemoglobin
Mean corpuscular hemoglobin (**MCH**)	Determines the amount of hemoglobin in a red blood cell
Mean corpuscular hemoglobin concentration (**MCHC**)	Determines the weight of hemoglobin in a red blood cell and compares it with the size of the cell (expressed as a percent)
Mean corpuscular volume (**MCV**)	Determines the size of red blood cells
Platelet (Plt) count	Determines the number of platelets in circulating blood
Red blood cell (RBC) count	Determines the number of red blood cells in circulating blood
Red cell distribution width (**RDW**)	Calculation to determine the differences in the size of red blood cells (expressed as a percent)
White blood cell (WBC) count	Determines the number of white blood cells in circulating blood

TABLE 4–2. **TESTS PERFORMED IN THE COAGULATION AREA OF THE HEMATOLOGY SECTION**

Test	Function
Activated partial thromboplastin time [**APTT (PTT)**]	Evaluates the intrinsic system of the coagulation cascade and monitors heparin therapy
Antithrombin III	Screening test for increased clotting tendencies
Bleeding time (**BT**)	Evaluates the function of platelets
Factor assays	Determine the amount of the coagulation factors in plasma
Fibrin degradation products (**FDP**)	Test for increased fibrinolysis (usually a STAT test drawn in a special tube)
Fibrinogen	Determines the amount of fibrinogen in plasma
Platelet aggregation	Evaluates the function of platelets
Prothrombin time (**PT**)	Evaluates the extrinsic system of the coagulation cascade and monitors coumadin therapy
Thrombin time (**TT**)	Determines the ability to convert fibrinogen to fibrin

CHEMISTRY SECTION

Terminology Associated with the Chemistry Section

Roots/Combining Forms	Meaning
amyl/o	starch
gluc/o, glyc/o	glucose

Suffixes	Meaning
-ase	enzyme
-ose	sugar
-prandial	meal

Key Terms	Definition
Albumin	Primary form of protein in plasma
Buffer	Chemical solution that controls pH
Centrifuge	Instrument that spins test tubes at high speeds to separate the cellular and liquid portions of blood
Cholesterol	Major blood lipid
Electrolytes	Ions in the blood (primarily sodium, potassium, chloride, and carbon dioxide)
Electrophoresis	Method of separation by electrical charge
Endogenous	Originating within the body
Enzyme	Protein that initiates chemical reactions
Exogenous	Originating outside the body
Globulin	Blood protein fraction containing antibodies
Glucose	Primary sugar in the body
Isoenzyme	Specific form of an **enzyme**
Jaundice, icteric	Appears yellow
Lithium	Chemical used to treat manic depression
Triglycerides	Blood fats
Urea	Waste product of protein metabolism
Uric acid	Waste product of purine metabolism

Abbreviations	Definition
A/G	**Albumin** to **globulin** ratio
ABG	Arterial blood gases
ALP (Alk Phos)	Alkaline phosphatase
ALT (SGPT)	Alanine aminotransferase
AST (SGOT)	Aspartate aminotransferase
BUN	Blood **urea** nitrogen
Ca	Calcium
CK (CPK)	Creatine kinase (creatine phosphokinase)
Cl	Chloride
CO_2	Carbon dioxide
EIA	Enzyme immunoassay
FBS	Fasting blood sugar
GGT	Gamma glutamyl transferase
GTT	Glucose tolerance test

Terminology Associated with the Chemistry Section
Continued

Abbreviations	Definition
HDL	High-density lipoprotein
K	Potassium
LD (LDH)	Lactic dehydrogenase
LDL	Low-density lipoprotein
Li	**Lithium**
Lytes	Electrolytes (**Na, K, Cl,** and **CO$_2$**)
mg/dL	Milligrams per deciliter
mmol/L	Millimoles per liter
Na	Sodium
P	Phosphorus
RIA	Radioimmunoassay
SMAC	Sequential multiple analyzer-computerized
TDM	Therapeutic drug monitoring
TIBC	Total iron-binding capacity
TP	Total protein
VLDL	Very–low-density lipoprotein
% (percent)	Parts per 100 units

The clinical chemistry section is the most automated area of the laboratory. Instruments are computerized and designed to perform single and multiple tests from small amounts of specimen. Figures 4–4 and 4–5 provide examples of the instrumentation and computerization utilized in the chemistry section.

The chemistry section may be divided into several areas such as general or automated chemistry, electrophoresis, toxicology, and immunochemistry. The **electrophoresis** area performs hemoglobin electrophoresis; protein electrophoresis on serum, urine, and cerebrospinal fluid; and **isoenzyme** detection. In toxicology, therapeutic drug monitoring (**TDM**) and the identification of drugs of abuse are performed. Examples of substances analyzed include alcohol, lead, salicylate, phenobarbital, dilantin, and cocaine. Immunochemistry uses the techniques of radioimmunoassay (**RIA**) and enzyme immunoassay (**EIA**) to measure substances such as digoxin, thyroid hormones, cortisol, vitamin B$_{12}$, folate, carcinoembryonic antigen, and CK isoenzymes.

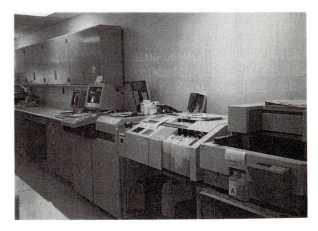

FIGURE 4–4. Example of clinical chemistry instrumentation.

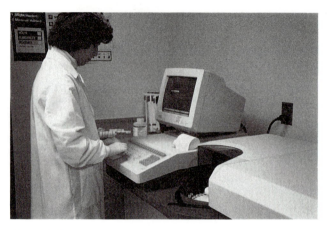

FIGURE 4–5. Technologist entering data into a computerized clinical chemistry analyzer.

Specimen Collection and Handling

Clinical chemistry tests are performed primarily on serum collected in serum separator tubes but may also be collected in tubes with red, green, gray, or dark-blue tops. Tests are also performed on plasma, urine, and other body fluids. Serum and plasma are obtained by **centrifugation**, which should be performed within 1 hour of collection.

Because many tests are performed on instruments that take photometric readings, differences in the appearance or color of a specimen may adversely affect the test results. Specimens of concern include hemolyzed specimens that appear red due to the release of hemoglobin from red blood cells, **icteric** specimens that are yellow from the presence of excess bilirubin, and lipemic specimens that are cloudy because of increased lipids. Fasting specimens must be drawn from patients who have not eaten for 8 to 12 hours.

Serum separator tubes contain an inert gel that prevents contamination of the specimen by red cells or their metabolites. Specimens must be allowed to fully clot prior to centrifugation to ensure complete separation of the cells and serum. Many chemistry tests require special collection and handling procedures, such as chilling and protection from light, and these tests are discussed in Chapter 15.

Tests Performed in the Chemistry Section

The tests most frequently performed in the chemistry section and their function are presented in Table 4–3.

Chemistry profiles are groups of tests used to evaluate a particular organ, body system, or the general health of a patient. The specific tests included in a profile will vary among institutions. Examples of common profiles are:

Profile	Tests
General health	Glucose, BUN, creatinine, Na, K, AST, LD, cholesterol, triglycerides, uric acid, total protein/albumin, bilirubin, Ca, and ALP
Liver	ALP, ALT, AST, bilirubin, and GGT
Myocardial infarction	AST, CK, CK isoenzymes, and LD
Coronary risk	Cholesterol, triglycerides, HDL, and LDL

TABLE 4–3. **TESTS PERFORMED IN THE CHEMISTRY SECTION**

Test	Function
Acid phosphatase	Elevated levels indicate prostatic cancer
Alanine aminotransferase [**ALT (SGPT)**]	Elevated levels indicate liver disorders
Albumin	Decreased levels indicate liver or kidney disorders or malnutrition
Alcohol	Elevated levels indicate intoxication
Alkaline phosphatase (**ALP**)	Elevated levels indicate bone or liver disorders
Ammonia	Elevated levels indicate severe liver disorders
Amylase	Elevated levels indicate pancreatitis
Arterial blood gases (**ABGs**)	Determine the acidity or alkalinity and gas pressures in blood
Aspartate aminotransferase [**AST (SGOT)**]	Elevated levels indicate recent myocardial infarction or liver disorders
Bilirubin	Elevated levels indicate liver or hemolytic disorders
Blood urea nitrogen (**BUN**)	Elevated levels indicate kidney disorders
Calcium (**Ca**)	Mineral associated with bone, musculoskeletal, or endocrine disorders
Cholesterol	Elevated levels indicate coronary risk
Creatine kinase [**CK (CPK)**]	Elevated levels indicate myocardial infarction or other muscle damage
Creatine kinase [CK (CPK)] isoenzymes	Determine the extent of muscle or brain damage
Creatinine	Elevated levels indicate kidney disorders
Creatinine clearance	Urine and serum test to measure glomerular filtration rate
Drug screening	Detects drug abuse and monitors therapeutic drugs
Electrolytes (Lytes)	Evaluate body fluid balance
Gamma glutamyl transferase (**GGT**)	Elevated levels indicate early liver disorders
Glucose	Elevated levels indicate diabetes mellitus
Glucose tolerance test (**GTT**)	Detects diabetes mellitus or hypoglycemia
Hemoglobin (Hgb) electrophoresis	Detects abnormal hemoglobins
High-density lipoprotein (**HDL**)	Assesses coronary risk
Lactic dehydrogenase [**LD (LDH)**]	Elevated levels indicate myocardial infarction or lung or liver disorders
Lead	Elevated levels indicate poisoning
Lipase	Elevated levels indicate pancreatitis
Lithium (**Li**)	Monitors antidepressant drug
Low-density lipoprotein (**LDL**)	Assesses coronary risk
Phosphorus (**P**)	Mineral associated with skeletal or endocrine disorders
Protein	Decreased levels associated with liver or kidney disorders
Total protein (**TP**)	Decreased levels indicate liver or kidney disorders
Triglycerides	Used to assess coronary risk
Uric acid	Elevated levels indicate kidney disorders or gout

BLOOD BANK SECTION

Terminology Associated with the Blood Bank Section	Key Terms	Definition
	Antibody	Protein produced by exposure to antigen
	Antigen	Substance that stimulates the formation of antibodies
	Antiserum	Serum containing antibodies
	Blood group	Classification based on the presence or absence of A or B antigens on the red blood cells
	Blood type	Classification based on the presence or absence of the Rh (D) antigen on the red blood cells
	Compatibility test/ crossmatch	Procedure that matches patient and donor blood prior to a transfusion

Terminology Associated with the Blood Bank Section
Continued

Key Terms	Definition
Cryoprecipitate	Component of fresh plasma that contains clotting factors
Fresh frozen plasma	Plasma collected from a unit of blood and immediately frozen
Immunohematology	The study of blood cell antigens and their antibodies
Packed cells (RBCs)	Blood from which the plasma has been removed
Platelet concentrate	Platelets from several units of blood combined in a single packet
Unit of blood	405 to 495 mL of blood collected from a donor for a transfusion

Abbreviations	Definition
Ab	Antibody
ABO	Blood groups
Ag	Antigen
AHG	Antihuman globulin
BB	Blood bank
CPD-A	Citrate phosphate dextrose adenine
DAT	Direct antihuman globulin (**AHG**) test
Rh	The D (Rhesus) antigen on red blood cells
T & C	Type and crossmatch
X-match	Crossmatch (compatibility test)

The blood bank (**BB**) is the section of the laboratory where blood is collected, stored, and prepared for transfusion. It is also called **immunohematology** because the testing procedures involve red blood cell **antigens (Ag)** and **antibodies (Ab)**.

In the blood bank, blood from patients and donors is tested for its **blood group (ABO)** and **Rh**, the presence and identity of abnormal antibodies, and its **compatibility** for use in a transfusion (Fig. 4–6). **Units** (pints) **of blood** are collected from donors, tested for the presence of blood-borne pathogens such as hepatitis viruses

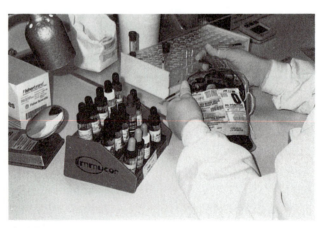

FIGURE 4–6. A technologist tests a unit of blood prior to transfusion.

and human immunodeficiency virus, and stored for transfusions (Fig. 4-7). Donor blood may also be separated into components including **packed cells**, platelets, **fresh frozen plasma**, and **cryoprecipitate**. These are stored separately and used for patients with specific needs. Patients may come to the blood bank to donate their own blood so that they can receive an autologous transfusion if blood is needed during their surgery.

Specimen Collection and Handling

Blood bank specimens are collected in plain red or pink top tubes. Serum separator tubes containing gel are not acceptable, as the gel will coat the red blood cells and interfere with testing. Hemolysis will also interfere with the interpretation of test results.

Patient identification is critical in the blood bank, and phlebotomists must carefully follow all patient identification and specimen labeling procedures to ensure that a patient does not receive a transfusion with an incompatible blood type.

Tests Performed in the Blood Bank Section

The tests most frequently performed in the blood bank section and their function are presented in Table 4-4.

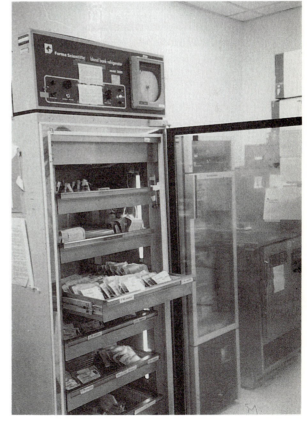

FIGURE 4-7. A blood bank refrigerator.

TABLE 4–4. **TESTS PERFORMED IN THE BLOOD BANK SECTION**

Test	Function
Antibody (Ab) screen	Detects abnormal antibodies
Direct antihuman globulin test (**DAT**) or direct Coombs	Detects abnormal antibodies on red blood cells
Group and type	ABO and Rh typing
Panel	Identifies abnormal antibodies
Type and **crossmatch (T & C)**	ABO, Rh typing, and compatibility test
Type and screen	ABO, Rh typing, and antibody screen

SEROLOGY (IMMUNOLOGY) SECTION

Terminology Associated with the Serology (Immunology) Section

Key Terms	Definition
Agglutination	Clumping of particles
Autoimmunity	Condition in which a person produces antibodies that react with the person's own antigens
Immunoglobulin	Another name for antibody
Immunology	The study of the immune system
Serology	The study of serum

Abbreviations	Definition
ANA	Antinuclear antibody
ASO	Antistreptolysin O
CMV	Cytomegalovirus
CRP	C-reactive protein
EBV	Epstein-Barr virus
FANA	Fluorescent antinuclear antibody
FTA-ABS	Fluorescent treponemal antibody — absorbed
HBsAg	Hepatitis B surface antigen
HCG	Human chorionic gonadotropin
HIV	Human immunodeficiency virus
Ig	Immunoglobulin
RA	Rheumatoid arthritis
RPR	Rapid plasma reagin
STS	Serological test for syphilis
VDRL	Venereal Disease Research Laboratory

The serology (immunology) section performs tests to evaluate the body's immune response, that is, the production of antibodies and cellular activation. Because the majority of tests performed in this section analyze for the presence of antibodies in serum, this section is frequently called serology rather than the broader term, immunology.

Tests in the serology section detect the presence of antibodies to bacteria, fungi, parasites, viruses, and antibodies produced against body substances (**autoimmunity**).

TABLE 4–5. **TESTS PERFORMED IN THE SEROLOGY (IMMUNOLOGY) SECTION**

Test	Function
Anti-**HIV**	Screening test for human immunodeficiency virus
Antinuclear antibody (**ANA**)	Detects nuclear autoantibodies
Antistreptolysin O (**ASO**) titer	Detects a previous streptococcus infection
C-reactive protein (**CRP**)	Elevated levels indicate inflammatory disorders
Cold agglutinins	Elevated levels indicate atypical pneumonia
Complement levels	Evaluate the function of the immune system
Cytomegalovirus antibody (**CMV**)	Detects cytomegalovirus infection
Epstein-Barr virus (**EBV**)	Detects infectious mononucleosis
Febrile agglutinins	Detect antibodies to microorganisms causing fever
Fluorescent antinuclear antibody (**FANA**)	Detects nuclear autoantibodies
Fluorescent treponemal antibody-absorbed (**FTA-ABS**)	Confirmatory test for syphilis
Hepatitis B surface antigen (**HBsAg**)	Detects the presence of hepatitis B surface antigen
Herpes simplex antibody	Screening test for herpes simplex infection
Human chorionic gonadotropin (**HCG**)	Hormone found in the urine and serum during pregnancy
Immunoglobulin (**IgG**, **IgA**, **IgM**) levels	Evaluate the function of the immune system
Monospot	Screening test for infectious mononucleosis
Rapid plasma reagin (**RPR**)	Screening test for syphilis
Rheumatoid arthritis (**RA**)	Detects autoantibodies present in rheumatoid arthritis
Rubella titer	Evaluates immunity to German measles
Veneral Disease Research Laboratory (**VDRL**)	Screening test for syphilis
Western blot	Confirmatory test for human immunodeficiency virus

Specimen Collection

Blood for serological testing is collected in plain red top tubes. Serum separator tubes are not used, as the gel can interfere with the antigen-antibody reactions.

Tests Performed in the Serology (Immunology) Section

The tests most frequently performed in the serology (immunology) section and their function are presented in Table 4–5.

MICROBIOLOGY SECTION

Terminology Associated with the Microbiology Section

Roots/Combining Forms	Meaning
bacill/o	rod
contag/i	unclean
febr/o	fever
immun/o	protection
myc/o	fungus
py/o, pur/o	pus

Terminology Associated with the Microbiology Section
Continued

Suffixes	Meaning
-cidal	pertaining to death
-coccus	spherical
-phylaxis	protection

Key Terms	Definition
Abscess	Collection of pus
Aerobe	Microorganism requiring oxygen to survive
Anaerobe	Microorganism that does not survive in oxygen
Antimicrobial	Substance that destroys or inhibits the growth of microorganisms
Bacillus	Rod-shaped bacterium
Bacteria	One-cell microorganism
Bacteriology	The study of bacteria
Carrier	Person with no symptoms who spreads a disease
Coccus	Spherical bacterium
Communicable	Capable of being transmitted
Culture	Laboratory procedure to detect the presence of microorganisms
Febrile	Pertaining to fever
Gram-negative	Refers to bacteria that stain red with Gram stain
Gram-positive	Refers to bacteria that stain blue with Gram stain
Gram stain	Stain used to classify bacteria
Isolation	Confinement to a designated area
Microbiology	The study of microorganisms
Microorganism	One-cell organism such as a bacterium, fungus, parasite, or virus
Mycology	The study of fungi
Mycosis	Fungal disease
Parasitology	The study of parasites
Pathogenic	Capable of causing disease
Sensitivity	Laboratory procedure to determine the susceptibility of microorganisms to antibiotics
Sepsis	Presence of pathogenic microorganisms
Spirochetes	Spiral-shaped microorganisms
Sterile	Free of microorganisms
Toxin	Poisonous substance
Virology	The study of viruses

Abbreviations	Definition
AFB	Acid-fast bacilli (tuberculosis)
C & S	Culture and sensitivity
GC	Gonorrhea
O & P	Ova and parasites
Staph	Staphylococcus
Strep	Streptococcus

Terminology Associated with the Microbiology Section
Continued

Abbreviations	Definition
TC	Throat culture
UTI	Urinary tract infection

The **microbiology** section is responsible for the identification of pathogenic microorganisms and for hospital infection control. In large laboratories the section may be divided into **bacteriology**, **mycology**, **parasitology**, and **virology**.

A **culture** and **sensitivity** (**C & S**) is the primary procedure performed in microbiology. It is used to detect and identify **microorganisms**, and to determine the most effective antibiotic therapy. Results are available within 2 days for most bacteria; however, cultures for tuberculosis and fungi may require several weeks for completion.

Identification of **bacteria** is based on morphology, **Gram stain** reactions, oxygen and nutritional requirements, and biochemical reactions. Fungi are identified by culture growth and microscopic morphology. Stool specimens are concentrated and examined microscopically for the presence of parasites, ova, or larvae. Viruses must be cultured in living cells, and most laboratories send viral specimens to specialized reference laboratories.

Specimen Collection and Handling

The majority of microbiology specimens are obtained from the blood, urine, throat, sputum, genitourinary tract, wounds, and feces. Correct identification of pathogens depends on proper collection and prompt transport to the laboratory for processing. Figures 4-8 and 4-9 provide examples of specimen processing in the microbiology section. Phlebotomists may be asked to transport specimens to the laboratory.

Phlebotomists are responsible for collecting blood cultures and may be required to obtain throat cultures (**TC**) and instruct patients in the procedure for collecting urine specimens for culture. Specific **sterile** techniques must be observed in the collection of culture specimens to prevent bacterial contamination. These procedures are covered in Chapters 15 and 19.

Tests Performed in the Microbiology Section

The tests most frequently performed in the microbiology section and their function are presented in Table 4-6.

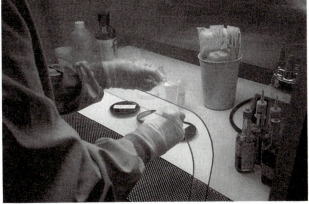

FIGURE 4-8. Technologist plating a culture and preparing a Gram stain.

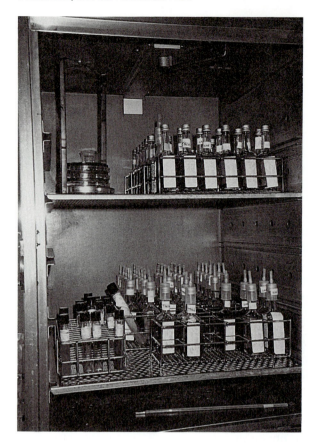

FIGURE 4–9. Incubation of blood cultures, tube media, and culture plates for bacterial growth.

TABLE 4–6. **TESTS PERFORMED IN THE MICROBIOLOGY SECTION**

Test	Function
Blood culture	Detects bacteria and fungi
Culture and sensitivity (C & S)	Detects microbial infection and determines antibiotic treatment
Fungal culture	Detects the presence of and determines the type of fungi
Gram stain	Detects the presence of and aids in the identification of bacteria
Occult blood	Detects nonvisible blood (performed on stool specimens)
Ova and parasites (**O & P**)	Detects parasitic infection (performed on stool specimens)

URINALYSIS SECTION

Terminology Associated with the Urinalysis Section	Key Terms	Definition
	Cast	Protein structure formed in the tubules of the kidney
	Glycosuria	Glucose in the urine
	Hematuria	Blood in the urine
	Ketonuria	Ketones in the urine
	Proteinuria	Protein (albumin) in the urine

Terminology Associated with the Urinalysis Section
Continued

Key Terms	Definition
Pyuria	Pus in the urine
Refractometer	Instrument to indirectly determine specific gravity by refractive index
Urinalysis	The physical, chemical, and microscopic analysis of urine

Abbreviations	Definition
Epi	Epithelial cell
hpf	High-power field
lpf	Low-power field
RBC/hpf or WBC/hpf	Number of red or white blood cells seen per microscopic high-power field
SG	Specific gravity
TNTC	Too numerous to count
Trich	Trichomonas vaginalis
UA	Routine urinalysis

Urinalysis may be a separate laboratory section or may be a part of the hematology or chemistry sections. Urinalysis is a routine screening procedure to detect disorders and infections of the kidney and to detect metabolic disorders such as diabetes mellitus and liver disease.

A routine urinalysis (**UA**) consists of physical, chemical, and microscopic examination of the urine. The physical examination evaluates the color, clarity, and specific gravity of the urine. The chemical examination is performed using chemical reagent strips to determine pH, glucose, ketones, protein, blood, bilirubin, urobilinogen, nitrite, and leukocytes (Fig. 4–10). The microscopic examination identifies the presence of cells, **casts**, bacteria, crystals, yeast, and parasites.

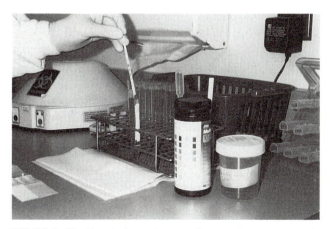

FIGURE 4–10. Chemical examination of urine using a reagent strip.

Specimen Collection and Handling

Phlebotomists may be requested to deliver urine specimens to the laboratory. This should be done promptly as many changes can take place in a urine specimen that sits at room temperature for longer than 1 hour. Different types of specimens are required for testing. Random specimens are most frequently collected for routine screening; however, a first morning specimen is more concentrated and may be required for certain tests. Other types of urine specimens include timed or 24-hour collections for quantitative chemistry tests, and midstream clean-catch and catheterized specimens for cultures.

Tests Performed in the Urinalysis Section

The primary test performed in the urinalysis section is the routine urinalysis. As shown in Table 4–7 the test has multiple parts.

TABLE 4–7. **ROUTINE URINALYSIS**

Test	Function
Color	Detects blood, bilirubin, and other pigments
Appearance	Detects cellular and crystalline elements
Specific gravity (**SG**)	Measures the concentration of urine
pH	Determines the acidity of urine
Protein	Elevated levels indicate kidney disorders
Glucose	Elevated levels indicate diabetes mellitus
Ketones	Elevated levels indicate diabetes mellitus or starvation
Blood	Detects red blood cells or hemoglobin
Bilirubin	Elevated levels indicate liver disorders
Urobilinogen	Elevated levels indicate liver or hemolytic disorders
Nitrite	Detects bacterial infection
Leukocyte esterase	Detects white blood cells
Microscopic	Determines the number and type of cellular elements

BIBLIOGRAPHY

Brown, BA: Hematology: Principles and Procedures, ed. 6. Lea & Febiger, Philadelphia, 1992.

Clerc, JM: An Introduction to Clinical Laboratory Science. CV Mosby, St Louis, 1992.

McKenzie, SB: Textbook of Hematology. Lea & Febiger, Philadelphia, 1988.

Walters, NJ, et al: Basic Medical Laboratory Techniques. Delmar Publishers, Albany, NY, 1986.

Study Questions   1. Interpret the following situations by defining the underlined words:

a. A patient with liver disease has <u>icteric</u> serum to be tested for <u>ALP</u> and <u>GGT</u>.

_____

_____

_____

b. You draw blood for a <u>PT</u>, <u>APTT</u>, and <u>CBC</u> on a <u>pre-op</u> patient.

_____

_____

_____

_____

c. A patient with <u>leukemia</u> has a low <u>Hgb</u>, <u>Hct</u>, and <u>RBC</u>, and a high <u>WBC</u>.

_____

_____

_____

_____

_____

d. A <u>C & S</u> is performed to determine if the patient has a <u>UTI</u>.

_____

_____

e. The <u>VDRL</u> and <u>RPR</u> are tests for syphilis, which is a <u>communicable</u> disease.

_____

_____

_____

f. The microbiology section includes <u>mycology</u> and performs tests for <u>AFB</u> and <u>O & P</u>.

_____

_____

_____

g. Tests for <u>HIV</u> are performed using <u>EIA</u> and tests for <u>HBsAg</u> are performed using <u>RIA</u>.

_____

_____

_____

_____

h. A request to the <u>BB</u> for a <u>type and screen</u> was made in the event the patient would need a transfusion.

_____

_____

2. To which laboratory departments would the following tests be taken:

a. Type and screen _____

b. C & S _____

c. Electrolytes _____

d. FBS _____

e. Sed rate _____

f. RPR and VDRL _____

g. Gram stain _____

h. Bilirubin _____

i. CBC _____

j. DAT _____

k. HIV _____

l. X-match _____

3. Define STS and give two examples of tests.

_____

_____

_____

4. Define autoimmune disease and give two examples of related tests.

_____

_____

_____

5. Define CRP and indicate a disorder identified by this test.

_____

_____

6. List the tests included in a liver profile.

a. _____

b. _____

c. _____

d. _____

e. _____

7. Name three areas of the chemistry section and give an example of a test performed in each.

   Area   **Test**

   a. _____   _____

   b. _____   _____

   c. _____   _____

8. Name the enzymes used to diagnose a myocardial infarction.

   _____

   _____

   _____

   _____

9. Name two tests performed in the coagulation area to monitor anticoagulant therapy.

   a. _____

   b. _____

10. Name the components of a CBC. Place a check-mark beside the components associated with red blood cells.

    a. _____   _____

    b. _____   _____

    c. _____   _____

    d. _____   _____

    e. _____   _____

    f. _____   _____

    g. _____   _____

    h. _____   _____

11. Differentiate between serum and plasma.

    _____

    _____

12. List three types of blood components prepared from whole blood.

    a. _____

    b. _____

    c. _____

13. Compare a type and screen request with a type and crossmatch request.

_____

_____

_____

14. Describe a situation where an autologous transfusion is performed.

_____

_____

15. Name eight chemical reactions tested in a routine urinalysis and state their clinical significance.

Reaction	**Significance**
a. _____	_____
b. _____	_____
c. _____	_____
d. _____	_____
e. _____	_____
f. _____	_____
g. _____	_____
h. _____	_____

16. Are the test results valid for a urine specimen that has sat at room temperature overnight? Why or why not?

_____

_____

17. List five types of urine specimens.

a. _____

b. _____

c. _____

d. _____

e. _____

18. How would you indicate the results of a Gram stain in which the bacteria stain red?

_____

19. Name four subsections of microbiology and give an example of a test performed in each.

Subsection	**Test Performed**
a. _____	_____
b. _____	_____
c. _____	_____
d. _____	_____

20. Name a microbiology test in which the phlebotomist would collect blood.

    _____

Terminology
Continued

Abbreviations	Definition
CDC	Centers for Disease Control
HBV	Hepatitis B virus
MSDS	Material Safety Data Sheets
NFPA	National Fire Protection Association
OSHA	Occupational Safety and Health Administration
PPE	Personal protective equipment

The healthcare setting contains a wide variety of safety hazards, many capable of producing serious injury or life-threatening disease. To work safely in this environment, the phlebotomist must learn what hazards exist, the basic safety precautions associated with them, and finally to apply the basic rules of common sense required for everyday safety. As can be seen in Table 5–1, some hazards are unique to the healthcare environment and others are encountered routinely throughout life. One must keep in mind that these hazards affect not only the phlebotomist but also the patient. Therefore phlebotomists must be prepared to protect both themselves and the patients.

TABLE 5–1. **TYPES OF SAFETY HAZARDS**

Type	Source	Possible Injury
Biologic	Infectious agents	Bacterial, fungal, viral, or parasitic infections
Sharp	Needles, lancets, and broken glass	Cuts, punctures, or blood-borne pathogen exposure
Chemical	Preservatives and reagents	Exposure to toxic, carcinogenic, or caustic agents
Radioactive	Equipment and radioisotopes	Radiation exposure
Electrical	Ungrounded or wet equipment and frayed cords	Burns or shock
Fire/explosive	Bunsen burners and organic chemicals	Burns or dismemberment
Physical	Wet floors, heavy boxes, and patients	Falls, sprains, or strains

BIOLOGIC HAZARDS

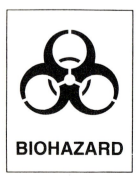

BIOHAZARD

The healthcare setting provides an abundant source of potentially harmful microorganisms including bacteria, fungi, parasites, and viruses. An understanding of the transmission (chain of infection) of microorganisms is necessary to prevent infection. The chain of infection requires a continuous link between three elements — a source, a method of transmission, and a susceptible host. The source refers to the location of the potentially harmful microorganisms and may be a person or a contaminated object. Microorganisms from the source must then be transferred to the host. This may occur through direct contact (host touches or is touched by the contaminated source), inhaling infected material (**aerosol** droplets released by an infected patient or an uncapped tube in a centrifuge), ingesting contaminated food or water (food poisoning), or by means of a **vector** (malaria transmitted by mosquitoes). Although patients are considered the most logical susceptible host, anyone can serve

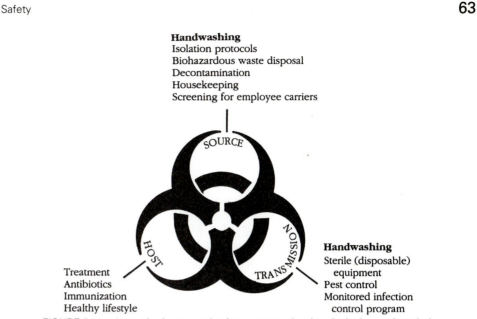

Handwashing
Isolation protocols
Biohazardous waste disposal
Decontamination
Housekeeping
Screening for employee carriers

SOURCE

HOST

TRANSMISSION

Treatment
Antibiotics
Immunization
Healthy lifestyle

Handwashing
Sterile (disposable)
equipment
Pest control
Monitored infection
control program

FIGURE 5–1. Chain of infection and safety pratices related to the biohaazard symbol.

as the host. Therefore safety precautions are designed for both healthcare workers and patients. Keep in mind that once the chain of infection is completed, the susceptible host becomes the new source. The ultimate goal of biologic safety is to prevent completion of the chain. Figure 5 - 1 utilizes the universal symbol for **biohazardous** material to illustrate the chain of infection and demonstrates how it can be broken by following prescribed safety practices.

Previously uninfected patients who become infected during hospitalization represent approximately 5% of the patient population. The term **nosocomial infection** designates an infection contracted by a patient during a hospital stay. Although some of these infections may be caused by visitors, the majority are the result of personnel not following infection control practices.

Handwashing

Notice the emphasis on handwashing in Figure 5 - 1. Hand contact represents the number one method of infection transmission. Phlebotomists have contact with numerous patients each day and without the observance of proper precautions such contact can provide an unlimited vehicle for the transmission of infection. It is essential to **change gloves and wash the hands between patients**.

The importance of handwashing continues away from the patient setting for the purpose of protecting coworkers, family and friends, and the phlebotomist. Hands should always be washed prior to leaving the laboratory, at any time when they have been knowingly contaminated, and before going to designated break areas, as well as before and after using bathroom facilities.

Correct routine handwashing technique includes:

1 Wetting hands with warm water
2 Applying soap, preferably antimicrobial
3 Rubbing to form a lather, create friction, and loosen debris
4 Thoroughly cleaning between the fingers and under fingernails and rings for at least 15 seconds

5 Rinsing hands in a downward position

6 Drying with a paper towel

7 Turning off faucets with the used paper towel to prevent recontamination

More stringent procedures are utilized in surgery and areas with highly susceptible patients.

Isolation Procedures

Preventing the spread of **infection** by isolation of the source can be accomplished through the use of protective barriers such as walls and doors in isolation rooms, and by wearing protective clothing, including gowns, masks, and gloves. The type of protective barriers used will vary, depending on the infectious agents present or the susceptibility of the patient. Isolation procedures may be specified for a particular room or for an entire hospital area, such as the nursery or a burn unit. Common isolation classifications are summarized in Table 5 – 2.

Phlebotomists need to be aware of particular hospital isolation practices and to be always alert to warning signs posted on the doors of patient rooms. Warning signs usually contain specific instructions for the type of protective apparel that should be worn.

TABLE 5–2. **ISOLATION CLASSIFICATIONS**

Type of Isolation	Conditions	Protective Apparel
Strict	Infectious diseases: chicken pox, measles, diphtheria, rabies, staphylococcal and streptococcal pneumonia	Gown, mask, and gloves
Respiratory	Air-borne infections: tuberculosis, mumps, whooping cough, and meningococcal meningitis	Mask and gloves for phlebotomy
Enteric	Organisms causing disease through ingestion: *Salmonella*, *Shigella*, *Yersinia*, and intestinal parasites	Gown and gloves
Drainage/secretion	Skin, wound, and surgical infections	Gown and gloves
Blood/body fluid	Blood-borne pathogens: hepatitis and HIV	Gloves (gown and face shield if performing more than phlebotomy)
Protective (reverse)	Immunocompromised patients: burns, nursery, and chemotherapy	Sterile gown, mask, gloves, and equipment

Personal Protective Equipment

Personal protective equipment (**PPE**) encountered by phlebotomists includes gowns, masks, gloves, and face shields. Fluid-resistant lab coats and gloves are worn with all patients. A mask or other face protection may be necessary when working with isolation patients or processing specimens in the laboratory.

Specific procedures must be followed when putting on and removing protective apparel. Protective clothing is donned prior to entering the room and, except for protective isolation, is removed prior to leaving the room. The removed clothing is placed in designated containers.

Gowns usually tie in the back and have long sleeves with tightly fitting cuffs. The gowns should be large enough to provide full body coverage, including closing in the back. Masks must be securely tied at both the top and bottom. To provide maximum effectiveness, be sure the side designated "outside" is facing outward. Gloves are put on last and are stretched over the cuffs of the gown. Protective apparel is removed in reverse order — gloves, mask, and gown. Care must be taken not to touch the contaminated outer surfaces of the apparel (Fig. 5 – 2).

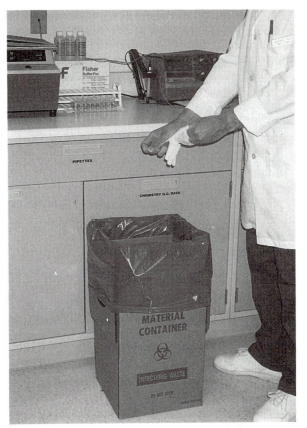

FIGURE 5–2. Removal of contaminated gloves.

When dealing with isolation situations special precautions must also be taken with phlebotomy equipment and specimens collected. Bring only the necessary equipment (not the phlebotomy tray) into the room; however, be sure to include duplicate collection tubes and enough supplies to perform a second venipuncture, should it be necessary. Tourniquets, gauze, alcohol pads, and pens may already be present in the room. All equipment taken into the room must be left in the room and, when appropriate, deposited in labeled waste containers. Specimens taken from the room should be cleaned of any blood contamination and placed in plastic bags located at the door. Bags should be folded open to allow tubes to be added without touching the outside of the bag with contaminated gloves or tubes. Double bagging is required when contaminated waste is removed from isolation rooms.

As with protective isolation apparel, the exception to these rules is protective isolation, which requires that all materials be removed from the room and does not require specimen bagging.

Universal Precautions

The primary biologic hazard associated with phlebotomy is exposure to blood-borne pathogens transmitted by blood-to-blood contact. Transmission may occur by accidentally puncturing oneself with a contaminated needle or lancet, or by passive contact through open skin lesions or mucous membranes of the eyes, nose, or mouth. Blood-borne **pathogens** of major concern are the hepatitis B virus (**HBV**) and the human immunodeficiency virus (HIV).

Because it is impossible to always know whether or not a patient's blood contains a blood-borne pathogen, the Centers for Disease Control (**CDC**) developed the guideline of **Universal Precautions** in 1988. Under universal precautions all patients should be assumed to be infectious for blood-borne pathogens. The guideline recommends wearing gloves when collecting and handling blood specimens, wearing face shields when there is a danger of blood splashing on mucous membranes, and disposing of all needles and sharp objects in puncture-resistant containers without recapping.

To protect workers further, the universal precautions guidelines were expanded in 1992 and enacted into law. These regulations are monitored and enforced by the Occupational Safety and Health Administration (**OSHA**). Under the Occupational Exposure to Blood-Borne Pathogens Standard all employers must have a written blood-borne pathogen exposure control plan available in the workplace and must provide necessary protection free of charge to employees. Specifics of the OSHA standard include:

1   Requiring all employees to practice universal precautions.
2   Providing lab coats, gowns, face shields, and gloves to employees, and laundry facilities for nondisposable protective clothing.
3   Providing sharps disposal containers and prohibiting recapping of needles.
4   Prohibiting eating, drinking, smoking, and applying cosmetics in the work area.
5   Labeling all biohazardous material and containers.
6   Providing immunization for the hepatitis B virus free of charge.
7   Establishing a daily work surface disinfection protocol. The **disinfectant** of choice for blood-borne pathogens is sodium hypochlorite (household bleach freshly diluted 1:10).
8   Providing medical follow-up to employees who have been accidentally exposed.
9   Documenting regular training of employees in safety standards.

All phlebotomists should become familiar with the blood-borne pathogen exposure control plan in their laboratories.

SHARP HAZARDS

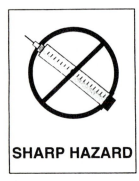

SHARP HAZARD

Exposure to sharp hazards is of particular concern to phlebotomists, as needles and lancets are the primary pieces of equipment associated with blood collection. They can present a very serious hazard to phlebotomists if proper safety precautions are not followed.

The number one personal safety rule in phlebotomy is to **never** manually recap a needle. Many safety devices are available for needle disposal and they provide a variety of safeguards. These include puncture-resistant containers that allow manual unscrewing or automatic removal of the needle from the holder, needle holders that become a sheathe, and needles that automatically resheathe. Phlebotomists should become proficient with the needle disposal equipment in their laboratory prior to drawing patients.

Lancets and butterfly apparatus are equally dangerous. They should be carefully disposed of in puncture-resistant containers immediately after use and should never be left lying on the work surface. Many lancets now have retractable points, and automatic needle covers have been developed for the butterfly apparatus.

Puncture-resistant containers with biohazard labels as shown in Figure 5–3 should always be available and conveniently located. Often they are attached to the

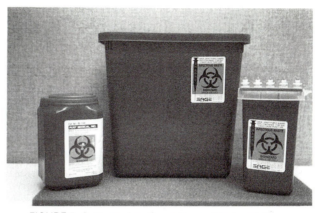

FIGURE 5–3. Examples of puncture-resistant containers.

walls in patient rooms. Do not reach into these containers when disposing of material as accidental puncture may occur from a previously discarded needle.

CHEMICAL HAZARDS

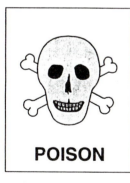

POISON

The same general rules for handling biohazardous materials apply to chemically hazardous materials; that is, to avoid getting these materials in or on your body, clothes, or work area. It should be assumed that every chemical in the laboratory is hazardous. When skin contact occurs, the best first aid is to flush the area with large amounts of water. Phlebotomists should know the location of emergency showers and eye wash stations located in the laboratory. Do not try to neutralize chemicals spilled on the skin.

Chemicals should never be mixed together unless specific instructions are followed, and they must be added in the order specified. This is particularly important when combining acid and water, as acid should always be added to water to avoid the possibility of splashing.

All chemicals and reagents containing hazardous ingredients in a concentration greater than 1% are required to have a Material Safety Data Sheet (**MSDS**) on file in the laboratory. By law, vendors must provide these sheets to purchasers; however, it is the responsibility of the laboratory to obtain and keep them available to employees. A MSDS contains information on physical and chemical characteristics; fire, explosion, reactivity, and health hazards; primary routes of entry; exposure limits and carcinogenic potential; precautions for safe handling; and spill clean-up and emergency first aid information. Containers of chemicals that pose a high risk must be labeled with a chemical hazard symbol.

OSHA requires all laboratories that use hazardous chemicals to have a written Chemical Hygiene Plan. The purpose of the plan is to detail appropriate work practices, procedures, methods of control, protective equipment, and special precautions that must be taken when working with particularly hazardous chemicals. Employees must receive documented training in the procedures detailed in the plan. They must also have access to the plan at all times.

Examples of required laboratory safety equipment and information are illustrated in Figures 5-4 and 5-5.

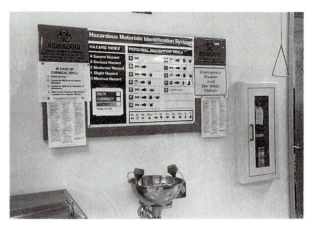

FIGURE 5-4. A laboratory safety equipment station.

RADIOACTIVE HAZARDS

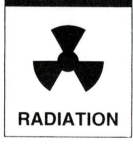

Phlebotomists may come in contact with **radioactivity** while drawing blood from patients in the radiology department, when drawing blood from patients receiving radioactive treatments, and in the laboratory when procedures using **radioisotopes** are performed.

The amount of radioactivity present in most medical situations is very small and represents little danger; however, the effects of radiation are related to the length of exposure. Persons working in a radioactive environment are required to wear measuring devices to determine the amount of radiation they are accumulating.

Phlebotomists should be familiar with the radioactive hazard symbol shown in the margin. This symbol must be displayed on the doors of all areas where radioactive material is present. Exposure to radiation during pregnancy presents a danger to the fetus and phlebotomists who are pregnant or think they may be should avoid areas with this symbol.

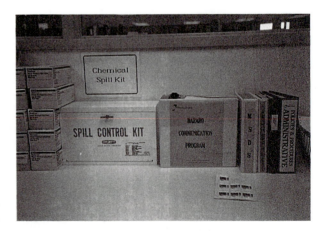

FIGURE 5-5. Laboratory safety supplies and information manuals.

ELECTRICAL HAZARDS

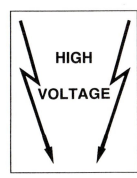

The healthcare setting contains a large amount of electrical equipment that phlebotomists are in contact with, both in the laboratory and in the patients' rooms. The same general rules of electrical safety observed outside the workplace apply. Keep in mind that the danger of water or fluid coming in contact with equipment is greater in the hospital setting.

Electrical equipment is closely monitored by designated hospital personnel; however, phlebotomists should be observant for any dangerous conditions, such as frayed cords and overloaded circuits, and should report them to the appropriate persons. Equipment that has become wet should be unplugged and allowed to dry completely before reusing.

When drawing blood, phlebotomists should avoid contact with electrical equipment in the room, as current from ungrounded equipment can pass through the phlebotomist and metal needle to the patient.

When a situation involving electrical **shock** occurs it is important to remove the electrical source immediately. This must be done without touching the person or the equipment because the current will pass on to you. Turning off the circuit breaker, unplugging the equipment, or moving the equipment using a nonconductive glass or wood object are safe procedures to follow.

FIRE/EXPLOSIVE HAZARDS

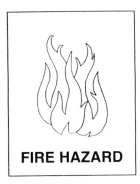

All healthcare institutions have posted evacuation routes and detailed plans to follow when a fire occurs. Phlebotomists should be familiar with these procedures and with the basic steps to follow when a fire is discovered. Initial procedures to follow are:

1 Pull the fire alarm and call the fire department.
2 Remove patients or other persons from any danger.
3 If possible, extinguish the fire using an appropriate fire extinguisher.
4 Close windows and doors when evacuating the area.
5 Evacuate, using stairs not the elevator, by the nearest exit.

The laboratory uses many chemicals that may be volatile or explosive and special procedures for their storage and handling are required. Designated chemicals are stored in explosion-proof cabinets or refrigerators and are used under vented hoods. Fire blankets must be available in the laboratory. Persons with burning clothes should be rolled in the blanket to smother flames.

When delivering specimens to laboratory sections that use open flames, phlebotomists should be aware of the flame location to avoid possible burns.

The National Fire Protection Association (**NFPA**) classifies fires with regard to the type of burning material and also classifies the type of fire extinguisher that is used to control them. This information is summarized in Table 5–3. The multipurpose ABC fire extinguishers are the most common but the label should always be checked before using.

The Standard System for the Identification of the Fire Hazards of Materials, NFPA 704, is a symbol system used to inform firefighters of the hazards they may encounter when fighting a fire in a particular area. The color-coded areas contain information relating to health, flammability, reactivity, use of water, and personal protection. These symbols are placed on doors, cabinets, and reagent bottles.

TABLE 5-3. **TYPES OF FIRES AND FIRE EXTINGUISHERS**

Fire Type	Composition of Fire	Type of Fire Extinguisher	Extinguishing Material
Class A	Wood, paper, or clothing	Class A	Water
Class B	Flammable organic chemicals	Class B	Dry chemicals, carbon dioxide, foam, or halon
Class C	Electrical	Class C	Dry chemicals, carbon dioxide, or halon
Class D	Combustible metals	None	Sand or dry powder
		Class ABC	Dry chemicals

PHYSICAL HAZARDS

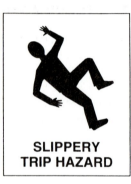

SLIPPERY TRIP HAZARD

These hazards are not unique to the healthcare setting and routine precautions observed outside the workplace apply. General precautions to consider are to avoid running in rooms and hallways; watching for wet floors; bending the knees when lifting patients and boxes; and maintaining a clean, organized work area. Phlebotomists should select comfortable, closed-toe shoes that provide maximum support.

BIBLIOGRAPHY

Baron, EJ, and Finegold, SM: Diagnostic Microbiology. CV Mosby, St. Louis, 1990.

Linne, JJ, and Ringsrud, KM: Basic Techniques in Clinical Laboratory Science. CV Mosby, St. Louis, 1992.

National Fire Protection Association: Hazardous Chemical Data, No. 49. NFPA, Boston, 1991.

Occupational Exposure to Blood-Borne Pathogens, Final Rule. Federal Register, 29(Dec 6), 1991.

Occupational Exposure to Hazardous Chemicals in Laboratories, Final Rule. Federal Register, 55(Jan 31), 1990.

Update, Universal Precautions for Prevention of Transmission of Human Immunodeficiency Virus, Hepatitis B Virus and Other Blood-Borne Pathogens in Health Care Settings. MMWR (Morb Mortal Wkly Rep), 37:377, 1988.

Study Questions

1. List an example of each of the following laboratory hazards.

   a. Biologic _____

   b. Sharp _____

   c. Chemical _____

   d. Radioactive _____

   e. Electrical _____

   f. Fire _____

   g. Physical _____

2. List four methods by which infection can be transferred from the source to the host.

   a. _____

   b. _____

   c. _____

   d. _____

3. When drawing blood from five patients in ICU, how many pairs of gloves should be used? _____

4. A patient who develops a staphylococcal pneumonia after entering the hospital has a _____ infection.

5. Indicate the correct order for putting on and removing protective apparel by placing a 1, 2, or 3 opposite the listed apparel.

	Putting On	**Removing**
a. Gown	_____	_____
b. Gloves	_____	_____
c. Mask	_____	_____

6. What type of isolation requires the phlebotomist to remove all items taken into the room? _____

7. The recommended disinfectant for blood and body fluid spills is

   _____ .

8. Under what conditions are face shields required to be worn in the laboratory?

   _____

   _____

9. Name two viruses transmitted by blood and body fluids.

   a. _____

   b. _____

10. When a caustic solution such as phenol is spilled on the skin, what is the recommended first aid?

_____

11. Differentiate between MSDS and NFPA regarding location in the laboratory and purpose.

_____

_____

_____

12. True or False. Water should always be added to acid. _____

13. Give an example of when a phlebotomist should avoid areas with a radiation symbol.

_____

14. List three ways to remove the source of an electrical shock.

a. _____

b. _____

c. _____

15. The first few things to do when a fire is discovered are to

_____

_____

_____

_____

_____

16. What type of fire can be extinguished using water?

_____

17. Match the following symbols with the numbered hazard they represent.

Symbol	Hazard

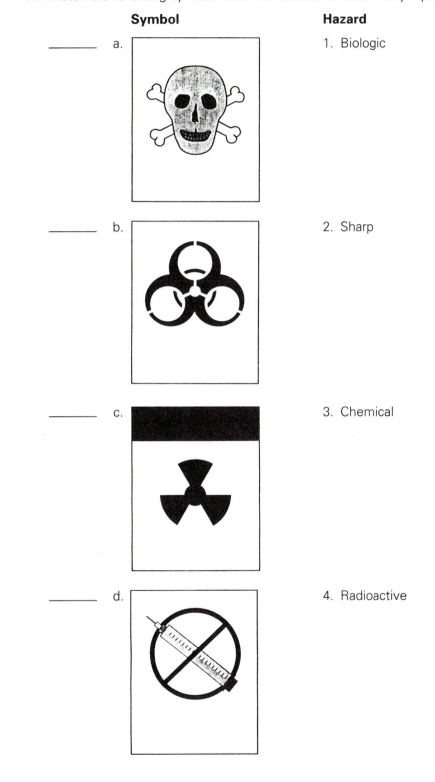

_____ a.

1. Biologic

_____ b.

2. Sharp

_____ c.

3. Chemical

_____ d.

4. Radioactive

18. After reading the Chemical Hygiene Plan and Blood-Borne Pathogen Exposure Control Plan for your training facility, state the name of the control officer responsible for each.

_____

_____

Laboratory Safety Exercise

Instructions
Explore the student laboratory or the area designated by the instructor and provide the following information.

1. Location of the fire extinguishers

   _____

   _____

2. State the instructions for operation of the fire extinguisher

   _____

   _____

   _____

3. Location of the fire blanket

   _____

4. Location of the eye wash station

   _____

5. Location of the emergency shower

   _____

6. Location of the first aid kit

   _____

7. Location of the master electrical panel

   _____

8. Location of the fire alarm

   _____

9. The emergency exit route

   _____

10. Location of the MSDS pertaining to phlebotomy

    _____

11. Location of the emergency spill kit

    _____

12. Location of the chemical hygiene plan

    _____

13. Location of the blood-borne pathogen exposure control plan

    _____

14. Locate an NFPA sign and list the following

    Location   _____

    Health Rating   _____

    Fire Rating   _____

    Reactivity Rating _____

15. What disinfectants are available for cleaning work areas?

    _____

    _____

RODUCTION TO THE BODY

inology
ued

Key Terms	Definition
Medial	Pertaining to the middle of a structure
Posterior, dorsal	Pertaining to the back of the body
Prone	Lying on the abdomen with the face down
Proximal	Closest to the point of attachment
Sagittal plane	Vertical plane dividing the body into right and left portions
Superficial	On the surface
Superior	Pertaining to a position above another structure
Supine	Lying on the back
Transverse plane	Horizontal plane dividing the body into upper and lower portions

Abbreviations	Definition
AP	Anterior-posterior
lat	Lateral
PA	Posterior-anterior

The phlebotomist, as well as all health professionals, must have knowledge of the basic anatomy and physiology of the body to communicate effectively in the medical setting.

The smallest functioning unit of the body is the cell. All cells are composed of a nucleus and cytoplasm contained within a membrane. There are many different types of cells and each has a specialized function and is capable of communicating with other cells throughout the body. Groups of specific cells with similar structure and function form the many types of body tissue. For example, muscle cells form muscle tissue and nerve cells form nerve tissue. Organs are then formed by the combination of various types of tissue and the organs are combined into the body systems.

ECTIONAL
RMS

Discussion of the anatomy and physiology of the body often refers to different body planes, directions, systems, cavities, and organs. An understanding of directional terms is necessary for the phlebotomist to perform procedures correctly and to communicate with other healthcare personnel. Directional terms are used to describe areas of the body in relation to other body structures.

To define the location of areas of the body, it is assumed that the body is in an anatomic position. Anatomic position describes the human body as standing erect, the eyes looking forward, the arms by the sides, and the palms of the hands and the toes pointed forward. It must be remembered, when studying anatomic illustrations, that the right and the left sides are opposite to your own.

SECTION II Body Systems (Anatomy, Physiology, and Terminology)

CHAPTER 6 # Introduction to the Body and Integumentary Sys

Learning Objectives

Upon completion of this chapter, the reader will be able to:

1 State the meaning of the roots and define the terms and abb associated with the body and the integumentary system.
2 Relate positions, directions, and planes of the body to phlebo
3 List the body cavities and the organs associated with each ca
4 List the major body systems.
5 Describe the function of the integumentary system.
6 Identify the layers of skin.
7 Name the accessory skin organs.
8 Describe the disorders associated with the integumentary sys
9 State the clinical correlations of laboratory tests associated wi integumentary system.

INTRODUCTION TO THE BODY

Terminology

Roots/Combining Forms	Meaning
anter/o	front, before
dist/o	distant
dors/o	back
later/o	side
medi/o	middle
poster/o	back, behind
proxim/o	near

Key Terms	Definition
Anterior, ventral	Pertaining to the front of the body
Bilateral	Pertaining to both sides of a structure
Distal	Farthest from the point of attachment
Frontal plane	Vertical plane dividing the body into the and the posterior (back) portion
Homeostasis	State of equilibrium in the body
Inferior, caudal	Pertaining to a position below another str
Lateral	Pertaining to a side of a structure

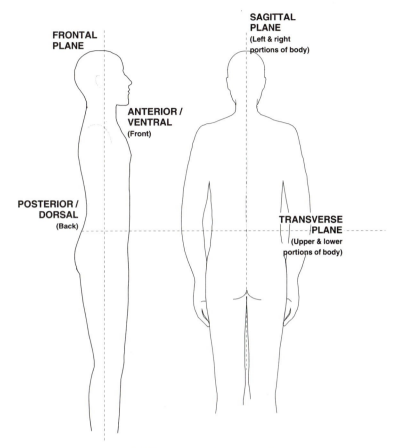

FIGURE 6–1. The planes of the body.

In describing areas of the body, the terms **anterior**, **posterior**, **superior**, **inferior**, **proximal**, **distal**, **lateral**, **medial**, **superficial**, and deep are used.

BODY PLANES

A plane is an imaginary flat surface that divides the body into front, back, right, left, upper, and lower sections to facilitate the identification and relationships of body structures. The body is divided into anterior (front or **ventral**) and posterior (back or **dorsal**) portions by the **frontal plane**. The **sagittal plane** divides the body vertically into right and left portions. The **transverse plane** is a cross-sectional plane. It divides the body horizontally into upper and lower portions. Refer to Figure 6–1 for the body planes.

BODY CAVITIES

Body cavities contain the internal organs. Two major cavities, the anterior and posterior, enclose five subcavities (Fig. 6–2). The anterior (ventral) cavity of the body is divided into the thoracic (chest), abdominal, and pelvic cavities. The posterior (dorsal)

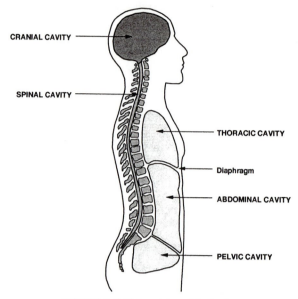

FIGURE 6–2. The cavities of the body.

cavity is divided into the cranial and spinal cavities. Table 6–1 lists the main organs contained in these cavities.

BODY SYSTEMS

Groups of organs working together make up the body systems. Each body system or unit has a common set of functions. The ability of the body systems to keep the body functioning normally, in spite of constantly changing conditions, is an essential function referred to as **homeostasis**. The major body systems are the integumentary, circulatory, lymphatic, skeletal, muscular, nervous, respiratory, digestive, urinary, endocrine, and reproductive. Laboratory tests to evaluate each of these body systems and the organs involved are discussed in the following chapters. By evaluating blood, urine, body fluids, and tissue specimens, the laboratory can provide the physician with the information necessary to assess the patient's condition, diagnose disorders, and treat the patient.

TABLE 6–1. **BODY CAVITIES AND THEIR ORGANS**

Plane	Cavity	Organ
Anterior	Thoracic	Lungs and heart
	Abdominal	Stomach, small and large intestines, spleen, liver, gallbladder, pancreas, and kidneys
	Pelvic	Bladder, colon, ovaries, and testes
Posterior	Cranial	Brain
	Spinal	Spinal cord

INTEGUMENTARY SYSTEM

Terminology Associated with the Integumentary System

Roots/Combining Forms	Meaning
carcin/o	cancer
cutane/o, dermat/o	skin
hidr/o	sweat
hist/o	tissue
hydr/o	water
kerat/o	hard tissue
melan/o	black
onych/o	nail
seb/o	sebum, oily secretion
squam/o	scalelike
trich/o	hair

Key Terms	Definition
Albino	Person who lacks the pigment melanin
Benign	Noncancerous
Dermis	Inner layer of skin
Epidermis	Outer layer of skin
Epithelium	Layer of skin cells
Erythema	Redness or inflammation of the skin
Keratin	Tough protein found in the outer skin, hair, and nails
Malignant	Cancerous
Melanin	Black pigment in the outer skin
Sebaceous gland	Oil-producing gland
Subcutaneous	Innermost layer of skin composed of connective tissue and fat

Abbreviations	Definition
Bx	Biopsy
KOH	Potassium hydroxide

The integumentary system is made up of the skin, hair, nails, and the sweat and sebaceous glands. The primary function of skin is protection of the body (Fig. 6-3). Skin, a sheetlike membrane, is the predominant organ of this system and is the largest organ of the body. The surface of skin is composed of dead, hardened cells, which are constantly sloughed off and replaced by new cells, which multiply underneath the dead cells. Dermatology is the branch of medicine specializing in the skin.

FUNCTION

Skin protects the body against invasion by microorganisms and environmental chemicals. In addition, it regulates temperature by insulating the body. Glands under the skin produce secretions to lubricate the skin and produce sweat to keep the

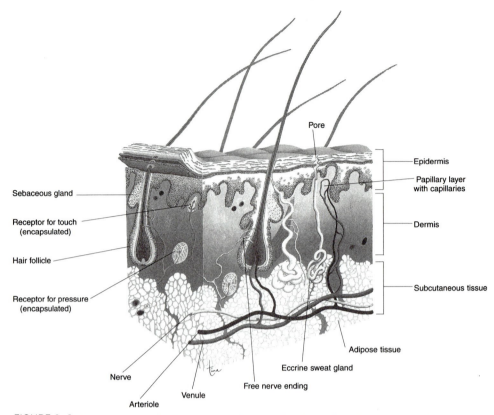

FIGURE 6–3. Cross-section of the skin. (Adapted from Scanlon, VC, and Sanders, T: Essentials of Anatomy and Physiology, ed. 2. FA Davis, Philadelphia, 1995, p. 89.)

body cool. Sensory organs are embedded in the skin to receive sensations such as pain, temperature, pressure, and touch.

COMPONENTS OF THE INTEGUMENTARY SYSTEM

Skin is composed of three layers, the epidermis, the dermis, and the subcutaneous. The outermost layer of skin is the **epidermis**, which is made up of stratified (layered) squamous **epithelium**, and keratinized (hardened) epithelium. This is the thinnest layer of skin and contains no blood vessels. In the innermost layer of the epidermis, cells undergo cell division (mitosis) to reproduce themselves, a process that allows the skin to repair itself when it is injured. **Melanin** is produced in the epidermis to give skin its color.

The **dermis** lies below the epidermis and is the living tissue of the skin. It is thicker than the epidermis and is composed of blood and lymph vessels, nerve fibers, hair follicles, sweat glands, sebaceous glands, and connective tissue. Dermal papillae are peglike projections that help bind the two skin layers together. These ridges and grooves form the fingerprints.

The **subcutaneous** layer is a connective tissue specializing in the formation of fat. It connects skin to the surface of muscles, protects the deep tissues of the body, and acts as a heat insulator.

Hair is composed of **keratin**, a hard protein substance. Hair follicles are small tubes or sheaths that hold the hair fibers from which the hair develops.

Nails consist of hard keratin plates and cover the ends of toes and fingers. Nails grow from the nail root located at the base of the nail plate.

Sweat glands are coiled glands, located in the dermis, with ducts extending up through the epidermis to small pores on almost all body surfaces. They produce a watery fluid called sweat, which functions to eliminate waste products and regulate body temperature.

Sebaceous glands are referred to as oil glands because they secrete an oil called sebum for the lubrication of hair and skin.

DISORDERS ASSOCIATED WITH THE INTEGUMENTARY SYSTEM

Acne

Acne occurs most commonly during adolescence. It is caused by an oversecretion of sebum, which causes blockage of the sebaceous gland ducts and the formation of pustules that rupture and cause infection.

Fungal Infections

Infections caused by the dermatophyte fungi include ringworm, athlete's foot, and jock itch. They can produce itching, scaling, and **erythema** and are referred to as tinea infections.

Impetigo

A highly contagious staphylococcus or streptococcus infection that is most frequently seen in younger children. It can start with erythema and develop into vesicles and yellow crusts.

Keloid

An enlarged thickened scar at the site of a surgical incision or skin wound that is produced by excess collagen formation.

Psoriasis

A chronic inflammatory skin disease characterized by itchy, scaly, red patches on the skin.

Skin Cancer

The most common skin carcinomas are squamous cell carcinoma, basal cell carcinoma, and **malignant** melanoma. Kaposi's sarcoma is also a form of skin cancer and is associated with acquired immunodeficiency syndrome.

LABORATORY TESTS

The most frequently ordered laboratory tests associated with the integumentary system and their clinical correlations are presented in Table 6 - 2.

TABLE 6–2. **LABORATORY TESTS ASSOCIATED WITH THE INTEGUMENTARY SYSTEM**

Test	Clinical Correlation
Culture and sensitivity (C & S)	Bacterial or fungal infection
Potassium hydroxide (**KOH**) prep	Fungal infection
Skin biopsy (**Bx**)	Malignancy

BIBLIOGRAPHY

Basmajian, JV: Grant's Method of Anatomy. Williams & Wilkins, Baltimore, 1971.

Chabner, D-E: The Language of Medicine. WB Saunders, Philadelphia, 1991.

Gylys, BA: Medical Terminology Simplified: A Programmed Learning Approach by Body Systems. FA Davis, Philadelphia, 1993.

Gylys, BA, and Wedding, ME: Medical Terminology: A Systems Approach, ed. 3. FA Davis, Philadelphia, 1995.

Scanlon, VC, and Sanders, T: Essentials of Anatomy and Physiology, ed. 2. FA Davis, Philadelphia, 1995.

Thibodeau, GA, and Patton, KT: The Human Body in Health and Disease. CV Mosby, St. Louis, 1991.

Study Questions
1. Using the basic terminology and the terminology from this chapter, define the following:

    a. Proximal   _____

    b. Bilateral   _____

    c. Posterior   _____

    d. Spinal   _____

    e. Thoracic   _____

    f. Dermatitis   _____

    g. Melanocyte   _____

    h. Subcutaneous   _____

    i. Intradermal   _____

2. Interpret the following situations by defining the underlined words:

    a. A skin <u>Bx</u> was sent to <u>histology</u> to diagnose <u>melanoma</u>.

    _____

    _____

    _____

    b. A <u>subcutaneous</u> injection was given by the <u>RN</u>.

    _____

    _____

    c. The teenager with <u>acne</u> was referred to a <u>dermatologist</u>.

    _____

    _____

3. Name the eleven body systems.

    a. _____

    b. _____

    c. _____

    d. _____

    e. _____

    f. _____

    g. _____

    h. _____

    i. _____

    j. _____

    k. _____

4. Name three body cavities located on the anterior surface of the body.

   a. _____

   b. _____

   c. _____

5. Explain the significance of the anatomic position

   _____

   _____

6. Name the three body planes and state how they divide the body.

   a. _____

   b. _____

   c. _____

7. Differentiate the layers of the skin.

   _____

   _____

   _____

8. List three functions of the skin.

   a. _____

   b. _____

   c. _____

9. Name the two types of skin glands and indicate their location and function.

Type	**Location**	**Function**
a. _____	_____	_____
b. _____	_____	_____

10. Name three common forms of skin cancer.

    a. _____

    b. _____

    c. _____

CHAPTER 7   Circulatory and Lymphatic Systems

Learning Objectives

Upon completion of this chapter, the reader will be able to:

1 State the meaning of the roots and suffixes, and define the terms and abbreviations associated with the circulatory and lymphatic systems.
2 Briefly describe the functions of the blood vessels, heart, and blood.
3 Differentiate between arteries, veins, and capillaries by structure and function.
4 Locate the femoral, radial, brachial, and ulnar arteries.
5 Locate the basilic, cephalic, median cubital, radial, and saphenous veins.
6 Trace the blood pathway through the heart and define the function of each chamber.
7 Identify the components of blood.
8 State the major function of red blood cells, white blood cells, and platelets.
9 Briefly explain the coagulation process.
10 Discuss the structures and function of the lymphatic system.
11 Explain the role of the immune system.
12 Describe the major disorders associated with the circulatory and lymphatic systems.
13 State the clinical correlations of laboratory tests associated with the circulatory and lymphatic systems.

CIRCULATORY SYSTEM

Terminology Associated with the Circulatory System

Roots/Combining Forms	Meaning
angi/o	vessel
ather/o	fatty substance
brachi/o	arm
cardi/o, coron/o	heart
electr/o	electricity
erythr/o	red
leuk/o	white
scler/o	hardening
thromb/o	clot
vas/o	pertaining to blood vessels

Suffixes	Meaning
-emia	pertaining to blood
-lysis	rupture

89

Terminology Associated with the Circulatory System
Continued

Suffixes	Meaning
-rrhage	bursting out
-stenosis	narrowing
-tension	pressure

Key Terms	Definition
Arteriole	Small arterial branch leading into a capillary
Artery	Blood vessel carrying oxygenated blood from the heart to the tissues
Atrium (pl. atria)	One of two upper chambers of the heart
Capillary	Small blood vessel connecting arteries and veins
Cardiovascular	Pertaining to the heart and blood vessels
Coumadin	Anticoagulant monitored by the prothrombin time
Diastole	Relaxation phase of the heartbeat
Embolus	Clot circulating in the blood stream
Endocardium	Inner lining of the heart
Endothelium	Layer of epithelial cells lining the blood vessels
Erythrocyte	Red blood cell
Fibrin	Protein substance produced in the coagulation process to form the foundation of a clot
Fibrinogen	Circulating protein converted to fibrin in the coagulation process (present in plasma but not in serum)
Heparin	Anticoagulant monitored by the activated partial thromboplastin time
Infarct	Death of a tissue (due to a lack of blood to the area)
Leukocyte	White blood cell
Lumen	Cavity of a tube or organ, such as a blood vessel
Myocarditis	Inflammation of the heart muscle
Pericardium	Membrane surrounding the heart
Prothrombin	Protein converted to thrombin in the coagulation process
Pulmonary circulation	Flow of blood from the heart to the lungs and back to the heart
Reticulocyte	Developing red blood cell
Systemic circulation	Flow of blood between the heart and the tissues
Systole	Contraction phase of the heartbeat
Thrombin	Enzyme that converts fibrinogen to fibrin
Thrombocyte (platelet)	Cell involved with clotting
Thrombus	Clot formed on the inner wall of a vein
Valve	Structure in veins and the heart that closes an opening so blood will flow in only one direction
Vascular	Pertaining to blood vessels
Vein	Blood vessel carrying deoxygenated blood from the tissues to the heart
Ventricle	One of two lower chambers of the heart
Venule	Small vein leading from a capillary

Terminology Associated with the Circulatory System Continued	Abbreviations	Definition
	BP	Blood pressure
	CHF	Congestive heart failure
	DIC	Disseminated intravascular coagulation
	ECG, EKG	Electrocardiogram
	H & H	Hemoglobin and hematocrit
	MI	Myocardial infarction
	PF3	Platelet factor 3

The circulatory (**cardiovascular**) system is the transportation system of the body. It is composed of blood vessels, the heart, and blood.

FUNCTION

The circulatory system performs the essential functions of delivering oxygen, nutrients, enzymes, hormones, and other substances to the cells and transporting waste products such as carbon dioxide and urea to organs where they can be expelled from the body. In the body's transportation system, blood cells are the vehicles, blood vessels are the roadways, and the heart provides the power. To facilitate this process the heart actually acts as two pumps with two separate circulations. The **pulmonary circulation** carries deoxygenated blood from the right ventricle of the heart to the lungs and returns oxygenated blood from the lungs to the left atrium of the heart. The **systemic circulation** carries blood from the left ventricle of the heart throughout the body.

BLOOD VESSELS

The vessels through which blood is transported are the arteries, veins, and capillaries. Arteries and veins are composed of three layers. The outer layer is a connective tissue called tunica adventitia. The middle layer is a smooth muscle tissue called tunica media. The inner layer is called the tunica intima and is composed of endothelial cells. The space within a blood vessel through which the blood flows is called the **lumen**. Capillary walls contain only a single layer of endothelial cells. Figure 7 – 1 shows the differences between arteries, veins, and capillaries.

    Arteries are large thick-walled blood vessels that carry oxygen-rich blood away from the heart. They are located deeper than veins and cannot be seen, but may be felt when pressed against a bone. The walls of arteries consist of tough connective tissue, elastic fibers, and an inner layer of endothelial cells. The thicker walls aid in the pumping of blood and give arteries the strength to resist the high pressure caused by the contraction of the heart ventricles. The elastic walls expand as the heart pushes blood through the arteries. The aorta is the largest artery and branches into smaller arteries. It receives oxygen-rich blood from the heart and distributes it to the arteries to flow throughout the body. The major arteries in the arm are the radial, brachial, and ulnar. The carotid artery is located near the side of the neck, and the femoral artery is located in the groin area. Figure 7 – 2 shows the major arteries in the body.

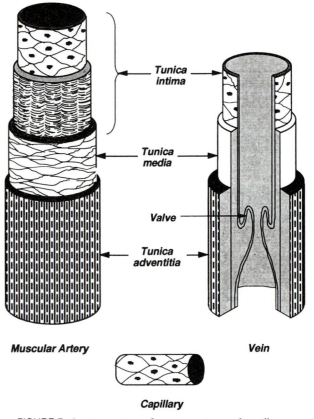

Muscular Artery   **Vein**

Capillary

FIGURE 7–1. Comparison of arteries, veins, and capillaries.

A pulse is the wave of increased pressure felt along arteries each time the heart ventricle contracts. The pulse rate is equal to the heart rate and can be felt by placing two fingers against an artery. The radial artery located near the thumb side of the wrist is the most common site for obtaining a pulse rate.

Arteries branch into smaller vessels called **arterioles** that are thinner than arteries and connect to capillaries.

Capillaries are vessels, one epithelial cell thick, that connect arterioles and venules. The blood in capillaries consists of a mixture of venous and arterial blood. The thin walls of capillaries allow the exchange of oxygen and carbon dioxide and nutrients between the blood and tissue cells.

Venules are small veins that fuse to become the larger veins, which carry blood back to the heart. **Veins** have thinner walls than arteries and carry oxygen-poor blood, carbon dioxide, and other waste products back to the heart. No gaseous exchange takes place in the veins, only in the capillaries. Vein walls have less elastic tissue and less connective tissue than arteries, and veins have **valves** to keep the blood flowing in one direction. Most blood tests are performed on venous blood. The main veins in the arm are the basilic, cephalic, and median cubital veins, as shown in Figure 7-3. These are the veins of choice for venipuncture. The saphenous vein is the principle vein in the leg. The largest veins, the superior and inferior vena cavae, carry

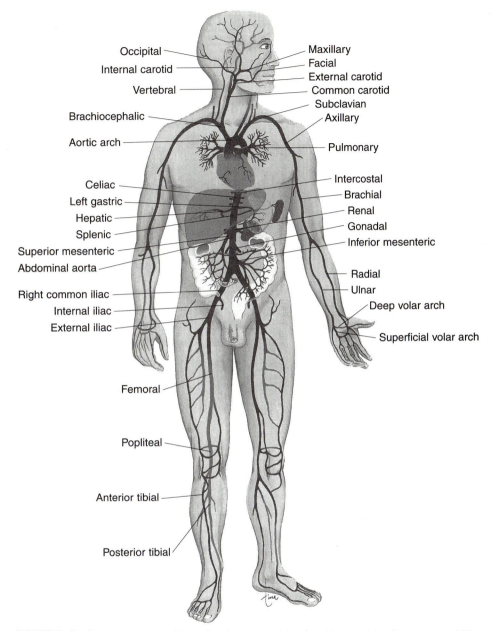

FIGURE 7–2. The major arteries. (From Scanlon, VC, and Sanders, T: Essentials of Anatomy and Physiology, ed. 2. FA Davis, Philadelphia, 1995, p. 288, with permission.)

the blood back to the right atrium of the heart. Figure 7‑4 shows the principle veins of the body.

HEART

The heart is a hollow muscular organ located in the thoracic cavity behind the sternum, between the lungs, and slightly to the left of the body midline. This muscu-

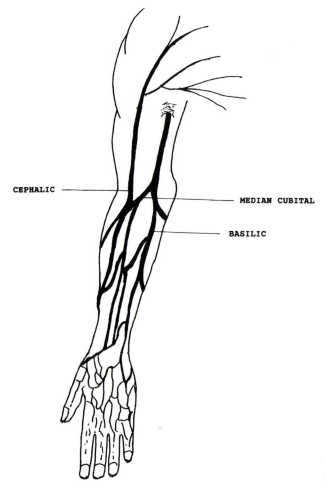

CEPHALIC

MEDIAN CUBITAL

BASILIC

FIGURE 7–3. Veins in the arm used for venipuncture.

lar organ is composed of four chambers, two upper chambers called **atria** and two lower chambers called **ventricles**. The heart is divided into the right and left halves by a partition called the septum. Valves are located between the chambers of the heart to prevent a back flow of blood and to keep the blood flowing in one direction.

The heart has three layers of tissue. The thin outer layer of the heart is called the epicardium. The walls of each heart chamber are composed of a thick cardiac muscle tissue called myocardium, and lining the cavities of the heart is a smooth tissue called **endocardium**. The **pericardium** is a fibrous membrane sac surrounding the heart to hold it in position. Cardiology is the branch of medicine specializing in the heart.

Pathway of Blood Through the Heart

The heart contracts and relaxes to pump deoxygenated blood through the heart to the lungs and bring oxygenated blood back to the heart to be distributed throughout the body. (Refer to Fig. 7–5 to follow the circulation of blood through the heart.)

Two large veins drain the body of deoxygenated blood. The superior vena cava and the inferior vena cava carry deoxygenated blood to the right atrium. The superior vena cava drains the upper portion of the body and the inferior vena cava car-

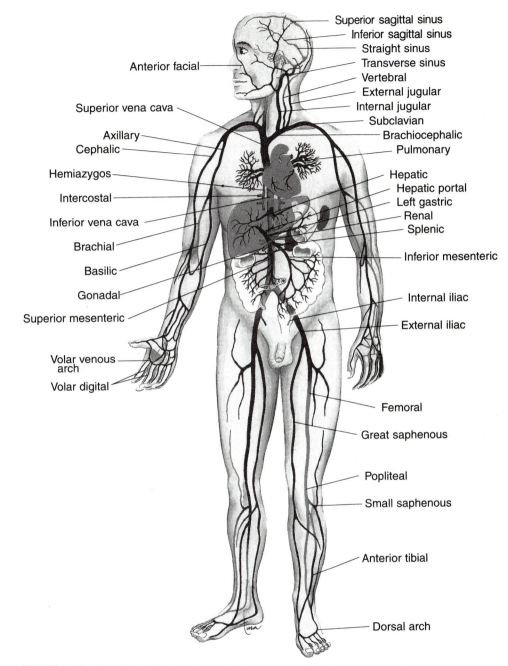

FIGURE 7–4. The principal veins. (From Scanlon, VC, and Sanders, T; Essentials of Anatomy and Physiology, ed. 2. FA Davis, Philadelphia, 1995, p. 289, with permission.)

ries blood from the lower portion of the body. The blood is pumped from the right atrium to the right ventricle through the tricuspid valve. The right ventricle contracts to pump the blood into the pulmonary artery. The pulmonary artery divides to carry blood to both lungs. The pulmonary artery is the only artery to carry deoxygenated blood. The blood releases carbon dioxide in the lung capillaries and acquires oxygen.

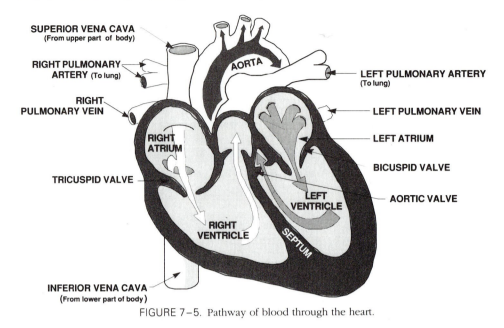

FIGURE 7–5. Pathway of blood through the heart.

The oxygenated blood is carried back to the heart via the pulmonary veins and enters the left atrium. Pulmonary veins are the only veins in the body that carry oxygenated blood. The left atrium contracts to force blood through the mitral valve into the left ventricle. The left ventricle contracts to pump blood into the aorta. The blood is carried throughout the body by arteries that branch off from the aorta, which is the largest artery of the body. The right and left coronary arteries branch off from the aorta to deliver blood carrying oxygen and nutrients to the heart.

The contraction of the heartbeat is called the **systole**. Systole occurs when the ventricles contract to force blood into the pulmonary artery and the aorta. The relaxation phase of the heartbeat is called the **diastole**. The ventricle walls relax and blood flows into the heart from the inferior and superior vena cavae and the pulmonary veins. A complete contraction phase and relaxation phase of the heart is called the cardiac cycle. The heart contracts approximately 72 times per minute. The number of heartbeats per minute is called the heart rate or pulse rate.

Blood pressure (**BP**) is a measure of the force of blood on the arterial walls during contraction and relaxation. It is measured in the brachial artery of the upper arm. A blood pressure cuff called a sphygmomanometer is placed over the upper arm and inflated to cut off the blood flow, while a stethoscope is used to listen for heart sounds. The cuff is slowly deflated until heart sounds are heard with the stethoscope, which has been placed over the brachial artery. The first heart sounds indicate the systolic pressure in the arteries during contraction of the ventricles. It is the top number of a pressure reading. The cuff is deflated until only a muffled sound is heard; this indicates the diastolic pressure during the relaxation of the ventricles and gives the lower number of a pressure reading. An average blood pressure for an adult is 120/80 mm Hg, representing a systolic pressure of 120 mm Hg and a diastolic pressure of 80 mm Hg.

Summary of Blood Circulation

1. Oxygen-poor blood from the vena cavae enters the right atrium of the heart.
2. The right atrium contracts to force the blood through the tricuspid valve to the right ventricle.
3. The right ventricle contracts to force the blood into the pulmonary artery, which divides to each lung.
4. The red blood cells release carbon dioxide and absorb oxygen in the lungs.
5. The oxygen-rich blood returns to the heart through the pulmonary veins and enters the left atrium.
6. The left atrium contracts to force the blood through the mitral valve into the left ventricle.
7. The left ventricle contracts to force the blood into the aorta.
8. The aorta divides into arteries, which branch into arterioles, to deliver blood throughout the body.
9. The arterioles connect to capillaries, where oxygen and nutrients leave the blood and carbon dioxide and waste products enter the blood.
10. The blood from the capillaries returns to the heart through venules, which fuse into larger veins.
11. The blood enters the heart through the largest veins, the superior vena cava and the inferior vena cava.

BLOOD

The average adult has 5 to 6 liters of blood. Blood is composed of a liquid portion, called plasma, and a cellular portion, called the formed elements.

The liquid portion of circulating blood (plasma) comprises approximately 55% of the blood and contains proteins (albumin, globulin, and fibrinogen), gases, salts, sugars, hormones, minerals, and vitamins dissolved in water.

The remaining 45% of the blood constitutes the cellular portion (formed elements) of the blood. These include **erythrocytes** (red blood cells), **leukocytes** (white blood cells), and **thrombocytes** (platelets). Blood cells are produced in the bone marrow, which is a spongy material that fills the inside of the major bones of the body. Cells originate from stem cells in the bone marrow, differentiate, and mature through several stages until they are released to the peripheral blood. To diagnose many blood disorders, a bone marrow aspiration is performed to remove the marrow and study the cells.

Erythrocytes

Erythrocytes or red blood cells (RBCs) contain hemoglobin, which carries oxygen to the tissue cells and carries carbon dioxide back to the lungs to be expelled. Hemoglobin is the main constituent of the RBC and consists of two parts, heme and globin. The heme portion requires iron for its synthesis.

Red blood cells mature through several stages in the bone marrow. Over a period of 5 to 7 days they become smaller and lose their nucleus. At this point they enter the blood as **reticulocytes** and continue to mature for 1 more day. A mature RBC is about 7.2 microns in diameter and is described as an anuclear, biconcave disk. An average number of RBCs is 4.2 to 6.2 million per microliter of blood, with men having slightly higher values than women. The normal life span for a RBC in the circulating blood stream is 120 days. After 120 days, macrophages in the liver and spleen remove the cells from the blood stream and destroy them. The iron is reused in new cells.

The surface of RBCs contains antigens that determine the blood group and blood type of an individual. As shown in Table 7–1 four ABO blood groups are recognized on the basis of the antigens present. Group A blood has the "A" antigen, group B has the "B" antigen, group AB has both "A" and "B" antigens, and group O has neither "A" nor "B" antigens on the cell membrane. Groups O and A are the most common and group AB is the least common blood group. Naturally occuring antibodies are also present in an individual's blood and will react with RBCs carrying antigens that are not present on the individuals own RBCs. If a person is transfused with a different blood group a transfusion reaction will occur because antibodies will destroy the donor RBCs containing their specific antigens. Misidentification of patients during phlebotomy is a major cause of transfusion reactions.

The presence or absence of the "D" antigen on the RBC membrane determines whether a person is Rh positive or negative. The "D" antigen is often referred to as the Rh factor and is present in approximately 85% of the population.

TABLE 7–1. **ABO BLOOD GROUP SYSTEM**

Blood Type	RBC Antigen	Plasma Antibodies
A	A	Anti-B
B	B	Anti-A
AB	A and B	Neither Anti-A nor Anti-B
O	Neither	Anti-A and Anti-B

Leukocytes

Leukocytes, or white blood cells (WBCs), provide immunity for the body by producing antibodies and destroying pathogens by phagocytosis. WBCs are produced in the bone marrow from a stem cell. They differentiate and mature through several stages before being released into the peripheral blood stream. The normal number of WBCs for an average adult is 4500 to 11,000 per microliter of blood. There are between 500 and 1000 RBCs for every WBC in the circulation. An increase in WBCs is called leukocytosis and is seen with infections or leukemia. A decrease in WBCs is called leukopenia and is caused by viral infections, exposure to radiation, or chemotherapy.

Five types of WBCs are present in the blood and are distinguished by their morphology, as shown in Figure 7–6. When stained with Wright's stain, cells are examined for granules in the cytoplasm, shape of the nucleus, and the size of the cell. A differential cell count is performed to determine the percentage of each type of WBC. Cells that have granules in their cytoplasm are collectively referred to as granulocytes and include the neutrophils, eosinophils, and basophils. The five normal types of WBCs are neutrophils, lymphocytes, monocytes, eosinophils, and basophils.

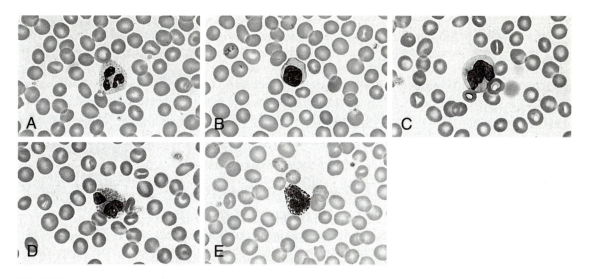

FIGURE 7-6. Normal white blood cells. *A*, Neutrophil; *B*, lymphocyte; *C*, monocyte; *D*, eosinophil; *E*, basophil. (Courtesy of Karen Lofsness, University of Minnesota, Minneapolis.)

Neutrophils (40%–60%)

Neutrophils are the most numerous leukocytes and their number increases in bacterial infections. The cytoplasm stains pink with fine granules and the nucleus stains dark purple. Neutrophils are called segmented or polymorphonuclear because the nucleus has two to five lobes.

Lymphocytes (20%–40%)

Lymphocytes are the second most numerous leukocytes. Their number is increased in viral infections and they play an important role in the immune system. The lymphocyte has a large round purple nucleus with a rim of sky-blue cytoplasm. Two main types of lymphocytes are present in the blood. The B lymphocyte develops in the bone marrow, becomes a plasma cell, and produces antibodies for defense against infections (humoral immunity). T lymphocytes mature in the thymus, act in delayed hypersensitivity reactions and graft rejection (cellular immunity), and assist B lymphocytes in the production of antibodies.

Monocytes (3%–8%)

Monocytes are the largest circulating leukocytes and act as powerful phagocytes or clean-up cells to digest foreign material. The cytoplasm has a fine blue-gray "ground glass" appearance with vacuoles, and the nucleus is large and irregular. The number of monocytes increases in intracellular infections and tuberculosis.

Eosinophils (1%–3%)

The cytoplasm of eosinophils is filled with granules that stain red-orange. Eosinophil numbers are increased in allergies, skin infections, and parasitic infections.

Basophils (0%–1%)   Basophils are the least common of the granulocytes. The cytoplasm contains large granules, which stain purple-black. The granules in basophils contain histamine, which is released in allergic reactions.

Thrombocytes   Thrombocytes or platelets are small, irregularly shaped disks formed from particles of a large cell in the bone marrow called the megakaryocyte. Platelets have a life span of 9 to 12 days and are essential for blood coagulation. The average number of platelets is 140,000 and 440,000 per microliter of blood.

COAGULATION   To recognize the importance of coagulation tests it is essential to understand how blood clots. A complex coagulation mechanism that involves blood vessels, platelets, and the coagulation factors maintains hemostasis. Hemostasis is the process of forming a blood clot when injury occurs and lysing the clot when the injury has been repaired. The process of coagulation occurs as primary hemostasis, secondary hemostasis, and fibrinolysis.

Primary Hemostasis   The function of primary hemostasis is to form a temporary platelet plug. It is called the **vascular** platelet phase because blood vessels and platelets are the first to respond to an injury. Blood vessels constrict to slow the flow of blood to the injured area. Platelets become activated, clumping together (platelet aggregation) and adhering to the injured blood vessel wall to stop bleeding. The bleeding time test evaluates primary hemostasis.

Secondary Hemostasis   Secondary hemostasis involves the interaction of the coagulation factors to convert the primary platelet plug to a stable fibrin clot. This interaction is called the coagulation cascade. In this cascade one factor becomes activated and activates the next factor in a specific sequence. Substances are released to activate the coagulation factors, which in combination with calcium and phospholipid from the platelets produce a fibrin clot to stabilize the platelet plug and stop bleeding. The coagulation cascade is divided into intrinsic and extrinsic systems, which come together in a common pathway (Fig. 7–7).

   The intrinsic system is initiated when large molecules in the circulatory system called contact factors are activated and platelets release the phospholipid, platelet factor 3 (**PF3**). The extrinsic system is activated by the release of tissue thromboplastin from an injured area. Both systems react with factors X and V to convert **prothrombin** (factor II) to thrombin. **Thrombin** is required to convert **fibrinogen** (factor I) to the fibrin that forms the basis of the fibrin clot.

   The intrinsic system is evaluated by the activated partial thromboplastin time test (APTT), which is also used to monitor **heparin** therapy. The prothrombin time test (PT) evaluates the extrinsic system and is used to monitor **coumadin** therapy.

Fibrinolysis   Fibrinolysis is the breakdown and removal of a clot once healing is complete. **Fibrin** in the clot is broken down into small fragments called fibrin degradation products (FDPs), which are cleared from the circulation by the liver. Fibrinolysis is monitored by the measurement of FDPs or D-dimers.

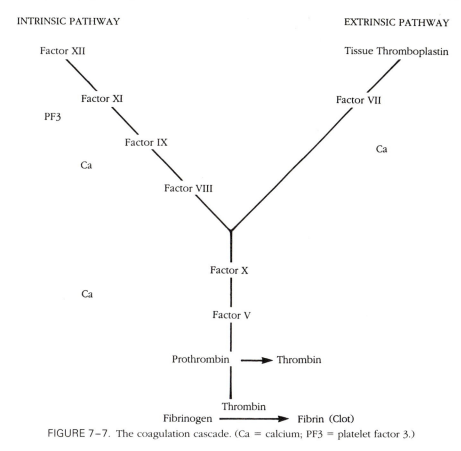

FIGURE 7–7. The coagulation cascade. (Ca = calcium; PF3 = platelet factor 3.)

DISORDERS ASSOCIATED WITH THE CIRCULATORY SYSTEM

Blood Vessels

Aneurysm

A weakness in an arterial wall that can burst and cause severe hemorrhaging.

Atherosclerosis

A condition often called "hardening of the arteries" caused by lipid buildup on the inside wall of blood vessels. The vessel eventually narrows and becomes plugged.

Varicose Veins

Swollen peripheral veins, caused by damaged valves that allow blood to collect in the veins.

Heart

Bacterial Endocarditis	An inflammation of the inner lining of the heart caused by a bacterial infection, usually streptococcal.
Congestive Heart Failure	A condition in which the left ventricle of the heart becomes weak and is unable to pump blood efficiently. Fluid accumulates in the lungs, creating pulmonary edema. **CHF** is a chronic disorder treated with digitalis.
Myocardial Infarction	Commonly known as a heart attack, **MI** is a major cause of death in middle to late adulthood. When a coronary artery is occluded by a blood clot or the buildup of fatty substances, blood cannot pass through the blood vessels to reach the cells of the heart muscle, and the heart tissue is damaged from the lack of oxygen.
Pericarditis	Bacteria, viruses, or trauma cause inflammation of the membrane surrounding the heart. Fluid accumulates in the pericardial cavity and severe chest pain may occur.
Rheumatic Heart Disease	An autoimmune disorder affecting heart tissue. It is usually seen in childhood following a streptococcal infection.

Blood

Anemia	A decrease in the number of red blood cells or the amount of hemoglobin in the circulating blood. A large variety of anemias exist, such as aplastic anemia, iron deficiency anemia, hemolytic anemia, pernicious anemia, sickle cell anemia, and thalassemia.
Leukemia	A marked increase in the number of white blood cells in the bone marrow and peripheral blood. Leukemias are named for the particular type of white blood cell that is increased, such as lymphocytic leukemia. An acute leukemia is characterized by the presence of immature cell forms and a chronic leukemia by mature cell forms.
Polycythemia	A condition caused by increased numbers of RBCs and other formed elements that give the blood a viscous consistency. Patients are often treated by periodic collection of a unit of blood, which is called therapeutic phlebotomy.

Coagulation

Disseminated Intravascular Coagulation	A condition in which spontaneous activation of the coagulation system by certain foreign substances entering the circulatory system results in rapid depletion of platelets and coagulation factors, producing a danger of hemorrhage. Fibrin degradation products are elevated.
Hemophilia	A hereditary disorder in which the lack of a clotting factor, most commonly factor VIII, causes excessive bleeding. It is inherited on the X chromosome and seen primarily in the male sex.
Thrombocytopenia	A decrease in the number of circulating platelets. As a result a platelet plug cannot be formed during primary hemostasis. This is frequently seen in patients receiving chemotherapy.

LABORATORY TESTS

The most frequently ordered laboratory tests associated with the circulatory system and their clinical correlations are presented in Table 7 – 2.

TABLE 7–2. **LABORATORY TESTS ASSOCIATED WITH THE CIRCULATORY SYSTEM**

Test	Clinical Correlation
Activated partial thromboplastin time [APTT(PTT)]	Coagulation disorders and heparin therapy
Antithrombin III	Clotting disorders
Aspartate aminotransferase [AST(SGOT)]	Recent myocardial infarction
Bleeding time (BT)	Platelet function
Bone marrow	Blood cell disorders
Cholesterol	Coronary heart disease
Complete blood count (CBC)	Infection, bleeding disorders, anemia, or leukemia
Creatine kinase [CK(CPK)]	Myocardial infarction
Creatine kinase isoenzymes (CK-MB)	Myocardial infarction
Fibrin degradation products (FDP)	Disseminated intravascular coagulation (**DIC**)
Fibrinogen	Coagulation disorders
Hemoglobin and hematocrit (**H & H**)	Anemia
Lactic dehydrogenase [LD(LDH)]	Myocardial infarction
Platelet aggregation	Platelet function
Prothrombin time (PT)	Coagulation disorders and coumadin therapy
Reticulocyte (Retic) count	Bone marrow function
Triglycerides	Coronary heart disease

LYMPHATIC SYSTEM

Terminology Associated with the Lymphatic System

Key Terms	Definition
B lymphocytes	Lymphocytes that transform into plasma cells to produce antibodies
Cell-mediated immunity	Immune response by T lymphocytes to directly destroy foreign antigens
Humoral immunity	Immune response that produces antibodies
Immune	Resistant to certain diseases
Interstitial fluid	Fluid located in the spaces between cells
Lymph	Fluid in the lymphatic vessels
Lymph node	Lymph tissue that filters lymph as it passes to the circulatory system
Lymph vessels	Structures that carry lymph throughout the body
Splenomegaly	Enlargement of the spleen
T lymphocytes	Lymphocytes that act directly on an antigen to destroy it

Abbreviations	Definition
AIDS	Acquired immunodeficiency syndrome
AZT	Azidothymidine (drug used to treat AIDS)
IM	Infectious mononucleosis

The lymphatic system is the body's "other" circulatory system. It consists of lymphatic vessels, called capillaries and veins, that extend throughout the body to carry lymph fluid, which is formed from **interstitial fluid**, the fluid that leaks from the blood capillaries and surrounds the body cells. **Lymph** consists of water, protein, salts, sugar, lymphocytes, monocytes, and waste products of metabolism that leak through the blood capillary walls into the tissue spaces. It does not contain platelets or red blood cells. Lymph flows through the lymphatic vessels and enters the circulatory system by passing through ducts that connect to veins in the upper chest.

FUNCTION

The lymphatic system drains fluid from the tissue spaces and transports the nutrients and waste products back to the blood stream. In addition the lymphatic system provides a defense mechanism against disease by storing lymphocytes and monocytes, which protect the body from foreign substances.

COMPONENTS OF THE LYMPHATIC SYSTEM

The lymphatic system consists of lymph vessels, right lymphatic duct, thoracic duct, lymph nodes, tonsils, adenoids, thymus gland, and spleen as shown in Figure 7-8.

Lymph capillaries carry the fluid from the interstitial spaces into larger lymph vessels called lymphatic venules and into veins, where it is emptied into two terminal vessels called the right lymphatic duct and the thoracic duct. The right lymphatic duct receives lymph from the upper right part of the body and the thoracic duct receives lymph from below the diaphragm and the left side of the body. The ducts empty the lymph into large veins in the neck region. Like blood veins, **lymph vessels** contain valves to permit the lymph to flow in only one direction toward the chest cavity. However, the lymph system has no pump of its own and the flow of lymph must depend on pressure from the circulatory system. Figure 7-9 shows the relationship between the lymphatic and circulatory systems.

As the lymph passes through the lymphatic vessels it is filtered by **lymph nodes** located along the lymphatic pathway. In addition to storing lymphocytes, lymph nodes filter and trap bacteria, foreign substances, and cancer cells. The nodes are located in the cervical (neck), axillary (armpit), inguinal (groin), and mediastinal (between the lungs) areas of the body. During infections, these nodes can swell and become tender.

The tonsils, adenoids, thymus gland, and spleen are composed of lymphoid tissue. The tonsils and adenoids are located in the throat and contain T and B lymphocytes to guard against infection at the entrance of the digestive and respiratory tracts. The thymus gland is located between the lungs and controls the immune system by changing lymphocytes produced in the bone marrow to T lymphocytes to provide cellular immunity. The spleen, the largest lymphatic organ, is located near the stomach. It filters and cleanses the lymph by removing cell debris, bacteria, parasites, and old red blood cells. During an infection the spleen may enlarge and the patient is said to have **splenomegaly**.

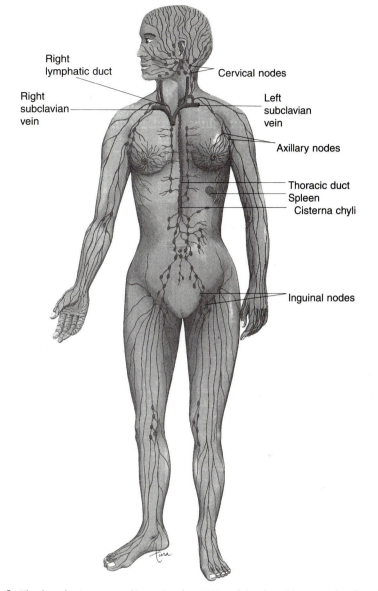

Right
lymphatic duct

Cervical nodes

Right
subclavian
vein

Left
subclavian
vein

Axillary nodes

Thoracic duct
Spleen
Cisterna chyli

Inguinal nodes

FIGURE 7–8. The lymphatic system. (From Scanlon, VC, and Sanders, T: Essentials of Anatomy and Physiology, ed. 2. FA Davis, Philadelphia, 1995, p. 313, with permission.)

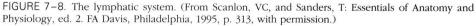

THE IMMUNE SYSTEM

The lymphatic system plays a major role in the body's immune system by recognizing foreign substances that are filtered through the lymph nodes and spleen and by maintaining a high concentration of B and T lymphocytes. Cells are recognized as "self" or foreign by the antigens present on the cell membrane. Cells containing foreign antigens are presented to B or T lymphocytes to activate an **immune** response. Immunology is the branch of medicine specializing in the immune system.

B lymphocytes are responsible for the production of antibodies (immunoglob-

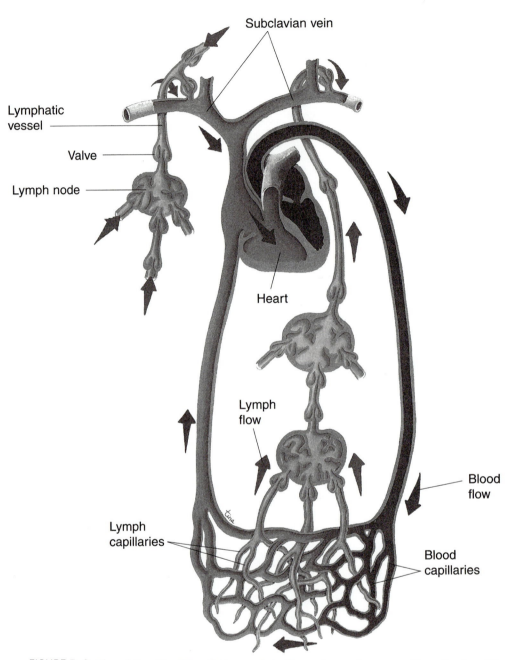

FIGURE 7–9. The relationship of lymphatic vessels to the cardiovascular system. (From Scanlon, VC, and Sanders, T: Essentials of Anatomy and Physiology, ed. 2. FA Davis, Philadelphia, 1995, p. 311, with permission.)

ulins) that combine with specific antigens to neutralize and destroy them. **Humoral immunity** results from this process and is the major immune response to bacterial infections.

T lymphocytes produce chemical substances (lymphokines), rather than antibodies, to destroy foreign antigens; they also differentiate into T helper and T suppressor cells to control the immune response. These processes that produce **cell-mediated immunity** are stimulated by the presence of intracellular microorganisms, transplanted tissue, and tumor cells.

DISORDERS ASSOCIATED WITH THE LYMPHATIC SYSTEM

Acquired Immuno-deficiency Syndrome

A syndrome caused by the blood-borne pathogen, human immunodeficiency virus (HIV), suppresses the immune response by destroying helper T cells. This allows opportunistic infections to be more easily contracted and increases the risk of developing cancer. Conditions frequently associated with **AIDS** are pneumocystosis and Kaposi's sarcoma.

Hodgkin's Disease

A malignant tumor of the lymph tissue located in the upper body producing enlarged lymph nodes, splenomegaly, fever, weakness, and loss of weight.

Infectious Mononucleosis

A disease caused by the Epstein-Barr virus characterized by enlarged lymph nodes, increased numbers of lymphocytes, fatigue, and a sore throat.

Lymphoma

A malignant tumor of the lymph nodes or lymphatic tissue located throughout the body. Burkitt's lymphoma and non-Hodgkin's lymphoma are examples.

Multiple Myeloma

A malignant proliferation of plasma cells in the bone marrow producing painful nodules and interference with the normal bone marrow functions. The subsequent impairment of hematologic and immune system functions and destruction of bone results in a poor prognosis.

LABORATORY TESTS

The most frequently ordered laboratory tests associated with the lymphatic system and their clinical correlations are presented in Table 7–3.

TABLE 7–3. **LABORATORY TESTS ASSOCIATED WITH THE LYMPHATIC SYSTEM**

Test	Clinical Correlation
Anti-HIV	Human immunodeficiency virus
Biopsy	Malignant lymphomas
Complement levels	Autoimmune disorders
Complete blood count (CBC)	Lymphomas or infectious mononucleosis
Monospot	Infectious mononucleosis (**IM**)
Protein electrophoresis	Multiple myeloma
Western blot	Human immunodeficiency virus

BIBLIOGRAPHY

Chabner, D-E: The Language of Medicine. WB Saunders, Philadelphia, 1991.

Gylys, BA: Medical Terminology Simplified: A Programmed Learning Approach by Body Systems. FA Davis, Philadelphia, 1993.

McKenzie, SB: Textbook of Hematology. Lea & Febiger, Philadelphia, 1988.

Scanlon, VC, and Sanders, T: Essentials of Anatomy and Physiology, ed. 2. FA Davis, Philadelphia, 1995.

Thibodeau, GA, and Patton, KT: The Human Body in Health and Disease. CV Mosby, St. Louis, 1991.

Study Questions

1. Using the basic terminology and the terminology from this chapter, define the following words:

   a. Hypertension _____

   b. Leukocyte _____

   c. Hemorrhage _____

   d. Carditis _____

   e. Atherosclerosis _____

   f. Coronary stenosis _____

   g. Electrocardiogram _____

   h. Cardiomegaly _____

   i. Pericarditis _____

   j. Thrombophlebitis _____

   k. Splenectomy _____

   l. Lymphoma _____

   m. Immunology _____

   n. Splenomegaly _____

   o. Immunity _____

2. Interpret the following situations by defining the underlined words:

   a. A cardiologist examining a patient in the CCU requests an EKG.

   _____

   _____

   _____

   b. A patient with a thrombus is given an anticoagulant to prevent blockage of the carotid.

   _____

   _____

   _____

   c. You are requested to draw a sample for PT and an APTT on a patient with an embolus.

   _____

   _____

   _____

d. A patient is admitted to the CCU with CHF. The RN gives an IM injection and starts IV fluids.

_____

_____

_____

_____

_____

e. A patient in the OR for coronary artery bypass surgery had an HDL and an H & H ordered.

_____

_____

_____

_____

f. A 23-year-old pregnant woman with DIC needs an FDP because she is hemorrhaging.

_____

_____

_____

g. An IM screen was ordered on a young man with splenomegaly and enlarged lymph nodes.

_____

_____

_____

h. A patient with AIDS caused by HIV was treated with AZT.

_____

_____

_____

i. A patient with lymphoma presented with anemia, leukopenia, and thrombocytopenia.

_____

_____

_____

_____

3. Differentiate the three major types of blood vessels.

   a. _____

   b. _____

   c. _____

4. Name the three cellular constituents of blood and state their function.

   a. _____

   b. _____

   c. _____

5. Name the artery that carries deoxygenated blood. _____

6. Label the indicated parts of the heart.

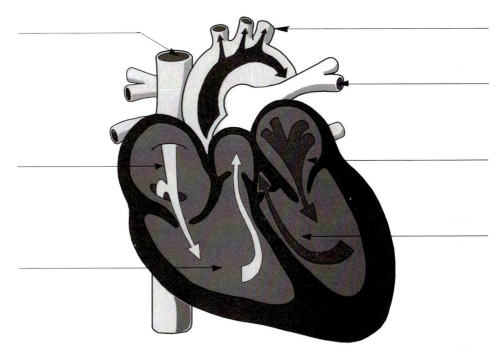

7. Starting with the vena cavae, trace the flow of blood through the heart. The pathway should include four chambers, two veins, two arteries, and one accessory organ.

   _____

   _____

   _____

   _____

   _____

   _____

   _____

   _____

8. What is the cell, formed from a B lymphocyte, that secretes antibodies?

_____

9. List two types of T lymphocytes.

a. _____

b. _____

10. What is cell-mediated immunity?

_____

_____

11. What is humoral immunity?

_____

_____

12. Another name for immunoglobulin is _____.

CHAPTER 8 Skeletal and Muscular Systems

Learning Objectives

Upon completion of this chapter, the reader will be able to:

1 State the meaning of the roots and suffixes and define the terms and abbreviations associated with the skeletal and muscular systems.
2 List the functions of the skeletal and muscular systems.
3 Explain the formation of bones, joints, and cartilage.
4 Name the four classifications of bones.
5 Locate the major bones of the body.
6 List and describe the appearance of the three main types of muscles.
7 Discuss the mechanism by which muscles provide movement.
8 Describe the disorders associated with the skeletal and muscular systems.
9 State the clinical correlations of laboratory tests associated with the skeletal and muscular systems.

SKELETAL SYSTEM

Terminology Associated with the Skeletal System

Roots/Combining Forms	Meaning
arthr/o	joint
chrondr/o	cartilage
cost/o	ribs
myel/o	bone marrow
orth/o	straight
oste/o	bone
synov/i	synovial membrane

Key Terms	Definition
Antecubital fossa	Indentation of the midarm opposite the elbow (location of the large veins used in phlebotomy)
Arthritis	Inflammation of the joints
Articulation	Joint
Bone marrow	Site of blood cell formation
Carpals, metacarpals	Bones of the wrists and hands
Cartilage	Flexible connective tissue surrounded by gel (located where bones come together)

4   Comminuted fractures are breaks in which the bone has splintered into many pieces.

5   An impacted fracture occurs when a bone fragment is driven into another bone.

6   A greenstick fracture indicates a bone that is partially bent and partially broken.

7   A pathological fracture is caused by a disease rather than mechanical stress.

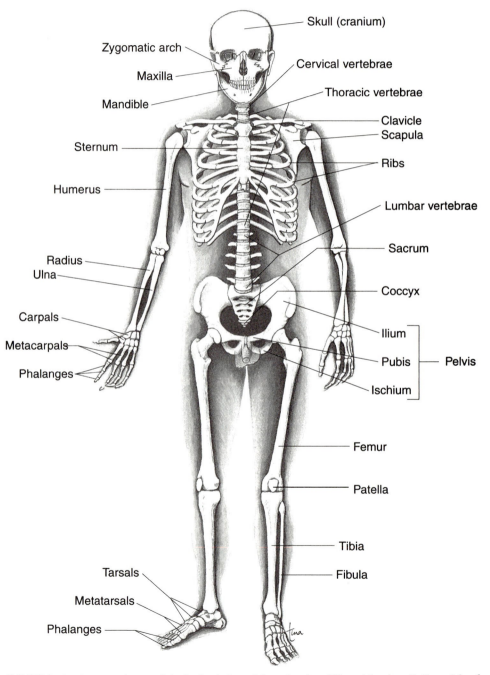

FIGURE 8–1. The major bones of the body. (Adapted from Scanlon, VC, and Sanders, T: Essentials of Anatomy and Physiology, ed. 2. FA Davis, Philadelphia, 1995, p. 109.)

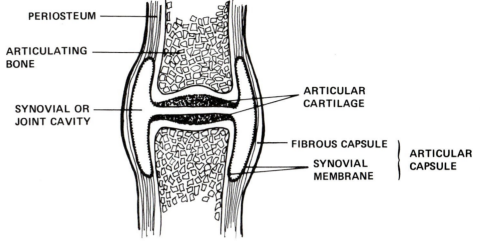

FIGURE 8-2. Synovial joint. (From Strasinger, SK: Urinalysis and Body Fluids, ed. 3. FA Davis, Philadelphia, 1994, p. 165, with permission.)

Gout A metabolic condition causing increased uric acid in the blood. Monosodium urate crystals form in the joints causing inflammation and pain.

Lyme Disease A disease caused by a spirochete bacterium carried by ticks. The synovial membranes become infected, producing inflammation of joints, and neurologic and cardiac symptoms may be present.

Osteoma A tumor of the bone that may be benign or malignant. Malignant tumors are called **sarcomas**, of which there are different types depending on the tissue affected. An osteosarcoma is a skeletal tumor and perhaps the most deadly. A fibrosarcoma is a tumor affecting the fibrous connective tissue. It may result in the appearance of excessive connective tissue in the **bone marrow**. Chrondosarcoma is a malignant tumor of the cartilage tissue. Ewing's sarcoma is a malignant bone tumor affecting the entire shaft of a long bone and is most frequently seen in young adult males. Sarcomas are treated with chemotherapy and radiation therapy.

Osteomalacia Often called rickets, this metabolic disorder causes softening of the bones as a result of the inability to absorb calcium due to a deficiency of vitamin D. It is seen in infants and children, and may result in bone deformity.

Osteomyelitis An inflammation of the bone caused by a bacterial infection. It is difficult to cure, as antibiotics are not readily absorbed by the bone. Osteomyelitis can be caused by improper microtechniques in phlebotomy.

Osteoporosis A common, serious bone disease in which the bones become brittle and easily broken due to decreased density. Causes of osteoporosis include a lack of protein, calcium, vitamin D, or high doses of corticosteroids, and the lack of estrogen in postmenopausal women.

Paget's Disease A metabolic disorder in which spongy bone is replaced by new abnormal bone. Bowing of the legs and deformity of the flat bones occur due to filling of the marrow spaces by abnormal, excess bone. Paget's disease usually affects adults over the age of 35.

Rheumatoid Arthritis

Chronic inflammation of the joints due to an autoimmune reaction involving the joint connective tissue. The inflammation causes painful swelling of the joint and can produce crippling deformities as it spreads from the inflamed synovial membrane to the cartilage of a joint. Diagnosis can be made with a blood test to detect the presence of the autoantibody (rheumatoid factor [**RF**]).

Scoliosis

Lateral curvature of the spine that gives the spine the shape of an "S." It can be congenital or can develop in the early teen years due to poor posture. Braces, casts, exercise, and sometimes surgery are necessary to treat this condition.

Spina Bifida

A congenital disorder in which abnormal closing of the vertebrae surrounding the spinal cord results in malformation of the spine.

Systemic Lupus Erythematosus

An autoimmune disease affecting the connective tissue and involving cartilage, bones, ligaments, and tendons. One of the hallmarks of the disease is the appearance of a red rash across the cheeks and the bridge of the nose (butterfly rash). Chronic inflammation of the joints leads to arthritis. **SLE** is usually seen in women of child-bearing years and is treated with corticosteroids.

LABORATORY TESTS

The most frequently ordered laboratory tests associated with the skeletal system and their clinical correlations are presented in Table 8–1.

TABLE 8–1. **LABORATORY TESTS ASSOCIATED WITH THE SKELETAL SYSTEM**

Test	Clinical Correlation
Alkaline phosphatase (ALP)	Bone disease
Antinuclear antibody (ANA)	Systemic lupus erythematosus
Calcium (Ca)	Bone disease
Fluorescent antinuclear antibody (FANA)	Systemic lupus erythematosus
Phosphorus (P)	Skeletal disease
Rheumatoid arthritis (RA)	Rheumatoid arthritis
Synovial fluid analysis	**Arthritis**
Uric acid	Gout

MUSCULAR SYSTEM

Terminology Associated with the Muscular System

Roots/Combining Forms	Meaning
fibr/o	fibrous connective tissue
my/o	muscle

Suffixes	Meaning
-asthenia	lack of strength
-trophy	development

Terminology Associated with the Muscular System Continued	**Key Terms**	**Definition**
	Abduction	Moving away from the middle of the body
	Adduction	Moving toward the middle of the body
	Atrophy	Lack of development
	Extension	Straightening of a limb
	Flexion	Bending of a limb

	Abbreviations	**Definition**
	CTS	Carpal tunnel syndrome
	MD	Muscular dystrophy
	Mg	Magnesium

The muscular system works in conjunction with the skeletal and nervous systems to provide body movement. Physical medicine (physical therapy) is the department specializing in neuromuscular system disorders.

FUNCTION

The three main functions of the muscular system are movement, posture, and heat production. The ability of the muscle to contract makes these functions possible.

Muscles attach to two bones. Muscles that produce movement are agonists and the opposing muscles are the antagonists. Muscles can contract but they cannot expand; therefore, it is necessary to have an opposing set of muscles to provide smooth movement. A muscle is attached to a bone that is stationary and to one which moves. The stationary bone is the origin of the muscle. The other end of the muscle is attached to a bone that moves. This is the insertion bone and the muscles are attached at the insertion point. As the muscle contracts and shortens, the insertion bone moves toward the stationary bone. In order to move the bone back, opposing muscles must contract. As one set of muscles contracts, the other set relaxes. Relaxation allows the muscle to return to its original shape. Tendons, which are cords of fibrous connective tissue, attach skeletal muscle to bones. The concept of muscular movement is illustrated in Figure 8-3.

Posture is maintained by a special type of contraction called tonic contraction, which shortens only a few muscles and does not allow movement. Muscles are held in position and resist the pull of gravity.

Body temperature is maintained by the heat that is produced during a contraction of the muscle fibers. The energy lost as heat during a muscle contraction maintains constant body temperature.

MUSCLE TYPES

Three types of muscle are found in the body and are shown in Figure 8-4. The muscle that attaches to bones is called *skeletal muscle* and is responsible for movement of the body. It can also be called a voluntary muscle because a person has control over its activity. It is further described as a striated muscle, which means that it will appear striped when examined microscopically.

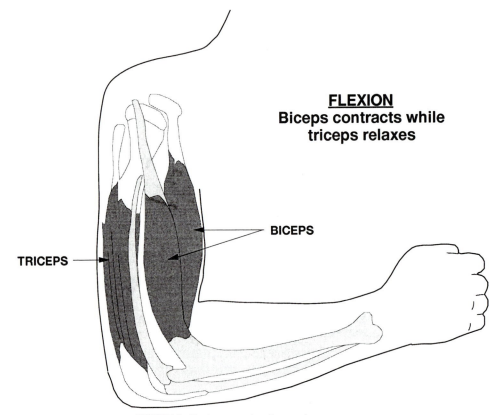

FIGURE 8–3. An example of muscular movement.

Smooth muscle is a nonstriated muscle, and under a microscope, it has a smooth appearance without stripes. This is the muscle found in the walls of veins and arteries and in internal organs such as the stomach and intestine. It is called an involuntary muscle because a person does not consciously control its actions. For example, food is digested and passed through the stomach and intestines without any conscious control.

Cardiac muscle is the muscle of the heart. Like skeletal muscle, it is a striated muscle. However, it is also an involuntary muscle because the heart muscle contracts to pump blood without any conscious control.

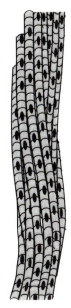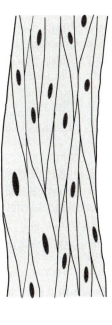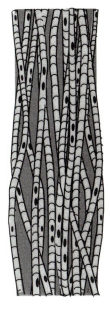

Skeletal / Striated   **Smooth / Unstriated**   **Cardiac**

FIGURE 8-4. The three types of muscle.

DISORDERS ASSOCIATED WITH THE MUSCULAR SYSTEM

Carpal Tunnel Syndrome

A condition caused by pressure on the median nerve as it passes through the ligaments, bones, and tendons to the wrist. It is characterized by pain and tingling in the fingers and hand, and may radiate to the shoulder. Treatment can range from immobilization of the wrist, to injection of an anti-inflammatory agent, to surgery.

Muscular Dystrophy

An inherited disorder in which muscles are replaced by fat and fibrous tissue and progressively weaken. The most common type is Duchenne type dystrophy, which begins in early childhood.

Myasthenia Gravis

An autoimmune disease of the muscle cells at the neuromuscular junction, in which nerve impulses cannot be transmitted to the muscle tissue. Weakness begins in the face and throat and spreads throughout the body.

Poliomyelitis

A viral infection of the nerves that control skeletal movement. Such infection results in muscle weakness and paralysis. Immunization during childhood is recommended.

LABORATORY TESTS

The most frequently ordered laboratory tests associated with the muscular system and their clinical correlations are presented in Table 8–2.

TABLE 8–2. **LABORATORY TESTS ASSOCIATED WITH THE MUSCULAR SYSTEM**

Test	Clinical Correlation
Aldolase	Muscle disease
Aspartate aminotransferase [AST (SGOT)]	Cardiac muscle damage
Calcium (Ca)	Musculoskeletal disease
Creatine kinase [CK (CPK)]	Muscle damage
Creatine kinase isoenzymes (CK-MM)	Muscle damage
Lactic dehydrogenase [LD (LDH)]	Cardiac muscle damage
Magnesium (**Mg**)	Musculoskeletal disease
Potassium (K)	Muscle function

BIBLIOGRAPHY

Chabner, D-E: The Language of Medicine. WB Saunders, Philadelphia, 1991.

Gylys, BA: Medical Terminology Simplified: A Programmed Learning Approach by Body Systems. FA Davis, Philadelphia, 1993.

Thibodeau, GA, and Patton, KT: The Human Body in Health and Disease. CV Mosby, St. Louis, 1991.

Study Questions

1. Using the basic terminology and the terminology in this chapter, define the following words:

   a. Arthritis _____

   b. Tendinitis _____

   c. Osteoma _____

   d. Subclavian _____

   e. Osteomyelitis _____

   f. Synovial fluid _____

   g. Myopathy _____

   h. Myosclerosis _____

   i. Myocardial _____

   j. Intramuscular _____

   k. Cardiomyopathy _____

   l. Myocardium _____

2. Interpret the following situations by defining the underlined words:

   a. A patient with a Fx of the tibia was referred to orthopedics.

   _____

   _____

   b. The rheumatologist requested an ESR and a RA test for a patient with rheumatoid arthritis.

   _____

   _____

   _____

   _____

   c. An ANA test was ordered on a patient to diagnose SLE.

   _____

   _____

   d. A patient with myalgia was given an IM injection for pain.

   _____

   _____

   e. The physician requested a CK on a patient brought to the ER with an MI.

   _____

   _____

   _____

f. A patient was referred to <u>PT</u> with symptoms of muscular <u>atrophy</u>.

_____

_____

3. What are the four main components of the skeletal system?

a. _____

b. _____

c. _____

d. _____

4. Name two tests performed in the chemistry section to evaluate the skeletal system.

a. _____

b. _____

5. The femur, tibia, and humerus belong to which classification of bones?

_____

6. Why is it important for phlebotomists to know the location of the major bones?

_____

_____

7. List two locations for the collection of bone marrow specimens.

a. _____

b. _____

8. The type of muscle lining the veins is _____

9. What attaches muscles to bone? _____

10. Describe the microscopic appearance of three types of muscle.

a. _____

b. _____

c. _____

11. Explain how movement of muscle occurs.

_____

_____

_____

_____

CHAPTER 9 Nervous and Respiratory Systems

Learning Objectives

Upon completion of this chapter, the reader will be able to:

1 State the meaning of the roots and suffixes and define the terms and abbreviations associated with the nervous and respiratory systems.
2 Describe the major parts, subdivisions, and cells of the nervous system.
3 Compare internal and external respiration.
4 List the six major components of the respiratory system and briefly describe their location and function.
5 Describe the pressure relationship between oxygen and carbon dioxide in the lungs and in the tissues.
6 Describe the disorders associated with the nervous and respiratory systems.
7 State the clinical correlations of laboratory tests associated with the nervous and respiratory systems.

NERVOUS SYSTEM

Terminology Associated with the Nervous System

Roots/Combining Forms	Meaning
cephal/o	head
cerebell/o	cerebellum
cerebr/o	cerebrum
encephal/o	brain
meningi/o	meninges
neur/o	nerve

Suffixes	Meaning
-algesia	excessive sensitivity to pain
-esthesia	nervous sensation
-kinesia	movement
-lepsy	seizure
-plegia	paralysis

Terminology Associated with the Nervous System
Continued

Key Terms	Definition
Acetylcholine	Neurotransmitter released at the ends of nerve cells
Afferent nerves	Nerves carrying impulses to the brain and spinal cord (sensory neurons)
Autonomic nervous system	System regulating the body's involuntary functions by carrying impulses from the brain and spinal cord to the muscles, glands, and internal organs
Axon	Fiber of nerve cells that carries impulses away from the cell body of the neuron
Central nervous system	Brain and spinal cord
Cerebellum	Back part of the brain responsible for voluntary muscle movements and balance
Cerebrospinal fluid	Fluid surrounding the brain and spinal cord
Cerebrum	Largest part of the brain (responsible for mental processes)
Dendrite	Fiber of nerve cells that carries impulses to the cell body of the neuron
Efferent nerves	Nerves carrying impulses away from the brain and spinal cord (motor neurons)
Lumbar	Pertaining to the lower back
Meninges	Protective membranes around the brain and spinal cord
Myelin sheath	Tissue around the axon of the peripheral nerves
Neuroglia	Connective tissue cells of the nervous system that do not carry impulses
Neuron	Nerve cell
Peripheral nervous system	All nerves outside the brain and spinal cord
Synapse	The point at which an impulse is transmitted from one neuron to another

Abbreviations	Definition
ALS	Amyotrophic lateral sclerosis
CNS	Central nervous system
CSF	Cerebrospinal fluid
CVA	Cerebrovascular accident
EEG	Electroencephalogram
LP	Lumbar puncture
MS	Multiple sclerosis
PNS	Peripheral nervous system

The communication system of the body is the nervous system consisting of the brain, spinal cord, and nerves. All other body systems are dependent on the nervous system for normal function. Nerve impulses cause muscles to contract to move bones, and enable us to hear, see, taste, think, and react. The specialized cell of the nervous system is the neuron, whose type varies depending on the function it performs. Neurology is the branch of medicine specializing in the nervous system.

FUNCTION

The complex nervous system provides four primary functions: communication between body functions, integration of body functions, control of body functions, and recognition of sensory stimuli. This is accomplished through electrical nerve impulses traveling via a nerve fiber and causing the release of chemical stimuli.

STRUCTURE

The nervous system is divided into the **central nervous system (CNS)** and the **peripheral nervous system (PNS)**. The central nervous system lies in the center of the body and consists of the brain and the spinal cord. The peripheral nervous system consists of nervous tissue located outside the skull and spinal column that extends out into the body and connects the brain and spinal cord to all parts of the body.

PERIPHERAL NERVOUS SYSTEM

The peripheral nervous system consists of two subdivisions, the autonomic and the voluntary nervous systems. The **autonomic** (involuntary) **nervous system** connects the central nervous system to glands, cardiac muscle, and smooth muscle throughout the body to regulate the involuntary functions of the body such as heart rate, contractions of the stomach, and gland secretions. The voluntary nervous system conducts nerve impulses from the central nervous system for conscious control of skeletal muscles and relays sensory information to the central nervous system.

Two types of cells are present in the peripheral nervous system. The main functioning cell that conducts nerve impulses is the neuron. The second type of cell is the **neuroglia**, which acts as nerve glue or connective support for neurons and does not conduct nerve impulses.

Different types of neurons are classified by the way they transmit impulses. Sensory neurons, also called **afferent** neurons, transmit impulses from the sensory organs to the brain and spinal cord. Motor, or **efferent**, neurons transmit impulses away from the brain and spinal cord to the muscles and glands to produce a response of either contraction or secretion. Interneurons or central neurons transmit impulses from sensory neurons to motor neurons.

A **neuron** consists of three main parts: dendrites, a cell body, and an axon. Several **dendrites** branch out to receive and carry impulses to the cell body. The **axon**, which is a single long projection, extends out and carries impulses away from the cell body. Axons are covered by a protective **myelin sheath** that acts as a special insulator and can accelerate electrical impulses. Because myelin is a white fatty substance, the axons have a white appearance and are therefore called the white matter. Gray matter consists of all the fibers, dendrites, and nerve cell bodies that are not covered with the myelin sheath and have a gray appearance. Figure 9–1 illustrates the sensory and motor neurons.

The point at which the axon of one neuron and the dendrite of another neuron come together is called a **synapse**. Nerve impulses are transmitted at the synapse.

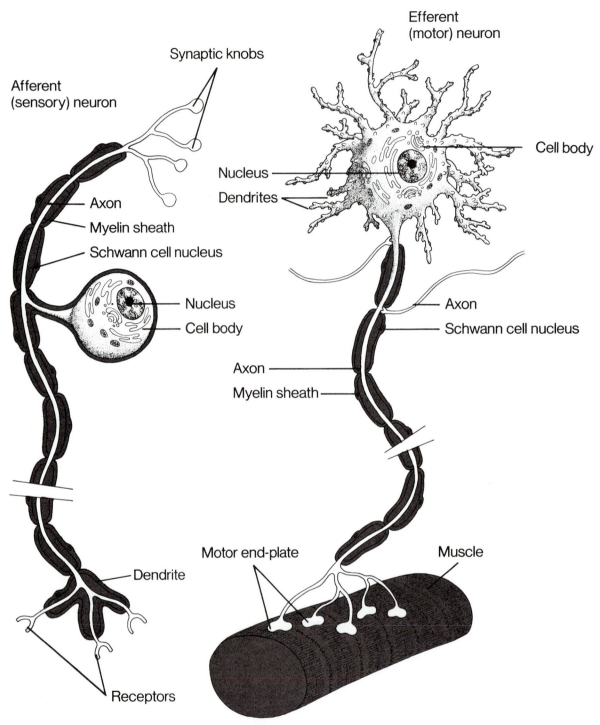

FIGURE 9–1. Sensory and motor neurons. (Adapted from Gylys, BA, and Wedding, ME: Medical Terminology: A Systems Approach, ed. 3. FA Davis, Philadelphia, 1995, p. 321.)

The nerve impulse from an axon stops at the synapse, chemical signals are sent across the gap, and the impulse then continues along the dendrites, cell body, and the axon of the next neuron.

CENTRAL NERVOUS SYSTEM

The brain and spinal cord make up the central nervous system. The brain is one of the largest organs in the body. It consists of four parts, the brain stem, **cerebellum**, diencephalon, and **cerebrum** and is the center for regulating body functions. The spinal cord, with its ascending and descending nerve track, is an extension of the brain and acts as a pathway for incoming and outgoing impulses. If one examines a cross-section of the spinal cord, the inner section is gray matter composed of dendrites and neuron cell bodies, while the outer region is white matter composed of myelinated nerve axons.

The skull bones provide protection for the brain, and the vertebrae provide protection for the spinal cord. An additional shock-absorbing protection is provided by the three layers of meninges that coat the brain and spinal cord. The **meninges** are spongy tissues filled with a special liquid called **cerebrospinal fluid (CSF)**, which acts as a cushion for the brain and the spinal cord. Normally cerebrospinal fluid is clear and colorless, but when the meninges become inflamed due to a bacterial or viral infection, a serious condition called meningitis exists and the fluid becomes cloudy. To diagnose meningitis, the physician must extract some CSF for laboratory analysis. A **lumbar puncture (LP)** is performed by inserting a needle between the vertebrae of the lower spine and aspirating fluid into a syringe. Three or four tubes of fluid are collected, each with approximately 1 milliliter of fluid. The first tube is tested in the chemistry section for substances such as glucose and protein. The specimen in the second tube is cultured in the microbiology section for infectious agents. The third tube is analyzed in the hematology section, where cell counts and cell identification are performed.

DISORDERS ASSOCIATED WITH THE NERVOUS SYSTEM

Alzheimer's Disease

A disease characterized by diminished mental capabilities including memory loss, anxiety, and confusion.

Amyotrophic Lateral Sclerosis

Also known as Lou Gehrig's disease. This disorder of the motor neurons in the brain and spinal cord produces weakness of skeletal and respiratory muscles.

Bell's Palsy

Paralysis and numbness of the face caused by inflammation of a facial nerve.

Cerebral Palsy

A childhood disease caused by damage to the brain during the prenatal period or during delivery. The condition is marked by partial paralysis and poor muscle coordination.

Cerebrovascular Accident

Commonly known as a stroke. This disorder can be caused by a hemorrhage from a cerebral artery or by arteriosclerosis, hardening of the arteries. A decrease in the flow of blood to the brain causes destruction of brain tissue due to lack of oxygen.

Epilepsy

A condition characterized by seizures ranging from mild alteration of consciousness to severe convulsions and caused by sudden abnormalities in brain function. Patients are treated with antiepileptic medications.

Meningitis

Inflammation of the meninges of the spinal cord and brain due to the presence of a microorganism. Severe headaches and a stiff neck are common symptoms.

Multiple Neuro-fibromatosis

An inherited disorder producing fibrous tumors throughout the body. Crippling deformities, such as those seen in the movie "The Elephant Man," are the result of these tumors.

Multiple Sclerosis

An autoimmune disorder characterized by destruction of the myelin sheath of the brain and spinal cord. As the myelin is destroyed it is replaced by hard plaquelike lesions that interfere with the transmission of nerve impulses. Motor control is diminished; muscle weakness, poor coordination, and paralysis may occur.

Parkinson's Disease

A disease of the elderly, caused by degeneration of the nerves responsible for movement. Patients experience stiffness of joints, tremors, unblinking eyes, and slowness of movement.

Shingles

The virus that causes chicken pox, *varicella-zoster*, remains dormant in the body and may reappear in the form of shingles and affect the peripheral nerves. Blisters and pain follow the course of the peripheral nerves at and above the waist.

LABORATORY TESTS

The most frequently ordered laboratory tests associated with the nervous system and their clinical correlations are presented in Table 9–1.

TABLE 9–1. **LABORATORY TESTS ASSOCIATED WITH THE NERVOUS SYSTEM**

Test	Clinical Correlation
Cerebrospinal fluid (CSF) analysis	
Cell count/differential	Neurological disorders or meningitis
Culture	Meningitis
Gram stain	Meningitis
Glucose	Meningitis
Protein	Neurological disorders or meningitis
Creatine kinase isoenzymes (CK-BB)	Brain damage

RESPIRATORY SYSTEM

Terminology Associated with the Respiratory System

Roots/Combining Forms	Meaning
cyan/o	blue
nas/o, rhin/o	nose
olfact/o	sense of smell
pector/o, thorac/o	chest
pneum/o	air, lung
pulmon/o	lung
trache/o	trachea, windpipe

Suffixes	Meaning
-capnia	carbon dioxide
-phonia	voice
-pnea	breathing
-ptysis	spitting

Key Terms	Definition
Apnea	Absence of breathing
Asphyxia	Severe lack of oxygen
Cyanosis	Bluish skin color due to lack of oxygen
Effusion	Accumulation of fluid
Nasopharynx	Area of the throat next to the nose
Pleura/pleural	Double-folded membrane surrounding each lung/ pertaining to the lungs
Thoracentesis	Surgical puncture of the **pleural** cavity
Tracheotomy	Emergency opening of the trachea to provide air

Abbreviations	Definition
COPD	Chronic obstructive pulmonary disease
ENT	Ear, nose, and throat specialty
IRDS	Infant respiratory distress syndrome
PPD	Purified protein derivative
SOB	Shortness of breath
T & A	Tonsillectomy and adenoidectomy
TB	Tuberculosis
URI	Upper respiratory infection

The respiratory system provides the oxygen that is crucial to the survival of all cells in the body. Equally important, the respiratory system removes carbon dioxide, a waste product of metabolism, from the body. Pulmonary medicine is the branch of medicine specializing in respiratory tract disorders.

FUNCTION

The function of the respiratory system is to exchange the gases, oxygen and carbon dioxide, between the circulating blood and the air. Oxygen (O_2) is a colorless, odorless, combustible gas found in the air, and carbon dioxide (CO_2) is a colorless, odorless, incombustible gas that is a waste product of metabolism.

Breathing moves air in and out of the lungs where the exchange of gases, called respiration, occurs. There are two types of respiration processes. External respiration is the exchange of air at the lungs and internal respiration is the exchange of gases between the blood and the cells of the body. In external respiration, the oxygen from the air enters the blood stream through capillaries in the lungs, and carbon dioxide leaves the blood stream and is expelled into the air by the lungs. In internal respiration, the oxygen is released from the red blood cells and enters the tissue cells, and carbon dioxide from the tissue cells is picked up by the red blood cells.

COMPONENTS OF THE RESPIRATORY SYSTEM

The organs of the respiratory system include the nose, pharynx, and larynx (which comprise the upper respiratory tract), and the trachea, bronchi, and lungs (which constitute the lower respiratory tract) (Fig. 9–2).

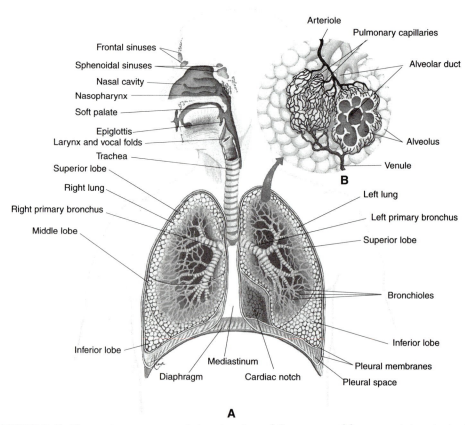

A

FIGURE 9–2. The respiratory system. *A*, Anterior view of the upper and lower respiratory tracts. *B*, Microscopic view of alveoli and pulmonary capillaries. (From Scanlon, VC, and Sanders, T: Essentials of Anatomy and Physiology, ed. 2. FA Davis, Philadelphia, 1995, p. 338, with permission.)

Air first enters the body through the nose, which acts as the primary filter. The nose moistens and warms the inhaled air, helps to produce sound, and contains the sensory organs for smell.

Air from the nose passes into the pharynx (throat), which is a tubelike structure that acts as a passageway for food and air. The pharynx divides into two branches, the larynx (voice box) and the esophagus. Food passes to the esophagus, which leads to the stomach, and air passes to the larynx, that leads to the lungs. Vocal cords, which determine the quality of voice sounds, are located in the larynx. A piece of cartilage, called the epiglottis, closes off the opening to the larynx, when food is swallowed, to prevent food from becoming lodged in the trachea.

From the larynx, the air passes to the trachea (windpipe), which provides the opening through which outside air can reach the lungs. The trachea divides into two main branches called primary bronchi that lead to the right and left lungs. These bronchi continue to subdivide into smaller and smaller treelike secondary branches, which extend to all parts of the lung. The smallest branches are called bronchioles. These subdivide into alveolar ducts, which have clusters of air sacs, called alveoli, located at their ends.

To exchange oxygen and carbon dioxide with the surrounding capillaries each lung is structured into millions of branches of alveoli. Effective gas exchange can take place between the alveoli and the surrounding capillaries because the walls of the alveoli and the capillaries are composed of a one-cell layer of epithelium. Figure 9-3 summarizes the pathway of air in the respiratory system.

NOSE

↓

PHARYNX

↓

LARYNX

↓

TRACHEA

↓

BRONCHI

↓

BRONCHIOLES

↓

ALVEOLI

↓

LUNG CAPILLARIES

↓

ARTERIES

↓

TISSUES

FIGURE 9-3. The pathway of respiration.

Blood transports oxygen and carbon dioxide via the hemoglobin in red blood cells. Hemoglobin with oxygen attached is called oxyhemoglobin and is carried to the tissues for use by the body cells. Carbon dioxide attaches to hemoglobin to form deoxyhemoglobin, which is carried to the lungs where the carbon dioxide is expelled.

Gaseous pressure determines how oxygen or carbon dioxide associates with (attaches to) or dissociates from (releases from) hemoglobin. The concentration of each gas in a particular site is expressed as a value called partial pressure. In the lungs, the partial pressure of oxygen (P_{O_2}) is high and the partial pressure of carbon dioxide (P_{CO_2}) is low. Therefore, in the lungs, oxygen is attached to hemoglobin and carbon dioxide dissociates from hemoglobin. In the tissues, the P_{O_2} is low and the P_{CO_2} is high so that oxygen dissociates from hemoglobin and carbon dioxide attaches to hemoglobin. Arterial blood gases are used to measure the partial pressure of oxygen and carbon dioxide in the blood.

DISORDERS ASSOCIATED WITH THE RESPIRATORY SYSTEM

Asthma

Obstruction of the bronchi due to swelling that may be caused by infections or allergies. It is accompanied by difficulty in breathing and by wheezing.

Bronchitis

Inflammation of the mucous membranes of the bronchial tubes. It causes a deep cough that produces sputum.

Chronic Obstructive Pulmonary Disease

Inflammation or obstruction of the bronchi over a long period of time. The result is the progressive, irreversible damage seen with chronic bronchitis and emphysema.

Emphysema

Destruction of the alveoli and bronchioles due to chronic inflammation caused by cigarette smoke or air pollutants. Shortness of breath (**SOB**) and enlargement of the chest cavity are symptoms.

Infant Respiratory Distress Syndrome

A condition affecting prematurely born infants and caused by a lack of surfactant in the alveolar air sacs in the lungs. Surfactant coats the alveolar walls to lower the surface tension so that air moves easily in and out of the lungs. Without surfactant, the alveoli collapse and breathing is difficult.

Lung Cancer

The most common cause of cancer deaths in men and women in the United States. It arises in the bronchi and can spread rapidly to other parts of the lung or body. Symptoms include coughing and sputum production. Radiation, chemotherapy, and removal of part or all of the lung are forms of treatment.

Pleurisy

Inflammation of the pleural membrane covering the chest cavity and the outer surface of the lungs. The symptoms are chest pain and difficult breathing.

Pneumonia

An acute infection of the alveoli (air sacs) of the lungs. The alveoli fill with fluid so that the air spaces are blocked and it is difficult to exchange oxygen and carbon dioxide. It is characterized by fever, chills, cough, and headache.

Pulmonary Edema

The accumulation of fluid in the lungs due to decreased pumping of blood through the lungs by the heart. This is a frequent complication of congestive heart failure.

Strep Throat

A streptococcal bacteria causes an inflammation of the pharynx that is characterized by a fever. Antibiotics are an effective treatment.

Tuberculosis

Tuberculosis (**TB**), caused by the bacteria *Mycobacterium tuberculosis*, usually affects the lungs. It is highly contagious, and transmitted by inhaling or swallowing infected droplets. Damage produced in the lung tissue decreases respiratory function.

Upper Respiratory Infection

Any infection of the nose, pharynx, or larynx, including the common cold. These infections include rhinitis, inflammation of the nasal mucosa, pharyngitis, inflammation of the pharynx (commonly called a sore throat), and laryngitis (inflammation of the larynx). The latter is marked by hoarseness or loss of voice.

LABORATORY TESTS

The most frequently ordered laboratory tests associated with the respiratory system and their clinical correlations are presented in Table 9 – 2.

TABLE 9–2. **LABORATORY TESTS ASSOCIATED WITH THE RESPIRATORY SYSTEM**

Test	Clinical Correlation
Arterial blood gases (ABGs)	Acid-base balance
Cold agglutinins	Atypical pneumonia
Electrolytes (Lytes)	Acid-base balance
Microbiological cultures, throat swabs, and bronchial washings	Microbial infection
Purified protein derivative (**PPD**)	Skin test for tuberculosis

BIBLIOGRAPHY

Chabner, D-E: The Language of Medicine. WB Saunders, Philadelphia, 1991.
Gylys, BA: Medical Terminology Simplified: A Programmed Learning Approach by Body Systems. FA Davis, Philadelphia, 1993.
Scanlon, VC, and Sanders, T: Essentials of Anatomy and Physiology, ed. 2. FA Davis, Philadelphia, 1995.
Thibodeau, GA, and Patton, KT: The Human Body in Health and Disease. CV Mosby, St. Louis, 1991.

Study Questions

1. Using the basic terminology and the terminology in this chapter, define the following:

   a. Analgesia _____

   b. Encephalitis _____

   c. Myelogram _____

   d. Neurology _____

   e. Anesthesia _____

   f. Bronchoscopy _____

   g. Dyspnea _____

   h. Hemothorax _____

   i. Oxyhemoglobin _____

   j. Nasopharyngitis _____

2. Interpret the following situations by defining the underlined words:

   a. A <u>LP</u> was performed on a patient to obtain <u>CSF</u> in order to diagnose <u>meningitis</u>.

   _____

   _____

   _____

   b. A <u>neurologist</u> examining a patient with <u>epilepsy</u> orders an <u>EEG</u>.

   _____

   _____

   _____

   c. A patient with a <u>CVA</u> due to a <u>thrombosis</u> had symptoms of <u>paralysis</u> in the left arm.

   _____

   _____

   _____

   d. A <u>CAT scan</u> was ordered on a patient to <u>R/O</u> <u>hemorrhage</u> or a tumor in the <u>CNS</u>.

   _____

   _____

   _____

   _____

e. A patient in the <u>ER</u> is given a <u>tracheotomy</u> to prevent <u>asphyxia</u> and <u>cyanosis</u>.

_____

_____

_____

_____

f. A request was made for a <u>PT</u> and <u>APTT</u> on a <u>pediatric</u> patient scheduled for a <u>T & A</u>.

_____

_____

_____

_____

g. A physician requested <u>ABGs</u> on a patient in the <u>OR</u> to determine P_{O_2} and P_{CO_2} values for evaluating <u>COPD</u>.

_____

_____

_____

_____

_____

h. A patient with a <u>URI</u> had symptoms of <u>rhinitis, laryngitis,</u> and <u>pharyngitis</u>.

_____

_____

_____

_____

3. What is the protective membrane surrounding the brain and spinal cord?

_____

_____

4. Name the components of the central nervous system.

_____

_____

5. What are the three major parts of the neuron?

a. _____

b. _____

c. _____

6. Name two types of neurons and describe their function.

   a. _____

   b. _____

7. What is the main body fluid analyzed by the laboratory to assess the nervous system? _____

8. What is a synapse?

   _____

   _____

9. List the organs of the respiratory system and their function.

   _____

   _____

   _____

   _____

   _____

   _____

10. Name the three functions of the nose.

   a. _____

   b. _____

   c. _____

11. Differentiate between external and internal respiration.

   _____

   _____

   _____

   _____

12. List two laboratory tests to evaluate the respiratory system.

   a. _____

   b. _____

13. What protective apparel should a phlebotomist wear when collecting blood from a patient with tuberculosis?

   _____

CHAPTER 10

Digestive and Urinary Systems

Learning Objectives

Upon completion of this chapter, the reader will be able to:

1 State the meaning of the roots and suffixes and define the terms and abbreviations associated with the digestive and urinary systems.
2 Describe the three major functions of the digestive system.
3 List the components of the gastrointestinal tract and the accessory organs of the digestive system.
4 Explain the process of mechanical and chemical digestion.
5 Identify and give the function of each component in the urinary system.
6 Describe the processes of filtration, reabsorption, and secretion in the formation of urine.
7 Describe the disorders associated with the digestive and urinary systems.
8 State the clinical correlations of laboratory tests associated with the digestive and urinary systems.

DIGESTIVE SYSTEM

Terminology Associated with the Digestive System

Roots/Combining Forms	Meaning
adip/o, lip/o, steat/o	fat
bil/i, chol/o	bile, gall
cholecyst/o	gallbladder
cirrh/o	yellow
dent/i, odont/o	tooth
enter/o	intestine
gastr/o	stomach
gingiv/o	gums
gloss/o, lingu/o	tongue
hepat/o	liver
lapar/o	abdomen
lith/o	stone
or/o, stomat/o	mouth
proct/o	rectum
sigmoid/o	sigmoid colon

Terminology Associated with the Digestive System
Continued

Suffixes	Meaning
-pepsia	digestion
-phagia	eating, swallowing

Key Terms	Definition
Alimentary tract	Digestive tract
Amino acids	"Building blocks" for protein
Appendectomy	Surgical removal of the appendix
Ascites	Abdominal swelling (caused by the accumulation of fluid in the peritoneal cavity)
Bowel	Intestine
Cholecystectomy	Surgical removal of the gallbladder
Diarrhea	Watery **stools**
Digestion	Breakdown of complex foods to simpler forms so they can be used by cells
Duodenum	First part of the small intestine
Dysentery	Diarrhea in which blood or mucus is present in the feces
Emesis	Vomit
Enteric	Pertaining to the intestinal tract
Feces/stools	Waste product of digestion/bowel movement (**BM**)
Hernia	Protrusion of an organ through a wall
Ileum	Last part of the small intestine
Jejunum	Second part of the small intestine
Nausea	Unpleasant sensation producing the urge to vomit
Peristalsis	Wavelike muscular contractions to propel material through the digestive tract
Rectum	End part of the colon

Abbreviations	Definition
BaE	Barium enema
BM	Bowel movement
CEA	Carcinoembryonic antigen
GB	Gallbladder
GI	Gastrointestinal
TPN	Total parenteral nutrition
UGI	Upper gastrointestinal

Food provides the energy needed for the growth, repair, and maintenance of body cells. A meal of meat and mashed potatoes with butter provides protein, carbohydrates, and fat. However, the body cells cannot absorb food in this complex form. The protein from meat must be broken down to amino acids, the carbohydrate from the potatoes must be broken down to a simple sugar (glucose), and the fat from the butter must be broken down to fatty acids and triglycerides. The digestive system provides the means to break down (digest) food into simple usable molecules and to eliminate waste products in the form of **feces**. Gastroenterology is the branch of medicine specializing in disorders of the digestive system.

FUNCTION

The digestive system performs three major functions: digestion, absorption of nutrients, and the elimination of waste products. **Digestion** occurs by both mechanical and chemical processes. The mechanical breakdown begins in the mouth, where the teeth and tongue physically alter the food before it is swallowed. The food continues to be mechanically digested by churning in the stomach, where it mixes with digestive fluids. Chemical breakdown of food is caused by digestive enzymes and acids that break down the larger molecules to smaller molecules. Enzymes in the saliva, gastric fluid, pancreatic fluid, and intestinal fluid speed up these chemical reactions and specific enzymes exist to break down carbohydrates, proteins, and fats. Carbohydrates such as starch are digested to simple sugars by the enzyme amylase, proteins are digested to **amino acids** by the protease enzymes, and fats are converted to fatty acids and glycerol by lipase. Other chemicals facilitate the process and help the food pass through the digestive tract.

The digestive products of food are absorbed through the walls of the small intestine into the blood and lymph, which transport nutrients to the other parts of the body to produce energy and nourish body cells. Sugars and amino acids are absorbed into the blood stream, and fat and triglycerides enter the lymphatic vessels.

Elimination of waste products is the third function of the digestive system. Unusable products of digestion are concentrated as feces in the large intestine, from which they are passed out of the body through the anus.

COMPONENTS OF THE DIGESTIVE SYSTEM

The digestive system (Fig. 10-1) consists of a gastrointestinal (**GI**) tract or **alimentary tract**, which is a continuous tube that begins with the mouth and ends at the anus. The organs of the gastrointestinal tract include the mouth, pharynx, esophagus, stomach, small intestine, large intestine, **rectum**, and anus. The pharynx and esophagus act as a passageway through which food is propelled to the stomach by wavelike muscular contractions called **peristalsis**. Digestion takes place in the mouth, stomach, and small intestine; absorption occurs in the small intestine. Elimination begins in the large intestine (colon) and ends at the anus.

Accessory organs that assist in the breakdown of food include the teeth, salivary glands, tongue, liver, gallbladder (**GB**), and pancreas. The teeth and tongue chew food; the salivary glands provide saliva to dissolve and moisten food and produce salivary amylase; the liver secretes bile to aid in fat digestion and absorption; the gallbladder stores bile; and the pancreas secretes the digestive enzymes, lipase, amylase, and trypsin, and produces insulin. The appendix does not function in the digestive process.

DISORDERS ASSOCIATED WITH THE DIGESTIVE SYSTEM

Appendicitis

Inflammation of the appendix producing acute pain in the right lower side. It is frequently treated by surgical removal of the appendix (**appendectomy**).

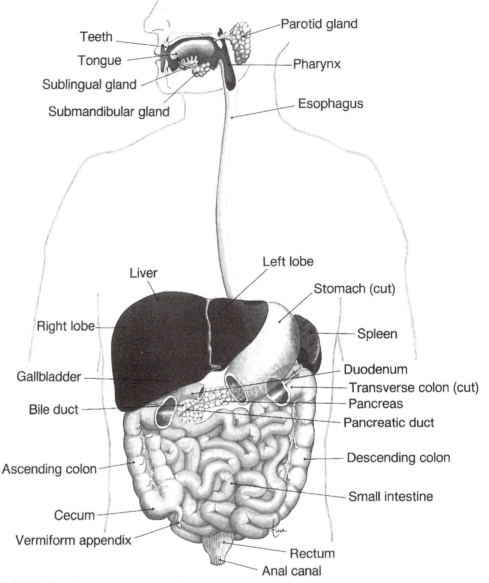

FIGURE 10–1. The digestive system. (From Scanlon, VC, and Sanders, T: Essentials of Anatomy and Physiology, ed. 2. FA Davis, Philadelphia, 1995, p. 361, with permission.)

Cholecystitis   Inflammation of the gallbladder that occurs when gallstones composed of crystal-lized bile and calcium block the bile duct and prevent the release of bile into the intestine.

Cirrhosis   Chronic inflammation resulting in degeneration of liver cells. The inflammation can be caused by alcoholism, hepatitis, or malnutrition and results in jaundice and liver failure.

Colitis   Inflammation of the colon that may be acute or chronic. It causes abdominal cramp-ing, **diarrhea**, and possible ulceration producing blood- and mucus-streaked stools.

Crohn's Disease	An autoimmune disorder producing chronic inflammation of the intestinal tract and accompanied by diarrhea and malabsorption.
Gastroenteritis	Inflammation of the stomach and intestinal tract producing **nausea**, vomiting, and diarrhea.
Hepatitis	An acute inflammation of the liver caused by exposure to toxins or the hepatitis viruses.
Pancreatitis	Inflammation of the pancreas that may be due to abdominal injury, alcoholism, drugs, or gallstones. Pancreatic digestive fluids accumulate in the pancreas producing tissue destruction.
Peritonitis	Inflammation of the lining of the abdominal cavity. It is frequently caused by a ruptured appendix or a perforated ulcer.
Ulcer	An open sore or lesion caused by increased acid secretion or bacterial infection in the gastric mucosa. Ulcers can occur in the stomach (gastric or peptic ulcer) or in the upper small intestine (duodenal ulcer). When untreated they may cause pain, hemorrhage, and perforation of the walls of the stomach or **duodenum**.

LABORATORY TESTS	The most frequently ordered laboratory tests associated with the digestive system and their clinical correlations are presented in Table 10–1.

TABLE 10–1. **LABORATORY TESTS ASSOCIATED WITH THE DIGESTIVE SYSTEM**

Test	Clinical Correlation
Alanine aminotransferase [ALT (SGPT)]	Liver disease
Alkaline phosphatase (ALP)	Liver disease
Ammonia	Severe liver disease
Amylase	Pancreatitis
Aspartate aminotransferase [AST (SGOT)]	Liver disease
Bilirubin	Liver disease or biliary obstruction
Carcinoembryonic antigen (**CEA**)	Carcinoma detection and monitoring
Carotene	Screening test for steatorrhea
Complete blood count (CBC)	Infection or appendicitis
Gamma glutamyl transferase (GGT)	Early liver disease
Gastrin	Gastric malignancy
Hepatitis B surface antigen (HBsAG)	Screening test for hepatitis B
Hepatitis antibodies for A, B, or C	Screening test for exposure to virus
Lipase	Pancreatitis
Occult blood	Gastrointestinal bleeding
Ova and parasites (O & P)	Parasitic infection
Stool culture	Stool pathogens

URINARY SYSTEM

Terminology Associated with the Urinary System

Roots/Combining Forms	Meaning
cyst/o	urinary bladder
nephr/o, ren/o	kidney
olig/o	scanty
ur/o, urin/o	urine

Suffixes	Meaning
-pexy	fixation
-tripsy	crushing
-uria	pertaining to urine

Key Terms	Definition
Azotemia	Increased nitrogenous waste products in the blood
Creatinine	Waste product of muscle metabolism
Cystoscope	Instrument for examining the interior of the bladder and urethra
Dysuria	Painful urination
Polydipsia	Excessive thirst
Polyuria	Marked increase in the urine flow
Renal	Pertaining to the kidney
Renal dialysis	Procedure to remove waste products from the blood when the kidneys are not functioning
Uremia	Increased urea in the blood
Urinary	Pertaining to the urinary tract
Urologist	Physician specializing in the male and female urinary tracts and the male genital tract

The **urinary** system removes waste products of metabolism, excess dietary chemicals, and excess water from the body in the form of urine. Urine is continually formed in the kidney and flows through the ureters to the bladder, where it is stored. When the bladder becomes full, muscles in the bladder wall squeeze urine into the urethra where it is expelled. Urology is the branch of medicine specializing in the male and female urinary tracts and the male genital tract. Nephrology is the branch of medicine specializing in the kidney.

FUNCTION

The kidney is the primary organ of the urinary system and functions to remove metabolic wastes from the blood stream, maintain the acid-base balance of the body, and regulate body hydration. The major waste product removed by the kidney is urea, a nitrogenous waste product from protein breakdown.

The acid-base and fluid balance of the body is regulated by the ability of the kidneys to reabsorb into the blood stream substances previously filtered from the blood. This reabsorption of filtered water and chemicals is called urine concentration.

The kidneys also produce hormones such as renin to control blood pressure, and erythropoietin to regulate the production of red blood cells.

COMPONENTS OF THE URINARY SYSTEM

The urinary system consists of two kidneys, two ureters, the urinary bladder, and the urethra. Refer to Figure 10–2.

The kidneys are bean-shaped organs containing an outer cortex region and an inner medulla region. The functioning unit of the kidney is the nephron, which consists of the Bowman's capsule, the glomerulus, the proximal convoluted tubule, the loop of Henle, the distal convoluted tubule, and collecting duct. Each kidney contains approximately one million nephrons, as illustrated in Figure 10–3. The

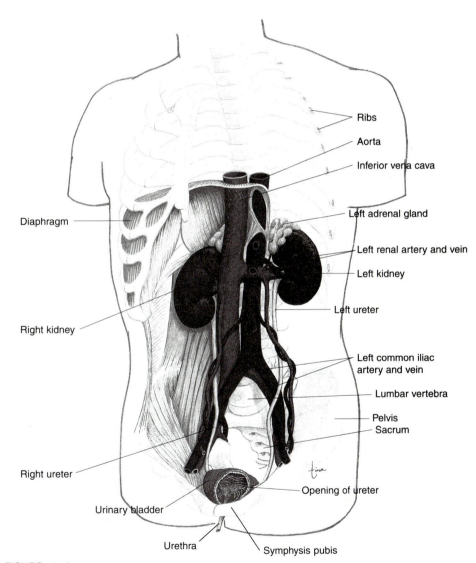

FIGURE 10–2. The urinary system. (Adapted from Scanlon, VC, and Sanders, T: Essentials of Anatomy and Physiology, ed. 2. FA Davis, Philadelphia, 1995, p. 416.)

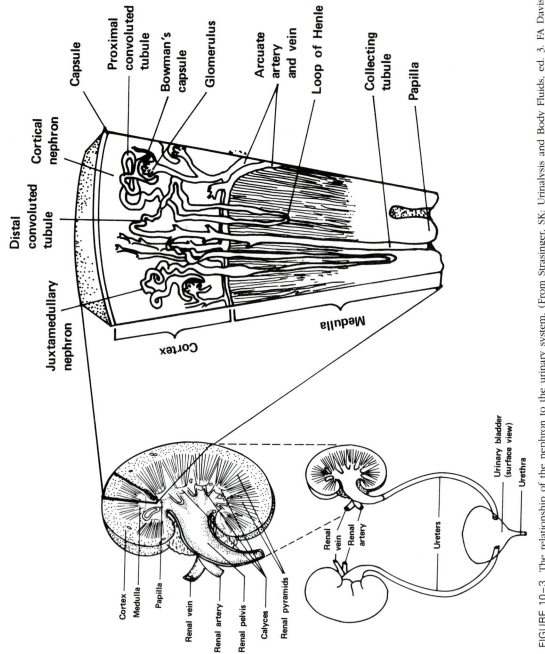

Distal convoluted tubule

Cortical nephron

Capsule

Proximal convoluted tubule

Bowman's capsule

Glomerulus

Arcuate artery and vein

Loop of Henle

Collecting tubule

Papilla

Juxtamedullary nephron

Cortex

Medulla

Cortex

Medulla

Papilla

Renal vein

Renal artery

Renal pelvis

Calyces

Renal pyramids

Renal vein

Renal artery

Ureters

Urinary bladder (surface view)

Urethra

FIGURE 10–3. The relationship of the nephron to the urinary system. (From Strasinger, SK: Urinalysis and Body Fluids, ed. 3. FA Davis, Philadelphia, 1994, p. 14, with permission.)

nephron controls the ability of the kidney to clear waste products from the blood and maintain the water and electrolyte balance of the body.

The two ureters are muscular tubes that carry urine from the kidney to the bladder.

The urinary bladder is an expandable sac located in the pelvis; it stores the urine formed by filtration of blood in the glomerulus of the nephron.

The urethra is a tube extending from the bladder to an external opening.

URINE FORMATION

Blood enters the kidney through the **renal** artery, which branches into arterioles leading to the nephrons and then into a collection of capillaries called the glomerulus. The filtration process takes place in the glomerulus, where small substances such as water, sodium and chloride ions, urea, creatinine, and uric acid are filtered out of the blood. Large proteins and cells remain in the blood.

Reabsorption of water, glucose, sodium, and other essential nutrients begins in the proximal convoluted tubule and continues in the descending and ascending loop of Henle. The final adjustment of urinary composition occurs in the distal convoluted tubule and collecting duct. Substances not filtered by the glomerulus are secreted by the tubules into the urinary filtrate.

The actual amount of urine produced is dependent upon the body's state of hydration and normally averages about 1000 mL every 24 hours. The amount of urine produced can be associated with certain disease states. A small amount of urine is termed oliguria, a large amount of urine is called **polyuria**, and the complete stoppage of urine flow is known as anuria.

DISORDERS ASSOCIATED WITH THE URINARY SYSTEM

Cystitis

Inflammation of the urinary bladder caused by a bacterial infection and most often seen in women.

Glomerulonephritis

A group of disorders in which there is inflammation of the glomerulus. It may be caused by an immune disorder or infection. Hypertension, albuminuria, renal failure, and **uremia** are characteristics of this disorder. Acute glomerulonephritis can be caused by a delayed immune response to a streptococcal infection.

Pyelonephritis

An inflammation of the renal pelvis and connective tissue of the kidney, usually caused by a bacterial infection.

Renal Calculi

Often called kidney stones, renal calculi are composed of calcium, uric acid, or other minerals that crystallize within the kidney. Small stones can sometimes pass through the urinary tract and be voided; however they may cause extreme pain. Lithotripsy, a process using high-energy sound waves, is a procedure used to crush larger stones so that surgery is not required.

Renal Failure   A complete cessation of renal function resulting in the need for **renal dialysis** and kidney transplantation.

Urinary Tract Infection   Any bacterial infection of the urinary tract including urethritis (inflammation of the urethra), cystitis (inflammation of the bladder), and pyelonephritis (inflammation of the kidney).

LABORATORY TESTS   The most frequently ordered laboratory tests associated with the urinary system and their clinical correlations are presented in Table 10-2.

TABLE 10-2. **LABORATORY TESTS ASSOCIATED WITH THE URINARY SYSTEM**

Test	Clinical Correlation
Blood urea nitrogen (BUN)	Kidney disease
Creatinine	Kidney disease
Creatinine clearance	Glomerular filtration
Culture and sensitivity (C & S)	Urinary tract infection
Electrolytes (Lytes)	Fluid and acid-base balance
Osmolality	Fluid balance
Protein	Kidney disorders
Renin	Hypertension
Routine urinalysis (UA)	Screening test for renal or metabolic disorders

BIBLIOGRAPHY

Chabner, D-E: The Language of Medicine. WB Saunders, Philadelphia, 1991.

Gylys, BA: Medical Terminology Simplified: A Programmed Learning Approach by Body Systems. FA Davis, Philadelphia, 1993.

Scanlon, VC, and Sanders, T: Essentials of Anatomy and Physiology, ed. 2. FA Davis, Philadelphia, 1995.

Strasinger, SK: Urinalysis and Body Fluids, ed. 3. FA Davis, Philadelphia, 1994.

Thibodeau, GA, and Patton, KT: The Human Body in Health and Disease. CV Mosby, St. Louis, 1991.

Study Questions

1. Using the basic terminology and the terminology in this chapter define the following:

   a. Appendicitis _____

   b. Colostomy _____

   c. Gastrectomy _____

   d. Gastroenteritis _____

   e. Gastroenterology _____

   f. Hepatomegaly _____

   g. Oliguria _____

   h. Cystoscopy _____

   i. Glomerulonephritis _____

   j. Hematuria _____

   k. Urology _____

   l. Nephrectomy _____

   m. Urethritis _____

   n. Nephrologist _____

   o. Proteinuria _____

2. Describe the following situations:

   a. A patient with <u>hepatitis</u> develops <u>cirrhosis</u> and appears <u>jaundiced</u> due to the accumulation of <u>bilirubin</u>.

   _____

   _____

   _____

   _____

   b. The lab receives a <u>stool</u> specimen for <u>O & P</u> from a patient suffering from <u>GI</u> distress and <u>diarrhea</u>.

   _____

   _____

   _____

   _____

   c. A request for an <u>amylase</u> and <u>lipase</u> is made by the physician to determine <u>pancreatitis</u>.

   _____

   _____

   _____

d. A <u>BaE</u> and a <u>CBC</u> are requested for a patient with <u>gastralgia</u> and <u>anemia</u> due to a suspected <u>gastric ulcer</u>.

_____

_____

_____

_____

_____

e. A patient with <u>cholecystitis</u> is scheduled for a <u>liver profile</u>.

_____

_____

f. A patient with <u>dysuria</u> was diagnosed with <u>renal calculi</u> and a <u>lithotripsy</u> was performed.

_____

_____

_____

g. A <u>GTT</u> was requested on a patient who complained of <u>polydipsia</u> and <u>polyuria</u>.

_____

_____

_____

h. After a <u>renal biopsy</u>, a <u>nephrectomy</u> was performed on the patient with <u>renal cell carcinoma</u>.

_____

_____

_____

i. A <u>UA</u> and <u>C & S</u> were ordered for a patient with <u>cystitis</u>. A <u>cystoscopy</u> was not indicated.

_____

_____

_____

_____

j. <u>Renal failure</u> as a result of <u>nephritis</u> led to <u>uremia</u> in the patient who consequently required <u>renal dialysis</u>.

_____

_____

_____

_____

3. List the organs of the gastrointestinal tract.

_____   _____

_____   _____

_____   _____

_____   _____

4. List the accessory organs of the digestive system

_____   _____

_____   _____

_____   _____

5. Name two processes of digestion.

a. _____

b. _____

6. Explain the function of the liver in digestion.

_____

7. Name three laboratory tests to assess liver function.

a. _____

b. _____

c. _____

8. Name three digestive enzymes.

a. _____

b. _____

c. _____

9. List the components of the urinary system.

_____

_____

_____

_____

10. What are the three steps in the process of urine formation?

    a. _____

    b. _____

    c. _____

11. In which part of the kidney does the filtration of the waste products from the blood occur? _____

12. What is the structure leading from the bladder to the external environment?

    _____

13. List two laboratory tests to evaluate the urinary system.

    a. _____

    b. _____

CHAPTER 11

Endocrine and Reproductive Systems

Learning Objectives

Upon completion of this chapter, the reader will be able to:

1 State the meaning of the roots and suffixes and define the terms and abbreviations associated with the endocrine and reproductive systems.
2 Describe the functions of the endocrine system.
3 Name the endocrine glands and the hormone secreted by each gland.
4 Explain the functions of the reproductive system.
5 List the organs of the male and female reproductive system.
6 Describe the disorders associated with the endocrine and reproductive systems.
7 State the clinical correlations of laboratory tests associated with the endocrine and reproductive systems.

ENDOCRINE SYSTEM

Terminology Associated with the Endocrine System

Roots/Combining Forms	Meaning
aden/o	gland
andr/o	male
cortic/o	cortex
crin/o	secrete
kal/o	potassium
natr/o	sodium
somat/o	body
ster/o	solid structure
thyr/o	thyroid gland

Suffixes	Meaning
-agon	assemble, gather together
-physis	growth
-tropin	stimulate

Key Terms	Definition
Adrenaline/ epinephrine	Hormone produced by the adrenal medulla to increase heart rate and blood pressure
Adrenocorticotropic hormone	Hormone produced by the anterior lobe of the pituitary gland to stimulate secretion of adrenal cortex hormones

Terminology Associated with the Endocrine System
Continued

Key Terms	Definition
Aldosterone	Hormone produced by the adrenal cortex to regulate electrolyte and water balance
Androgen	Male hormone produced by the testes and adrenal cortex
Antidiuretic hormone/ vasopressin	Hormone secreted by the posterior pituitary gland to stimulate retention of water by the kidney
Calcitonin	Hormone produced by the thyroid gland to reduce calcium levels in the blood
Cortisol	Hormone produced by the adrenal cortex to regulate the use of sugars, fats, and proteins by cells
Endocrine	Pertaining to ductless glands that secrete hormones directly into the blood stream to affect other organs
Follicle-stimulating hormone	Hormone produced by the anterior pituitary gland to stimulate estrogen secretion and egg production by the ovaries, and sperm production by the testes
Growth hormone/ somatotropin	Hormone produced by the anterior pituitary gland to stimulate growth of the bones and tissues
Hormone	Substance produced by a ductless gland and transported to parts of the body via the blood to control and regulate body functions
Hyperglycemia	Elevated glucose levels in the blood
Insulin	Hormone produced by pancreatic islets to promote the utilization of glucose by the body
Luteinizing hormone	Hormone produced by the anterior pituitary gland to stimulate ovulation
Melanocyte- stimulating hormone	Hormone produced by the anterior pituitary gland to stimulate pigmentation of the skin
Natremia	Sodium in the blood
Noradrenalin/ norepinephrine	Hormone secreted by the adrenal medulla to constrict blood vessels and increase blood pressure
Oxytocin	Hormone secreted by the posterior pituitary gland to stimulate contraction of the uterus at delivery and the release of milk into the breast ducts
Parathyroid hormone	Hormone produced by the parathyroid gland to regulate calcium levels in the blood
Thyroid-stimulating hormone	Hormone produced by the anterior pituitary gland to stimulate secretion of thyroid hormones
Thyroxine/ triiodothyronine	Hormone produced by the thyroid gland to stimulate energy metabolism of cells

Abbreviations	Definition
ACTH	Adrenocorticotropic hormone
ADH	Antidiuretic hormone
DI	Diabetes insipidus
DM	Diabetes mellitus

Terminology Associated with the Endocrine System Continued	Abbreviations	Definition
	FSH	Follicle-stimulating hormone
	GH	Growth hormone
	I	Iodine
	LH	Luteinizing hormone
	MSH	Melanocyte-stimulating hormone
	PRL	Prolactin
	TSH	Thyroid-stimulating hormone
	T3	Triiodothyronine
	T4	Thyroxine
	17-OH	17-Hydroxycorticosteroids

The **endocrine** system provides a communication system for the body. Unlike the nervous system, which commands and controls with nerve impulses, the endocrine system provides slower control by secreting chemical substances into the blood. These chemical substances are called hormones and act to communicate, regulate, and control body functions. Hormones are secreted directly into the blood stream by ductless glands called endocrine glands. These glands are located throughout the body and each performs a specific function. Endocrinology is the branch of medicine specializing in the study of endocrine glands.

FUNCTION

Body activities such as metabolism, growth and development, and reproduction are regulated by hormones. **Hormones** maintain homeostasis by regulating electrolyte balance, acid-base balance, and energy balance. Severe abnormalities such as dwarfism, gigantism, and sterility can be caused by hormonal imbalance.

Hormones bind to receptor sites located on the cell membrane of a target organ and, once bound, cause specific chemical reactions to occur. Each hormone has a specific receptor, so that the binding of a hormone to a receptor is like a key fitting into a lock.

ENDOCRINE GLANDS

The endocrine glands include the thyroid gland, four parathyroid glands, two adrenal glands, pancreas, pituitary gland, two female ovaries, two male testes, thymus, and the pineal gland (Fig. 11 – 1).

The right and left lobes of the thyroid gland are located on either side of the throat. The gland is responsible for the secretion of **calcitonin** to regulate the amount of calcium in the blood and of the hormones **thyroxine (T4)** and **triiodothyronine (T3)** to regulate cell metabolism. Iodine is necessary for production of the thyroid hormones.

The four oval parathyroid glands are located behind the thyroid gland. They secrete **parathyroid hormone** to regulate calcium and phosphorus levels in the blood.

The two small adrenal glands are located above each kidney. The outer portion

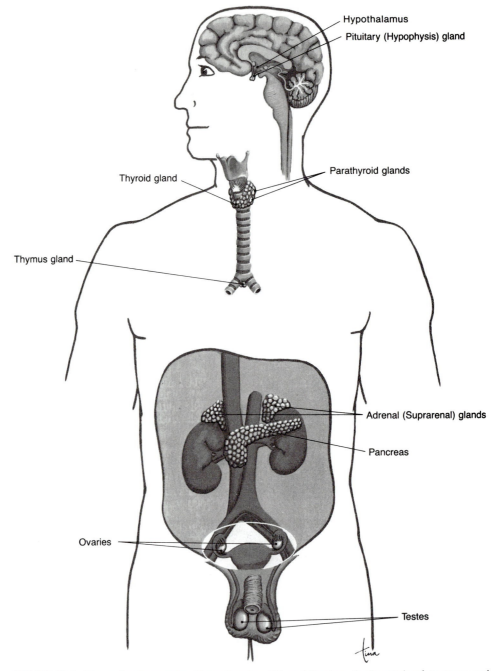

FIGURE 11–1. The endocrine system. (From Scanlon, VC, and Sanders, T: Essentials of Anatomy and Physiology, ed. 2. FA Davis, Philadelphia, 1995, p. 219, with permission.)

of the adrenal gland is called the adrenal cortex and the inner portion is the adrenal medulla. The adrenal cortex secretes the hormones **aldosterone** to regulate sodium and potassium levels in the blood, **cortisol** (hydrocortisone) to suppress inflammation and regulate the metabolism of proteins and carbohydrates, and the sex hormones (**androgen**, estrogen, and progesterone) to produce sex characteristics.

The adrenal medulla produces the catecholamine hormones: **adrenaline (epinephrine)** to increase cardiac activity, and **noradrenalin (norepinephrine)** to constrict blood vessels and increase the blood pressure. These hormones help the body react in stressful situations.

The pancreas, located behind the stomach, has specialized cells called the islets of Langerhans to produce insulin and glucagon. **Insulin** regulates blood sugar levels by transporting glucose from the blood to the body cells to decrease circulating blood sugar, and glucagon has the ability to convert glycogen (stored glucose) to sugar if increased blood sugar is needed.

The pituitary gland is located at the base of the brain and is divided into anterior and posterior portions. The anterior pituitary gland secretes **growth hormone (GH)** to stimulate growth of bone and tissue, **thyroid-stimulating hormone (TSH)** to stimulate the thyroid gland, **adrenocorticotropic hormone (ACTH)** to stimulate the adrenal cortex to secrete cortisol, **follicle-stimulating hormone (FSH)** and **luteinizing hormone (LH)** to stimulate ovulation and hormone secretion, prolactin (**PRL**) to promote growth of breast tissue, and **melanocyte-stimulating hormone (MSH)** to influence skin pigmentation. The posterior pituitary gland secretes **antidiuretic hormone (ADH)**, which stimulates water reabsorption to maintain body hydration, and **oxytocin** to stimulate uterine contraction and milk production in the mammary glands. Figure 11 – 2 illustrates the many functions of the pituitary gland.

The two small ovaries are located in the lower abdominal region of the female body. The hormones estrogen and progesterone are secreted by the ovaries and the adrenal cortex for the maintenance of the female reproductive system and the development of secondary female sex characteristics.

The two testes glands produce spermatozoa, and the male hormone testosterone, which is responsible for the development of male sex characteristics.

The thymus gland is located behind the sternum in the chest. It is responsible for producing the hormone thymosin, which is necessary for the development of the immune system in newborns and is active throughout childhood. The thymus decreases in activity and size with age.

The pineal gland is located in the center of the brain. It secretes melatonin to influence ovary and testes maturation and regulates the body's internal clock.

DISORDERS ASSOCIATED WITH THE ENDOCRINE SYSTEM

Acromegaly

Marked enlargement of the hands, feet, face, and jaw due to hypersecretion of growth hormone.

Addison's Disease

Decreased adrenal cortex function resulting in decreased blood sugar levels, muscle weakness, weight loss, nausea, low blood pressure, and dehydration.

Cushing's Disease

Hyperfunction of the adrenal cortex with increased cortisol secretion due to increased adrenal cortex stimulation by ACTH from the pituitary gland. Patients de-

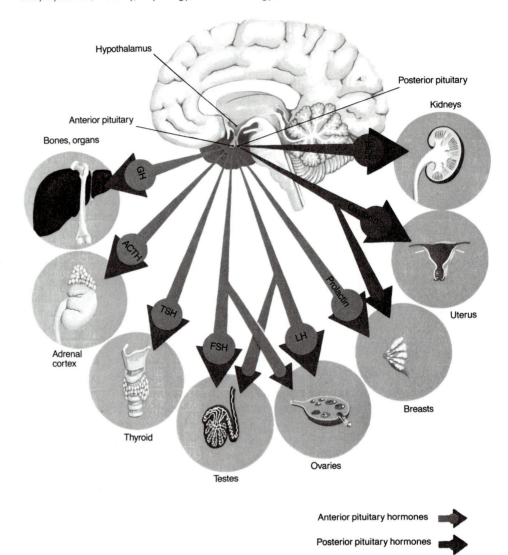

FIGURE 11–2. Hormones of the pituitary gland and their target organs. (From Scanlon, VC, and Sanders, T: Essentials of Anatomy and Physiology, ed. 2. FA Davis, Philadelphia, 1995, p. 223, with permission.)

velop a "moon face" and a buffalo hump on the thoracic region of the back due to redistribution of fat.

Diabetes Insipidus

Inadequate production or function of antidiuretic hormone that results in excessive urination and thirst.

Diabetes Mellitus

A condition caused by insulin insufficiency or malfunction that prevents sugar from leaving the blood and entering the body cells. **Hyperglycemia** is present and glucose may be found in the urine.

Dwarfism	Abnormally small body size that can be due to decreased secretion of growth hormone. Bones of these patients are underdeveloped.
Gigantism	A condition resulting from excess production of growth hormone, which causes a marked increase in body size.
Graves' Disease	Excess production of thyroid hormone that causes hyperthyroidism and increased cellular metabolism. Characteristics of this disorder include exophthalmus (a protrusion of the eyeballs due to swelling behind the eyes), nervousness, and weight loss.
Hyperinsulinism	A tumor of the pancreas may cause increased secretion of insulin, and consequently decreased blood sugar level.
Hypoglycemia	Decreased blood glucose level that is associated with nervousness, headaches, confusion, and sometimes convulsions and coma.
Myxedema	A condition resulting from decreased secretion of thyroid hormones (hypothyroidism), in which the lowered metabolic rate leads to fatigue, weight gain, loss of hair, and mental apathy.

LABORATORY TESTS	The most frequently ordered laboratory tests associated with the endocrine system and their clinical correlations are presented in Table 11 – 1.

TABLE 11–1. **LABORATORY TESTS ASSOCIATED WITH THE ENDOCRINE SYSTEM**

Test	Clinical Correlation
Calcium (Ca)	Parathyroid function
Catecholamines	Adrenal function
Cortisol	Adrenal cortex function
Follicle-stimulating hormone (FSH)	Ovarian function
Glucose	Pancreatic function
Glucose tolerance test (GTT)	Diabetes mellitus or hypoglycemia
Growth hormone (GH)	Pituitary gland function
Insulin	Pancreatic function and glucose metabolism
Phosphorus (P)	Parathyroid function
Thyroid function (T3, T4, TSH) studies	Thyroid function

REPRODUCTIVE SYSTEM

Terminology Associated with the Reproductive System	Roots/Combining Forms	Meaning
	amni/o	amnion
	colp/o	vagina
	episi/o	vulva
	gynec/o	female
	hyster/o	uterus, womb

Premenstrual Syndrome

Symptoms of depression, fatigue, mood swings, weight gain, and nervousness occurring 7 to 14 days before menstruation.

Sexually Transmitted Diseases

Diseases transmitted by sexual contact, including chlamydia infection, gonorrhea, genital herpes, syphilis, trichomoniasis, and AIDS.

Toxic Shock Syndrome

An infection, usually caused by staphylococcus, which may occur in women using superabsorbent tampons during menstruation. A toxin produced by the bacteria causes a decrease in blood pressure and the symptoms seen in systemic shock.

LABORATORY TESTS

The most frequently ordered laboratory tests associated with the reproductive system and their clinical correlations are presented in Table 11 – 2.

TABLE 11–2. **LABORATORY TESTS ASSOCIATED WITH THE REPRODUCTIVE SYSTEM**

Test	Clinical Correlation
Culture and sensitivity (C & S)	Microbial infection
Estradiol	Ovarian or placental function
Estrogen	Ovarian function
Fluorescent treponemal antibody absorbed (FTA-ABS)	Syphilis
Human chorionic gonadotropin (HCG)	Pregnancy
Pap smear (**Pap**)	Cervical or vaginal carcinoma
Prostate-specific antigen (**PSA**)	Prostatic cancer
Prostatic acid phosphatase (**PAP**)	Prostatic cancer
Rapid plasma reagin (RPR)	Syphilis
Semen analysis	Fertility, or the effectiveness of a vasectomy
Testosterone	Testicular function
Venereal Disease Research Laboratory (VDRL)	Syphilis

BIBLIOGRAPHY

Chabner, D-E: The Language of Medicine. WB Saunders, Philadelphia, 1991.
Gylys, BA: Medical Terminology Simplified: A Programmed Learning Approach by Body Systems. FA Davis, Philadelphia, 1993.
Thibodeau, GA, and Patton, KT: The Human Body in Health and Disease. CV Mosby, St. Louis, 1991.

Study Questions   1. Using the basic terminology and the terminology in this chapter, define the
following words:

a. Pancreatitis   _____

b. Endocrinologist _____

c. Acromegaly   _____

d. Hyperglycemia   _____

e. Hypothyroidism   _____

f. Amniocentesis   _____

g. Gynecology   _____

h. Hysterectomy   _____

i. Endometriosis   _____

j. Vasectomy   _____

2. Interpret the following situations by defining the underlined words:
a. An <u>FBS</u> was requested on a patient to <u>R/O</u> <u>hypoglycemia</u>.

_____

_____

_____

b. A test for <u>GH</u> was requested for a patient with symptoms of <u>dwarfism</u>.

_____

_____

c. A <u>T3, T4,</u> and <u>TSH</u> were requested on a patient with <u>hyperthyroidism</u>.

_____

_____

_____

_____

d. <u>LH</u> and <u>FSH</u> levels in a blood sample were determined by <u>RIA</u>.

_____

_____

_____

e. A blood test for a <u>PSA</u> level was ordered on a 60-year-old man with
<u>prostatic hyperplasia</u> to check for suspected <u>prostatic carcinoma</u>.

_____

_____

_____

   f. <u>GC</u> and <u>HSV</u> tests were requested for a patient with <u>PID</u> and a history of <u>STD</u>.

    _____

    _____

    _____

    _____

   g. An <u>RPR</u>, <u>VDRL</u>, and <u>FTA-ABS</u> were ordered on a patient with <u>syphilis</u>.

    _____

    _____

    _____

    _____

   h. An <u>HCG</u> was ordered to test for pregnancy in a patient scheduled for the <u>OR</u>.

    _____

    _____

3. What are the substances secreted by endocrine glands called?

  _____

4. Name three laboratory tests to evaluate thyroid function.

  a. _____

  b. _____

  c. _____

5. Name two laboratory tests associated with diabetes mellitus.

  a. _____

  b. _____

6. Which organ produces insulin and what is its major function?

  _____

  _____

7. Name two disease states associated with abnormal thyroid function.

  a. _____

  b. _____

8. Match one item in column A with one item in column B. Use an answer only once.

	Column A	**Column B**
a. _____	Acid phosphatase	1. Male sex hormone
b. _____	Ovulation	2. Female gonad
c. _____	Ovary	3. Test for prostate cancer
d. _____	Semen analysis	4. Monthly discharge of blood
e. _____	Spermatozoa	5. Release of ovum from ovary
f. _____	Hysterectomy	6. Hormone produced in pregnancy
g. _____	HCG	7. Male sex cell
h. _____	Menstruation	8. Removal of the uterus
i. _____	Testosterone	9. Test for fertility

SECTION III Phlebotomy Techniques

CHAPTER 12

Venipuncture Equipment

Learning Objectives

Upon completion of this chapter, the reader will be able to:

1 Define the terms and abbreviations associated with venipuncture equipment.
2 List 10 items that may be carried on a phlebotomist's tray.
3 Differentiate among the various needle sizes as to gauge and purpose.
4 Discuss methods to safely dispose of contaminated needles.
5 Differentiate between a vacuum collection tube, a syringe, and winged infusion apparatus, and know the advantages and disadvantages of each.
6 Identify the types of vacuum tubes by color code, and state the anticoagulants and additives present, any special characteristics, and the purpose of each.
7 State the mechanism of action, advantages, and disadvantages of the anticoagulants EDTA, sodium citrate, potassium oxalate, and heparin.
8 List the correct order of draw for vacuum tubes, and the correct order of fill for tubes collected by syringe.
9 Describe three types of tourniquets.
10 Name two substances used to cleanse the skin prior to venipuncture.
11 Discuss the use of sterile gauze, bandages, gloves, and slides when performing venipuncture.

Terminology

Key Terms	Definition
Antiglycolytic agent	Substance that prevents the breakdown of glucose
Antiseptic	Substance that destroys or inhibits the growth of microorganisms
Bacteriostatic	Capable of inhibiting the growth of bacteria
Bevel	Area of the needle point that has been cut on a slant
Butterfly	Winged infusion set used for small veins
Gauge	Unit of measure assigned to the diameter of a needle
Labile	Biologically or chemically unstable
Thixotropic gel	Substance that undergoes a temporary change in viscosity during centrifugation
Vacutainer	Becton Dickinson trade name for an evacuated blood collection tube

Abbreviations	Definition
ACD	Acid citrate dextrose
EDTA	Ethylenediaminetetraacetic acid

Terminology Continued	**Abbreviations**	**Definition**
	PST	Plasma separator tube
	SPS	Sodium polyanetholesulfonate
	SST	Serum separator tube

The first step in learning to perform a venipuncture is knowledge of the needed equipment. An adequate amount of necessary equipment is essential at all times when performing venipuncture. Therefore, this chapter will cover the types of equipment used when performing venipunctures with evacuated systems, syringes, and winged infusion sets. Discussion will include the advantages and disadvantages of the various pieces of equipment, the situations in which they are used, and when appropriate, the mechanisms by which the equipment works.

Equipment necessary to perform venipunctures includes needles, needle disposal containers, needle holders, collection tubes, syringes, winged infusion sets, tourniquets, **antiseptic** cleansing solutions, gauze pads, bandages, and gloves.

ORGANIZATION OF EQUIPMENT

Equipment for phlebotomy is usually organized in a collection tray similar to the one shown in Figure 12–1. In outpatient settings the phlebotomy tray or a more permanent arrangement is located at the drawing station (Fig. 12–2). The phlebotomy tray provides a convenient way for the phlebotomist to carry equipment to the patients' rooms. Except in isolation situations, the tray is carried into the patient's room. It should be placed on a solid surface, such as a night stand, and not on the patient's bed where it could be knocked off. Only the needed equipment should be brought directly to the patient's bed.

The duties of a phlebotomist include the cleaning, disinfecting, and restocking of the phlebotomy trays and of outpatient drawing stations. Trays should be totally emptied and disinfected on a weekly basis. Trays also contain equipment for performing the microcollection techniques to be discussed in Chapter 16.

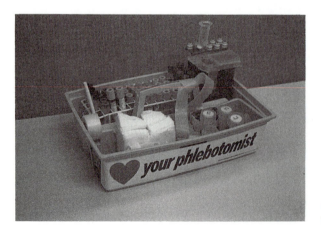

FIGURE 12–1. Phlebotomy collection tray.

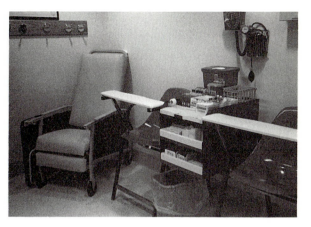

FIGURE 12–2. Phlebotomy drawing station, including a reclining chair.

NEEDLES

All needles used in venipuncture are disposable and are used only once. Needle size varies by both length and gauge (diameter). For routine venipuncture 1-inch and 1.5-inch lengths are used.

Needle **gauge** refers to the diameter of the needle bore. Needles vary from large (16-gauge) needles used to collect units of blood for transfusion to much smaller (23-gauge) needles used for very small veins. Notice that the smaller the gauge number the bigger the diameter of the needle. Needles with gauges smaller than 23 are available, but they can cause hemolysis when used for drawing blood specimens. They are most frequently used for injections and intravenous (IV) infusions.

Manufacturers package needles individually in sterile containers that are color-coded by gauge for easy identification.

As shown in Figure 12–3, needle structure varies to adapt to the type of collection equipment being used. All needles consist of a **beveled** point, shaft, lumen, and

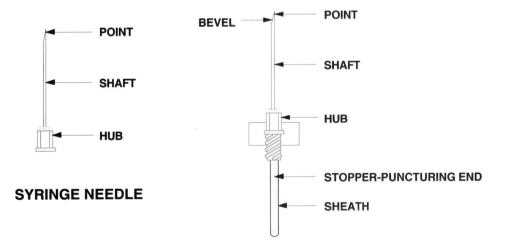

SYRINGE NEEDLE

EVACUATED TUBE NEEDLE

FIGURE 12–3. Needle structure.

hub. Needles should be visually examined prior to use to determine if any structural defects, such as nonbeveled points or bent shafts, are present.

The most frequently used needles in the clinical laboratory are those for evacuated collection systems. These are often referred to as **Vacutainer** needles (Becton Dickinson, Franklin Lakes, NJ). They are double-ended needles designed so that one end is for phlebotomy and the other end punctures the rubber stopper of the collection tube. Vacutainer needles are designated as single-draw and multi-draw needles. Single-draw needles have a visible stopper-puncturing needle and are used when only one tube of blood is required. Multi-draw needles have the puncturing needle covered by a rubber sheath that is pushed back when a tube is attached and returns to full needle coverage when the tube is removed. This prevents leakage of blood when tubes are being changed. The increased possibility of blood contamination when using single-draw needles, even when only one tube of blood is being drawn, has caused most institutions to use multi-draw needles for all venipunctures. However, phlebotomists should check the type of needle when working in an unfamiliar setting.

Needles used with syringes are attached to a plastic hub designed to fit onto the barrel of the syringe. They are also individually packaged, sterile, and color-coded as to gauge size. Routinely used syringe needles range from 20- to 23-gauge with 1-inch and 1.5-inch lengths. An advantage when using syringe needles is that blood will appear in the hub of the needle when the vein has been successfully entered.

NEEDLE DISPOSAL SYSTEMS

To protect phlebotomists from accidental needle sticks by contaminated needles, a means of safe disposal must be available whenever phlebotomy is performed. In recent years, due to the increased concern over exposure to blood-borne pathogens many disposal systems have been developed.

Needle disposal systems include basic needle recapping devices, puncture-resistant containers for manual unscrewing of the needle, needle holders that become disposable puncture-resistant shields, and automatic needle removal devices (Fig. 12–4). Phlebotomists should become familiar with the types of disposal systems used in their institutions. They should also remember that the rubber-sheathed puncturing end of a vacuum tube needle causes many accidental punctures.

Under no circumstances should a needle be recapped without using a safety device.

NEEDLE ADAPTERS

Needles used in the evacuated tube collection systems are designed to be screwed into an adapter that holds the collection tube. Adapters are made of clear, rigid plastic and may be reused, or they may be designed to act as a safety shield for the used needle in which case they are discarded. Nondisposable adapters must be disinfected whenever they become visibly contaminated.

Adapters are available to accommodate collection tubes of different sizes. To provide proper puncturing of the rubber stopper and maximum control, tubes should fit securely in the adapter. The Hemogard Vacutainer System (Becton Dickinson, Franklin Lakes, NJ) has standardized the diameter of all its collection tubes to 13 mm to allow use of a single adapter.

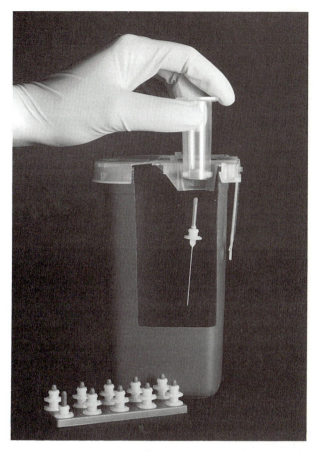

FIGURE 12–4. AutoDrop Needle disposal system. (Courtesy of Sage Products, Inc., Crystal Lake, IL.)

The flared ends of the needle adapters aid the phlebotomist during the transfer of tubes in multiple-draw situations. A marking near the top of the adapter indicates the distance an evacuated tube may be advanced into the stopper-puncturing needle without entering the tube and losing the vacuum (Fig. 12 – 5).

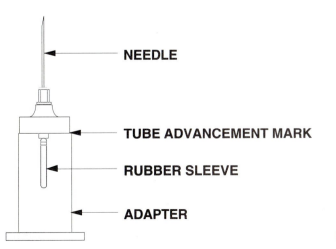

NEEDLE

TUBE ADVANCEMENT MARK

RUBBER SLEEVE

ADAPTER

FIGURE 12–5. Needle adapter.

COLLECTION TUBES

The primary tubes used for blood collection are evacuated (vacuum) tubes, often referred to as Vacutainers (Becton Dickinson, Franklin Lakes, NJ), although they are also available from other manufacturers. Use of vacuum tubes with their corresponding needles and adapters provides a means of collecting blood directly into the tube, thereby minimizing accidental contact with blood by the phlebotomist. Laboratory instrumentation is also available for direct sampling from the vacuum tubes, providing additional protection for laboratory workers.

The amount of blood collected in a vacuum tube ranges from 2 to 15 mL and is determined by the size of the tube and the amount of vacuum present. As shown in Figure 12–6, a wide variety of sizes is available to accommodate both adult and pediatric patients. When selecting the appropriate size tube, the phlebotomist must consider the amount of blood needed and the size and condition of the patient's veins. Using a 23-gauge needle with a large vacuum tube can produce hemolysis, because red blood cells are damaged when the large amount of vacuum causes them to be rapidly pulled through the small lumen of the needle. Therefore, if it is necessary to use a small-gauge needle, the phlebotomist should collect two small tubes instead of one large tube.

Most vacuum tubes are sterile and many are silicon coated to prevent cells from adhering to the tube, or to prevent the activation of clotting factors in coagulation studies. Information about the characteristics of a tube is contained on the write-on label attached to the tube and should be verified by the phlebotomist when special collection procedures are needed. Tubes may also contain anticoagulants and additives.

As shown in Figure 12–7, vacuum tubes have thick rubber stoppers with a thinner central area to allow puncture by the Vacutainer needle. To aid the phlebotomist in identifying the many types of vacuum tubes, the tops are color-coded. Color-coding for routinely used tubes is uniform among manufacturers, and instructions for sample collection usually refer to the tube color.

Example: Draw one red top, one light-blue top, and one lavender top tube.

Two types of color-coded tops are available. Rubber stoppers may be colored, or a color-coded plastic shield may cover the stopper, as with the Hemogard Vacutainer System. Removing the rubber stoppers from vacuum tubes can be hazardous to laboratory workers because an aerosol of blood can be produced if the stopper is

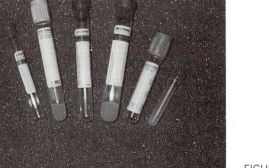

FIGURE 12–6. Examples of evacuated tubes.

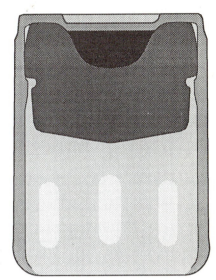

FIGURE 12–7. Cut-away view of a vacuum tube stopper (Hemogard closure). (Adapted from Product Literature, Becton Dickinson, Franklin Lakes, NJ.)

quickly "popped off." Stoppers should be covered with a gauze pad and slowly loosened with the opening facing away from the body. Hemogard closures provide additional protection by allowing the stoppers to be easily twisted and pulled off and have a shield over the stopper.

Principles of Color-Coded Tubes

Color-coding indicates the type of specimen that will be obtained when a particular tube is used. As discussed in Chapter 4, tests may be run on plasma, serum, or whole blood. Tests may also require the presence of preservatives, inhibitors, clot activators, or barrier gels. To produce these necessary conditions some tubes will contain anticoagulants or additives, and others will not. Phlebotomists must be able to relate the color of the collection tubes to the types of specimens needed and to any special techniques, such as tube inversion, that may be required. This section discusses the routinely used tubes with regard to anticoagulants, additives, types of tests for which they are used, and special handling required.

Lavender top tubes contain the anticoagulant **EDTA**, sodium or potassium ethylenediaminetetraacetic acid, in either liquid or powdered form. Coagulation is prevented by the binding of calcium in the specimen to sites on the large EDTA molecule, thereby preventing the participation of the calcium in the coagulation cascade (Fig. 12–8). All tubes containing anticoagulants or additives should be inverted immediately after drawing to ensure uniform mixing with the specimen. Lavender top tubes should be gently inverted eight times. When using powdered anticoagulants, the bottom of the tube should be gently tapped to loosen the powder from the tube prior to drawing the specimen.

For hematology procedures that require whole blood, such as the complete blood count (CBC), EDTA is the anticoagulant of choice because it maintains cellular integrity better than other anticoagulants, inhibits platelet clumping, and does not interfere with routine staining procedures. Lavender top tubes cannot be used for coagulation studies because EDTA interferes with factor V and the thrombin-fibrinogen reaction.

Light-blue top tubes contain the anticoagulant sodium citrate, which also prevents coagulation by binding calcium. Centrifugation of the anticoagulated light-blue

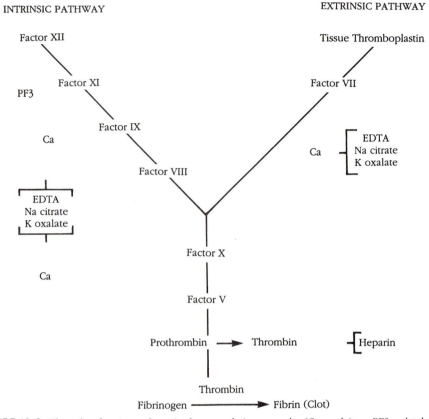

FIGURE 12–8. The role of anticoagulants in the coagulation cascade. (Ca = calcium; PF3 = platelet factor 3.)

top tubes provides the plasma used for coagulation tests. Sodium citrate is the required anticoagulant for coagulation studies because it preserves the **labile** coagulation factors. Tubes should be inverted eight times.

The ratio of blood to the liquid sodium citrate is critical and should be 9 to 1 (example: 4.5 mL blood and 0.5 mL sodium citrate). Therefore, light-blue top tubes must be completely filled to ensure accurate results. When drawing coagulation tests on patients with polycythemia or hematocrit readings over 55% the amount of anticoagulant must be decreased to maintain the 9 to 1 ratio, because the lower volume of plasma in these patients will be diluted by the standard volume of sodium ·citrate. Likewise the amount of anticoagulant must be increased for severely anemic patients because of the larger amount of plasma.

A special light-blue top tube containing thrombin and a soybean trypsin inhibitor must be used when drawing blood for determinations of certain fibrin degradation products.

Black top tubes containing sodium citrate are used for Westergren sedimentation rates. They differ from light-blue top tubes in that they provide a ratio of blood to liquid anticoagulant of 4 to 1.

Red/gray rubber stoppers and *gold* Hemogard closures are found on tubes containing a clot activator and a separation gel. They are frequently referred to as serum separator tubes (**SST**). Clot activators such as glass particles, silica, and celite increase platelet activation, thereby shortening the time required for clot formation.

Tubes should be inverted five times to expose the blood to the clot activator. A non-reactive **thixotropic gel** that undergoes a temporary change in viscosity during centrifugation is located at the bottom of the tube. As shown in Figure 12–9, when the tube is centrifuged, the gel forms a barrier between the cells and serum to prevent contamination of the serum with cellular materials. To produce a solid separation barrier, specimens must be allowed to clot completely before centrifuging. Specimens should be centrifuged as soon as clot formation is complete.

Serum separator tubes are used for most chemistry tests and prevent contamination of the serum by cellular chemicals. They are not suitable for use in the blood bank.

Green top tubes contain the anticoagulant heparin combined with either sodium, lithium, or ammonium ion. Heparin prevents clotting by inhibiting thrombin in the coagulation cascade (Fig. 12–8). Green top tubes are used for chemistry tests performed on plasma including ammonia, carboxyhemoglobin, and STAT electrolytes. Interference by sodium and lithium heparin with their corresponding chemical tests and by ammonium heparin in blood urea nitrogen (BUN) determinations must be avoided. In general lithium heparin has been shown to produce the least interference. Tubes should be inverted eight times. Green top tubes are not used for hematology because heparin interferes with the Wright's stained blood smear.

Light-green top tubes containing lithium heparin and a separation gel are called plasma separator tubes (**PST**) and are available with Hemogard closures. They are well suited for potassium determinations because heparin prevents the release of potassium by platelets during clotting and the gel prevents contamination by red blood cell potassium.

Red top tubes are often referred to as "plain" vacuum tubes because they contain no anticoagulants or additives. Blood drawn in red top tubes clots by the normal coagulation process in about 30 minutes. Centrifuging then yields serum as the liquid portion. Red top tubes are used for serum chemistry tests, serology tests, and in blood bank, where both serum and red blood cells are used. There is no need to invert red top tubes.

A *plain pink top* tube is also available and is used specifically for blood bank in some facilities. Using a designated tube for blood bank is believed to help prevent testing of specimens from the wrong patient.

Yellow/gray rubber stoppers and *orange* Hemogard closures are found on tubes containing the clot activator, thrombin. Notice, in Figure 12–8, that thrombin

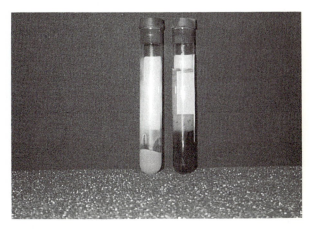

FIGURE 12–9. Serum separator tubes before and after collection and centrifugation.

is generated near the end of the coagulation cascade; addition of thrombin to the tube results in faster clot formation, usually within 5 minutes. Tubes should be inverted eight times. Tubes containing thrombin are used for STAT serum chemistry determinations and for patients receiving anticoagulant therapy.

Gray top tubes are available with a variety of additives and anticoagulants for the primary purpose of preserving glucose. All gray top tubes contain a glucose preservative (**antiglycolytic agent**), either sodium fluoride or lithium iodoacetate. Sodium fluoride maintains glucose stability for 3 days and iodoacetate for 24 hours. Sodium fluoride and iodoacetate are not anticoagulants; therefore, if plasma is needed for analysis, an anticoagulant must also be present and the tubes must be inverted eight times. In gray top tubes the anticoagulant is potassium oxalate which, like EDTA and sodium citrate, prevents clotting by binding calcium. When monitoring patient glucose levels, tubes for the collection of plasma and serum should not be interchanged. Sodium fluoride will interfere with some enzyme analyses; therefore, gray top tubes should not be used for other chemical analyses.

Blood alcohol levels are drawn in gray top tubes containing sodium fluoride that inhibits microbial growth, which could produce alcohol as a metabolic endproduct. Tubes with or without potassium oxalate can be used, depending on the need for plasma or serum in the test procedure.

Dark-blue top tubes are used for toxicology, trace metal, and nutritional analyses. Because many of the elements analyzed in these studies are significant at very low levels, the tubes must be chemically clean and the rubber stoppers are specially formulated to contain the lowest possible levels of metal. Dark-blue top tubes are available plain or with sodium heparin or disodium EDTA to conform to a variety of testing requirements.

Brown top tubes with Hemogard closures are available for lead determinations. They are certified to contain less than 0.1 μg/mL of lead.

Yellow top tubes are available for two different purposes and contain different additives. Yellow stoppers and yellow Hemogard closures are found on tubes containing the red blood cell preservative, acid citrate dextrose (**ACD**). Specimens drawn in these tubes are used for cellular studies in the blood bank.

Sterile yellow top tubes containing the anticoagulant, sodium polyanetholesulfonate (**SPS**), are used to collect specimens to be cultured for the presence of microorganisms. SPS aids in the recovery of microorganisms by inhibiting the actions of complement, phagocytes, and certain antibiotics. Yellow top tubes should be inverted eight times.

Evacuated tubes are summarized in Table 12 – 1.

Order of Draw

When collecting multiple specimens and specimens for coagulation tests, the order in which tubes are drawn can affect some test results. As shown in Figure 12 – 8, the extrinsic pathway of the coagulation cascade is initiated by the presence of tissue thromboplastin. Release of tissue thromboplastin from the skin as it is punctured can result in its presence in the first tube collected, and this could interfere with coagulation tests. Therefore, a light-blue top tube should not be drawn first. If only a coagulation test is ordered, it is recommended that a small red top tube be drawn first; it can be discarded if it is not needed.

Transfer of anticoagulants among tubes due to possible contamination of the stopper-puncturing needle must be avoided. This is why the red top tube is drawn before the coagulation tube and why tubes containing other anticoagulants are

TABLE 12–1. **SUMMARY OF EVACUATED TUBES***

Stopper Color	Anticoagulant/ Additive	Laboratory Use
(1) Lavender (2) Lavender	Ethylenediaminetetra- acetic acid (EDTA)	Whole blood for hematology tests
(1) Light-blue (2) Light-blue	Sodium citrate 0.105M or 0.129M	Plasma for coagulation tests
(1) Red/gray (2) Gold	Clot activator and thixotropic gel	Serum separator tube for chemistry tests
(1) Green (2) Green	Sodium heparin, lithium heparin, or ammonium heparin	Plasma chemistry tests
(1) Red (2) Red	None	Serum for tests in chemistry, blood bank, and serology
(1) Yellow/gray (2) Orange	Thrombin	STAT serum chemistry tests
(1) Gray (2) Gray	Potassium oxalate/ sodium fluoride, iodoacetate/ lithium heparin, or iodoacetate	Glucose tests (Glycolytic inhibitors stabilize values for up to 24 hours with iodoacetate and 3 days with fluoride. Oxalate and heparin produce plasma.)
(1) Dark-blue (2) Dark-blue	Sodium heparin, EDTA, or none	Trace elements, toxicology, and nutrient analyses (Special stopper provides a minimum of external contamination.)
(1) Brown (2) Brown	Sodium heparin	Lead determinations (Tube is certified to contain less than 0.01 µg/mL [ppm] lead.)
(1) Yellow (2) Yellow	Sodium polyanethole- sulfonate (SPS)	Blood cultures

*NOTE: (1) Conventional Stopper and (2) Hemogard Closure.

drawn after the light-blue top tube. Also tubes containing EDTA, which can bind calcium and iron, should not be drawn prior to a tube for chemistry tests on these substances.

When sterile specimens, such as blood cultures, are to be collected, they must be considered in the order of draw. Such specimens are always drawn first to prevent contamination.

Summarizing the above discussion, the order of draw for multiple tubes using the vacuum tube system is:

1 Sterile specimens
2 Plain tubes (red)
3 Coagulation tubes (light-blue)
4 Other anticoagulants and additives in this order: green–heparin; lavender–EDTA; yellow/gray or orange–clot activator; red/gray–serum separator; and gray–oxalate/fluoride

The order changes when tubes are being filled from a syringe because the portion of blood possibly contaminated by tissue thromboplastin is the first portion to enter the syringe and, therefore, as shown in Figure 12–10, is the last to be expelled. The order of tube fill from a syringe is:

1 Sterile specimens
2 Coagulation tubes
3 Other anticoagulants and additives (EDTA, heparin, and oxalate/fluoride)
4 Plain and serum separator tubes

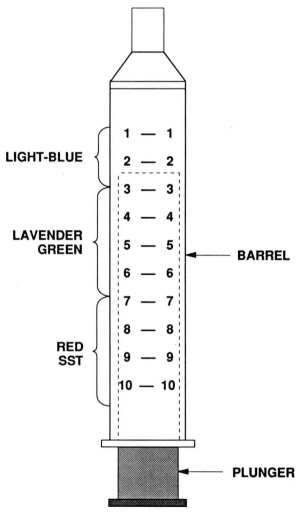

FIGURE 12–10. Diagram of a syringe, illustrating the order of tube fill.

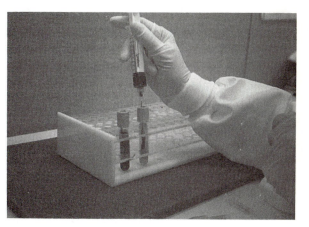

FIGURE 12–11. Transfer of blood from a syringe to an evacuated tube. (Note how the phlebotomist directs the blood against the side of the tube.)

SYRINGES

Syringes are often preferred over vacuum tubes when drawing blood from patients with small or fragile veins. The phlebotomist is able to control the suction pressure on the vein by slowly withdrawing the syringe plunger.

Syringes routinely used for venipuncture range from 2 to 10 mL, and a size corresponding to the amount of blood needed should be used. Syringes consist of a plunger, and a barrel graduated in milliliters or cubic centimeters (Fig. 12 – 10). The technique for use of syringes in discussed in Chapter 14.

Blood drawn in a syringe is transferred to appropriate evacuated tubes. It is acceptable to puncture the rubber stopper with the syringe needle and allow the blood to be drawn, but not forced, into the tube. Care must be taken to avoid hemolysis and needle punctures. As shown in Figure 12 – 11, the tube should be placed in a rack, not held in the free hand, and the needle should be angled toward the side of the tube for gentler transfer of the blood.

WINGED INFUSION SETS

Winged infusion sets, or **"butterflies"** as they are routinely called, are used for the infusion of IV fluids and for performing venipuncture from very small veins. Butterfly needles used for phlebotomy are usually 23-gauge with lengths of 1/2 to 3/4 inch. Plastic attachments to the needle that resemble butterfly wings are used for holding the needle during insertion and to secure the apparatus during IV therapy (Fig. 12 – 12). They also provide the ability to lower the needle insertion angle when working with very small veins. To accommodate the dual purpose of venipuncture and infusion the needle is attached to a flexible plastic tubing that can then be attached to an IV setup, syringe, or specially designed Vacutainer adapter.

TOURNIQUETS

Tourniquets are used during venipuncture to make it easier to locate patients' veins. They do this by impeding venous but not arterial blood flow in the area just below where the tourniquet is applied.

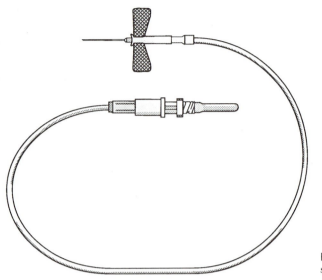
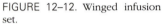

FIGURE 12–12. Winged infusion set.

The most frequently used tourniquets are flat latex strips (Fig. 12–13). They are inexpensive and may be disposed of between patients, or reused if disinfected. Tourniquets with Velcro and buckle closures are easier to apply but are more difficult to decontaminate.

Blood pressure cuffs can be used as tourniquets. They are used primarily for veins that are difficult to locate. The cuff should be inflated to a pressure below the patient's systolic blood pressure reading and above the diastolic reading. This allows blood to flow into but not out of the affected veins.

The application of tourniquets and their effects on blood tests are discussed in Chapters 13 and 14.

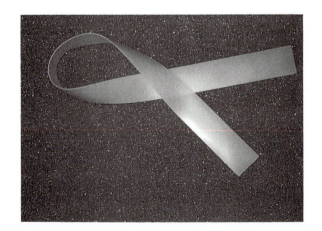

FIGURE 12–13. Latex strip tourniquet.

PUNCTURE SITE PROTECTION SUPPLIES

The primary antiseptic used for cleansing the skin in routine phlebotomy is 70% isopropyl alcohol. This is a **bacteriostatic** antiseptic used to prevent contamination by normal skin bacteria during the short period of time required to perform collection of the specimen.

For collections that require additional sterility, such as blood cultures and arterial punctures, the stronger antiseptics iodine or chlorhexidene gluconate (for patients allergic to iodine) are used to cleanse the area. To prevent skin discomfort, iodine should always be removed from the patient's skin with alcohol after a phlebotomy procedure.

Sterile $2'' \times 2''$ gauze pads are used for applying pressure to the puncture site after the needle has been removed. Gauze pads can also serve as additional protection when folded in quarters and placed under a bandage. Bandages or adhesive tape are placed over the puncture site when the bleeding has stopped. Patients should be instructed to remove the bandage in about an hour.

ADDITIONAL SUPPLIES

Phlebotomists must have an adequate supply of gloves at all times. Gloves are required for phlebotomy and must be changed after each patient. To provide the maximum manual dexterity, they should fit securely.

Clean glass slides may be needed to prepare blood films for certain hematology tests. This procedure will be discussed in Chapter 17.

The final piece of equipment needed by the phlebotomist is a pen for labeling tubes, initialing computer-generated labels, or noting unusual circumstances on the requisition form.

BIBLIOGRAPHY

Calam, RR, and Cooper, MH: Recommended "Order of Draw" for collecting blood specimens into additive-containing tubes. Clin Chem 28:1399, 1982.

National Committee for Clinical Laboratory Standards Approved Standard H1-A3: Evacuated Tubes for Blood Specimen Collection. NCCLS, Villanova, PA, 1991.

National Committee for Clinical Laboratory Standards Approved Guideline H21-A2: Collection, Transport and Processing of Blood Specimens for Coagulation Testing and Performance of Coagulation Assays. NCCLS, Villanova, PA, 1991.

National Committee for Clinical Laboratory Standards Tentative Standard H24-T: Additives to Blood Collection Devices: Heparin. NCCLS, Villanova, PA, 1988.

National Committee for Clinical Laboratory Standards Tentative Standard H35-T: Additives to Blood Collection Devices: EDTA. NCCLS, Villanova, PA, 1992.

Study Questions   1. State a purpose for which a phlebotomist would use each of the following:

      a. 16-gauge needle _____

      b. 21-gauge needle _____

      c. 23-gauge needle _____

  2. Using a 25-gauge needle to perform phlebotomy may cause

      _____ .

  3. List three parts common to all needles.

      a. _____

      b. _____

      c. _____

  4. How do evacuated tube systems accommodate both adult and pediatric patients?

      _____

      _____

      _____

  5. How does the anticoagulant in a green top tube work?

      _____

  6. Name three anticoagulants that prevent clotting by binding calcium and the color-coded top associated with them.

      Anticoagulant   **Color-Coded Top**

      a. _____   _____

      b. _____   _____

      c. _____   _____

  7. What is the purpose of sodium fluoride in a gray top tube?

      _____

  8. Why is EDTA the anticoagulant of choice for the CBC?

      _____

      _____

  9. The stopper color of the tube that must always be completely filled is

      _____ .

  10. What is the purpose of tapping a vacuum tube containing dried anticoagulant prior to using it?

      _____

11. Which of the following tubes will clot first: red, red/gray, or yellow/gray?

_____

12. Using the numbers 1 through 5, list the order of draw using a vacuum tube system for the following tests:

a. _____ CBC

b. _____ Blood culture

c. _____ Plasma glucose

d. _____ Serum iron

e. _____ Coagulation studies

13. List the order of tube fill from a syringe for the tests in study question 12.

a. _____

b. _____

c. _____

d. _____

e. _____

14. Under what circumstances should the amount of anticoagulant in a light-blue top tube be decreased?

_____

15. Why are dark-blue top tubes used for collecting trace metal analyses?

_____

16. List an advantage and a disadvantage of syringe use.

_____

_____

17. When are winged infusion sets used in phlebotomy?

_____

_____

18. Syringes are graduated in _____.

19. When a blood pressure cuff is used as a tourniquet, how should the pressure be adjusted?

_____

_____

20. List two antiseptics used in venipuncture and state a situation when each is used.

Antiseptic   **Used For**

a. _____   _____

b. _____   _____

21. Fill in the blanks in the following chart.

Tube Color	Anticoagulant/ Additive	Test	Department
Red	None	RPR	Serology
	EDTA		
		Prothrombin	
Pink			
		Ammonia	
	Sodium fluoride		
Brown			

Venipuncture Equipment Selection Exercise

INSTRUCTIONS
State or assemble (if requested) the appropriate equipment for the situations described in this exercise. Include the number and color of evacuated tubes, needle size, syringe size, or butterfly if appropriate. Instructors may specify the inclusion of other supplies.

1. Collection of a CBC from a 35-year-old woman.

   _____

   _____

   _____

2. Collection of a CBC from a 3-year-old boy.

   _____

   _____

   _____

3. Collection of a STAT CBC and electrolytes from a 40-year-old man.

   _____

   _____

   _____

4. Collection of a cholesterol from the hand of an obese patient.

   _____

   _____

   _____

5. Collection of a PTT from an elderly patient.

   _____

   _____

   _____

6. Assemble the equipment to collect a type and crossmatch on a 50-year-old man.

   _____

   _____

   _____

7. Assemble the equipment to collect a cardiac risk profile and ESR from a patient with fragile veins.

   _____

   _____

   _____

8. Assemble the equipment to collect a lead level from a 2-year-old patient.

_____

_____

_____

NAME _____

Evaluation of Equipment Selection and Assembly

Rating System
2 = Satisfactorily performed
1 = Needs improvement
0 = Incorrect/did not perform

_____ 1. Collects all necessary equipment and supplies

_____ 2. Selects appropriate tubes for requested tests

_____ 3. Selects correct number of tubes or syringe size

_____ 4. Correctly attaches needle to adapter or syringe

_____ 5. Does not uncap needle prematurely

_____ 6. Advances tube correctly into adapter or checks plunger movement

_____ 7. Arranges supplies and extra tubes conveniently

Total Points _____

Maximum Points = 14

COMMENTS:

CHAPTER 13 Routine Venipuncture

Learning Objectives

Upon completion of this chapter, the reader will be able to:

1. Define the terms associated with routine venipuncture.
2. List the required information on a requisition form.
3. Discuss the appropriate procedure to follow when greeting and reassuring a patient.
4. Describe correct patient identification procedures.
5. Describe patient preparation and positioning.
6. Correctly assemble venipuncture equipment and supplies.
7. Name and locate the three most frequently used veins for venipuncture.
8. Correctly apply a tourniquet.
9. Describe vein palpation.
10. Discuss the venipuncture site cleansing procedure.
11. Correctly perform a routine venipuncture using an evacuated tube system.
12. Safely dispose of contaminated needles and supplies.
13. List the information required on a specimen tube label.

Terminology

Key Terms	Definition
Hematoma	Discoloration produced by leakage of blood into the tissues
Hemoconcentration	Increase in the ratio of formed elements to plasma
ID band	Bracelet worn by patients that contains specific identification information
Palpation	Examination by touch
Petechiae	Small red spots appearing on the skin

The most frequently performed procedure in phlebotomy is the venipuncture, and the ability to perform this technique in an organized, patient-considerate manner is the key to success as a phlebotomist. Each phlebotomist develops his or her own style for dealing with patients and performing the actual venipuncture. Administrative protocols vary among institutions and, of course, every patient is different; however, many basic rules are the same in all situations. These basic rules must be followed to ensure the safety of the patient and the phlebotomist, produce specimens that are representative of the patient's condition, and create an efficient phlebotomy service for the institution.

In this chapter the routine venipuncture technique is presented for the beginning phlebotomist in the recommended step-by-step procedure. The procedure is outlined again in Chapter 14 with a presentation of the complications that may occur at each step.

REQUISITIONS

All phlebotomy procedures begin with the receipt of a test requisition form generated by or at the request of a physician. The requisition is essential to provide the phlebotomist with the information needed to correctly identify the patient, organize the necessary equipment, collect the appropriate specimens, and provide legal protection. Phlebotomists should not collect a specimen without a requisition form.

The method by which a phlebotomist receives a requisition varies with the setting. Requisitions from outpatients may be hand carried by the patient, or requests may be telephoned to the central processing or accessioning area by the physician's office staff, where a requisition form is generated by the laboratory staff. Inpatient requisitions may be delivered to the laboratory, sent by pneumatic tube system, or entered into the hospital computer at the nursing station and printed out by the laboratory computer. In emergency situations, the phlebotomy request may be telephoned to the laboratory and the requisition form picked up by the phlebotomist at the patient site.

Phlebotomists should carefully examine all requisitions for which they are responsible prior to leaving the laboratory. They should check to be sure that all requisitions for a particular patient are together so that all tests are collected with one venipuncture. They must be sure they have all the necessary equipment.

The actual format of a requisition form may vary. Patient information may be handwritten or imprinted by an imprinter on color-coded forms with test check-off lists for different departments. There may be multiple copies for purposes of record keeping and billing. Computer-generated forms can include not only the patient information and tests requested but also tube labels and bar codes for specimen processing, the number and type of collection tubes needed, and special collection instructions. Figure 13–1 shows a sample computer-generated requisition form with accompanying labels.

Requisitions must contain certain basic information to ensure that the specimen drawn and the test results are correlated to the appropriate patient and that these can be correctly interpreted with regard to any special conditions, such as the time of collection. This information includes:

1 *Patient's Name and Identification Number* (The identification number may be a hospital-generated number that is also present on the patient's wrist ID band and all hospital documents or, in an outpatient setting, may be a laboratory-assigned number or the patient's social security number.)
2 *Patient's Location*
3 *Ordering Physician's Name*
4 *Tests Requested*
5 *Date and Time of Specimen Collection* (When the specimen is collected, the phlebotomist must write the actual date and time on the requisition and the specimen label. Most hospitals have adopted the military time system because they operate continuously for 24 hours.)

```
***************** F A U Q U I E R    H O S P I T A L ********************

Pt# 279377        TRAINING, PATIENT #1        Room-Bed: 9999-99

                                         Current Dt-Tm: 01/26/94-12:26

Diag: TRAINING USE                       Age 45Y        Sex: M

Order # 0315      Svc To: LB             Dr: VON ELTEN, S.

Svc. Code  CBC    COMPLETE BLOOD COUNT   Freq: ONCE      Pt. Type:1

Sp. Inst:                                # TODAY: 1      By:  LBAS



      Start Date-Time: 01/26/94       Stop Date-Time: 01/26/94
                       12:26                          12:26

***** ORDER STATUS *****              *** COLLECTION STATUS ***
*                     *               *                       *
*         NEW         *               *                       *
*                     *               *     PRIORITY [ R ]     *
***********************               *                       *
                                      *                       *
                                      *                       *
                                      *************************
```

```
600  9999-99  A#1481  | P#279377.      A#1481 | A#1481  A#1481  P#279377      A#1481
TRAINING, PATIENT #1  | TRAINING, PATIENT #1  | 279377  279377  TRAINING, PATIENT #1
  R#8540    45Y   M   |   45Y M     0315/CBC  |                   45Y  M   0315/CBC
P#279377       01/26  | 01/26                 |                  01/26
            1226 ROUT | 1226 ROUT             | A#1481  A#1481  1226ROUT
   LAV         ONCE   | 9999-99               | 279377  279377  9999-99
VON ELTEN, S.         | LAV                   |                  LAV
```

FIGURE 13–1. Sample requisition form and label. (Courtesy of Anita Sutherland, MT(ASCP), The Fauquier Hospital, Warrenton, VA.)

Other information that may be present includes:

Patient's Date of Birth
Special Collection Information (such as fasting specimen)
Special Patient Information (such as areas that should not be used for venipuncture)
Number and Type of Collection Tubes

GREETING THE PATIENT

When approaching patients, phlebotomists should introduce themselves, say that they are from the laboratory, and explain that they will be collecting a blood specimen. In the outpatient setting the patient usually knows what is about to occur (Fig. 13-2). When entering a patient's room it is polite to knock lightly on the open or closed door. If the curtain is closed around the bed, speak to the patient first through the curtain. This will avoid any embarrassment if the patient happens to be bathing or using the bedpan. In the hospital setting a variety of other circumstances may be present that require additional consideration when greeting the patient. These will be discussed in Chapter 14.

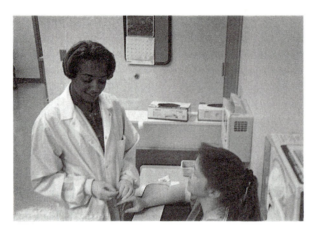

FIGURE 13–2. A phlebotomist greeting a patient in an outpatient setting.

PATIENT IDENTIFICATION

The most important procedure in phlebotomy is correct identification of the patient. Serious diagnostic or treatment errors and even death can occur when blood is drawn from the wrong patient. Ideally, identification is made by comparing information obtained verbally and from the patients wrist **identification (ID) band** with the information on the requisition form (Fig. 13 – 3).

Verbal identification is made after the patient greeting by asking the patient to state his or her full name. Always have patients state their names. Do not ask "Are you John Jones?" because many patients have a tendency to say "yes" to anything. In an outpatient setting, comparison of verbal information with the requisition form may be the only means of verifying identification. Asking the patients' date of birth or asking them to spell their name may be helpful in this situation.

Verbal identification is followed by examining the information on the patient's wrist ID band, which should always be present on hospitalized patients. Information on the wrist ID band should include patient's name, hospital identification number, date of birth, and physician. All information on the wrist ID band should match the information on the requisition form. Particular attention should be paid to the hospital identification number, as it is possible for two patients to have the same name,

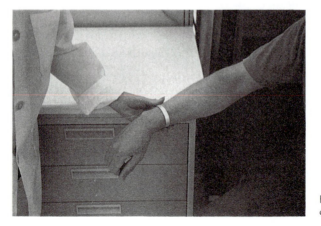

FIGURE 13–3. Phlebotomist checking a wrist ID band.

date of birth, and physician; however, they could not have the same identification number.

It is absolutely essential that identification of hospitalized patients be made from an ID band attached to the patient. Wrist bands are sometimes removed when IV fluids are being administered in the wrist or when fluids have infiltrated the area. They should be reattached to the patient's ankle. Ankle bands are frequently used with pediatric patients and newborns. A wrist band lying on the bedside table cannot be used for identification — it could belong to anyone. Likewise, a sign over the patient's bed or on the door cannot be relied on because the patient could be in the wrong bed.

PATIENT PREPARATION AND POSITIONING

When patient identification is completed the patient must be positioned conveniently and safely for the procedure and given an explanation of the procedure.

Blood should never be drawn from a patient who is in a standing position. Outpatients are seated at a drawing station as shown in Figure 12-2. In some drawing stations, the movable arm serves the dual purposes of providing a solid surface for the patient's arm and preventing a patient who faints from falling out of the chair. Phlebotomists should always be alert for any changes in the patient's condition while the procedure is being performed. Some patients know that they experience difficulties during venipuncture and provisions should be made to allow them to lie down for the procedure.

It may be necessary to move hospitalized patients slightly to make their arms more accessible, or to place a pillow or towel under the patient's arm for better support. If bed rails are lowered, they must always be returned to the raised position prior to leaving the room.

Patients should remove any objects such as gum or a thermometer from their mouths prior to performance of the venipuncture.

Reassurance of the patient actually begins with the greeting and continues throughout the procedure. Phlebotomists should demonstrate both concern for the patient's comfort and confidence in their ability to perform the procedure. Patients should be given a brief explanation of the procedure, including any nonroutine techniques that will be used, such as the additional site preparation performed when collecting blood cultures. They should not be told that the procedure will be painless.

Patients often question the phlebotomist about what tests are being performed or why their blood is being drawn so frequently. The best policy is to politely suggest that they ask their physician these questions. Even listing the names of tests can cause problems, as many medical books are available to the general public. Erroneous conclusions may be reached by the patient, since many tests have several diagnostic purposes; or the patient may misunderstand the test name and look up an inappropriate test associated with a very severe condition.

The phlebotomist's conversation with the patient should include verifying that the appropriate pretest preparation such as fasting or abstaining from medications has occurred. When these procedures have not been followed, this should be reported to the nursing station prior to drawing the blood. If the specimen is still required, the irregular condition, such as "nonfasting" should be written on the requisition form and the specimen.

tourniquet can only be applied for 1 minute; therefore, after the vein is located the tourniquet is removed while the site is being cleansed and is reapplied immediately before the venipuncture.

Veins are located by sight and by touch (referred to as **palpation**). The ability to feel a vein is much more important than the ability to see a vein — a concept that is often difficult for beginning phlebotomists to accept. Palpation is performed using the index finger to probe the antecubital area with a pushing rather than a stroking motion. The pressure applied by palpating locates deep veins; distinguishes veins, which feel like spongy cords, from rigid tendon cords; and differentiates veins from arteries, which produce a pulse (Fig. 13 – 7B). The thumb should not be used to palpate as it has a pulse beat. Once an acceptable vein is located, palpation is used to determine the direction and depth of the vein to aid the phlebotomist during needle insertion.

CLEANSING THE SITE

When an appropriate vein has been located, the tourniquet is released and the area cleansed using 70% isopropyl alcohol. Cleansing is performed with a circular motion starting at the inside of the venipuncture site (Fig. 13 – 8). For maximum bacteriostatic action to occur the alcohol should be allowed to dry on the patient's arm rather than being wiped off with a gauze pad. Performing a venipuncture before the alcohol has dried will cause a stinging sensation for the patient and may produce hemolysis in the specimen.

If additional palpation of the vein is needed after the cleansing process, the phlebotomist should use alcohol to cleanse the gloved end of the finger to be used.

While the alcohol is drying, the phlebotomist can make a final survey of the supplies at hand to be sure everything required for the procedure is present. The tourniquet is then reapplied and the suitability of the vein confirmed.

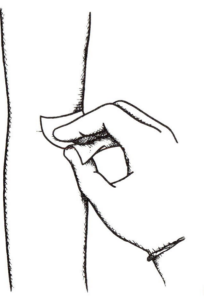

FIGURE 13 – 8. Cleansing the puncture site.

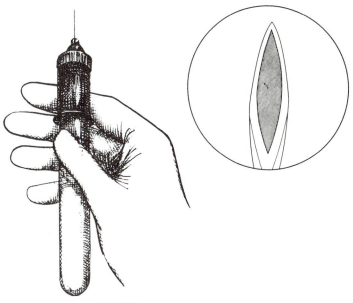

FIGURE 13–9. Needle inspection.

EXAMINATION OF PUNCTURE EQUIPMENT

Immediately prior to entering the vein the plastic cap of the needle is removed and the point of the needle is visually examined for any defects such as a nonpointed or rough (barbed) end (Fig. 13-9). The needle is then positioned for entry into the vein with the bevel facing up.

Visual examination cannot detect all defective vacuum tubes; therefore, extra tubes should be near at hand. It is not uncommon for the vacuum in a tube to be lost.

PERFORMING THE VENIPUNCTURE

The needle holder or syringe is held securely in the dominant hand with the thumb on top and the remaining fingers below. After insertion is made the fingers can be braced against the patient's arm to provide stability while tubes are being moved in the holder, or the plunger of the syringe is being pulled back. Figure 13-10 demonstrates the correct positioning of the hands during the venipuncture. Refer to these diagrams during the following discussion. Figure 13-11 provides additional illustration.

Use the thumb of the nondominant hand to anchor the selected vein while inserting the needle (Fig. 13-10A). Notice that the thumb is placed 1 or 2 inches below the insertion site. Anchoring the vein above and below the site using the thumb and index finger is not an acceptable technique, as sudden patient movement could cause the index finger to be punctured. A vein that moves to the side is said to have "rolled." Patients often state that they have "rolling veins"; however, all veins will roll if they are not properly anchored. What the patients are really saying is that their blood has been drawn by phlebotomists who were not anchoring the veins well enough. As mentioned previously the median cubital vein is the easiest to anchor and the basilic vein the most difficult. In general the closer a vein is to the surface the more likely it is to roll.

When the vein is securely anchored, the needle is inserted, bevel up, at an angle

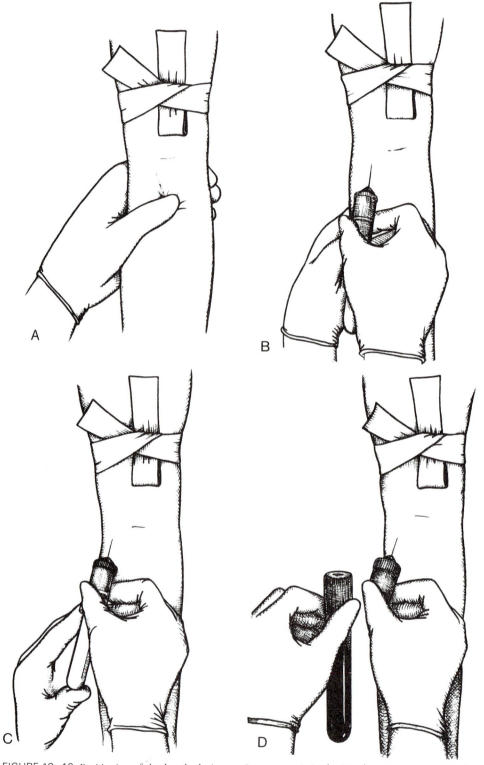

FIGURE 13–10. Positioning of the hands during venipuncture. *A*, Anchoring the vein. *B*, Inserting the needle (15- to 30-degree angle). *C*, Advancing the tube onto the needle. *D*, Removing the tube from the adapter.

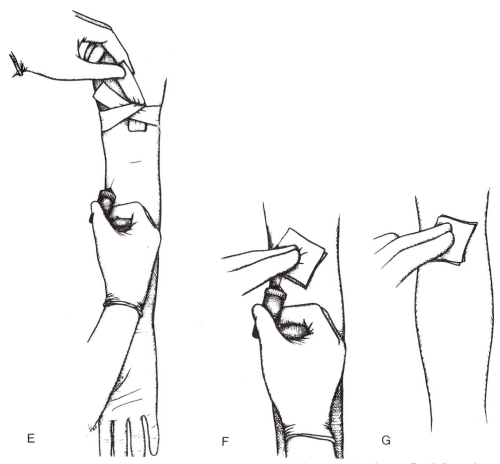

FIGURE 13–10. Continued. *E*, Removing the tourniquet before removing the needle. *F*, Removing the needle. *G*, Applying pressure to the puncture site.

of 15 to 30 degrees depending on the depth of the vein (Fig. 13-10*B* and Fig. 13-11*A*). This should be done in a smooth movement so the patient only briefly feels the stick. The phlebotomist is usually able to tell when the vein has been entered by feeling a lessening of resistance to the needle movement.

Once the vein has been entered, the hand anchoring the vein can be moved and used to push the vacuum tube completely into the holder or to pull back on the syringe plunger (Fig. 13-10*C* and Fig. 13-11*B*). Some phlebotomists prefer to change hands at this point so that the dominant hand is free for performing the remaining tasks. This method of operating is usually better suited for use by experienced phlebotomists because holding the needle steady in the patient's vein is often difficult for beginners.

The hand used to hold the needle assembly should remain braced on the patient's arm. This is of particular importance when vacuum tubes are being inserted or removed from the holder, as a certain amount of resistance is encountered and can cause the needle to be pushed through or pulled out of the vein. Tubes should be gently eased on and off the puncturing needle using the flared ends of the adapter as an additional brace (Fig. 13-11*C*).

To prevent any chance of blood refluxing back into the needle, tubes should be held at a downward angle while they are being filled. Be sure to follow the pre-

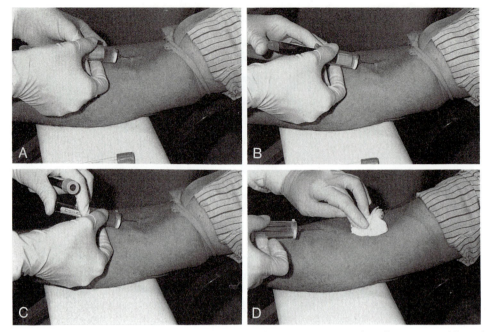

FIGURE 13–11. Performing the venipuncture. *A*, Needle insertion. *B*, Sample collection. *C*, Additional sample collection. *D*, Removal of needle, followed immediately by pressure to the puncture site.

scribed order of draw when multiple tubes are being collected, and allow the tubes to fill completely before removing them. Mixing of evacuated tubes should be done as soon as the tube is removed, before another tube is placed in the assembly. The few seconds that this requires does not cause additional discomfort to the patient and ensures that the specimen will be acceptable.

When the last tube has been filled, it is removed from the assembly and mixed prior to completing the procedure (Fig. 13-10*D*). Failure to remove the vacuum tube prior to removing the needle results in blood dripping from the end of the needle so that there is unnecessary contamination and possible damage to the patient's clothes.

REMOVAL OF THE NEEDLE

Before removing the needle, remove the tourniquet by pulling on the free end and tell the patient to relax his or her hand (Fig. 13-10*E*). Failure to remove the tourniquet prior to removing the needle may produce a **hematoma**.

Place folded sterile gauze over the venipuncture site and withdraw the needle; apply pressure to the site as soon as the needle is withdrawn (Figs. 13-10*F* and *G* and Fig. 13-11*D*). Do not apply pressure while the needle is still in the vein. To prevent blood from leaking into the surrounding tissue and producing a bruise (hematoma), pressure must be applied until the bleeding has stopped. The arm should be held in a raised, outstretched position. Bending the elbow to apply pressure allows blood to more easily leak into the tissue. A patient who is capable can be asked to apply the pressure, thereby freeing the phlebotomist to dispose of the used needle and label the specimen tubes. If this is not possible the phlebotomist must apply the pressure and perform the other tasks after the bleeding has stopped.

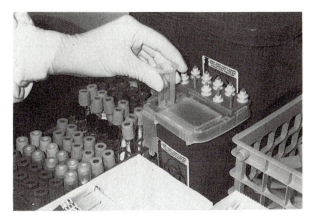

FIGURE 13–12. Needle disposal.

DISPOSAL OF THE NEEDLE

Upon completion of the venipuncture, the first thing the phlebotomist must do is dispose of the contaminated needle in an appropriate sharps container located at the site where the venipuncture has been performed (Fig. 13–12). As discussed in Chapter 12, the method by which this is done will depend on the type of disposal equipment selected by the institution. Remember, manual two-handed recapping of the needle is not acceptable. One-handed scooping of the cap onto the needle should only be used in extenuating circumstances.

LABELING THE TUBES

Tubes must be labeled at the time of specimen collection, prior to leaving the patient's room or accepting another requisition. Tubes are labeled by writing with a pen on the attached label or by applying a computer-generated label (Fig. 13–13). Tubes should not be labeled before the specimen is collected, as this could result in confusion of specimens when more than one patient is being drawn.

Information on the specimen label should include patient's name and identification number, date and time of collection, and the phlebotomist's initials. Additional information may be present on computer-generated labels. Specimens for the blood bank may require an additional label obtained from the patient's ID band.

Specimens requiring special handling, such as cooling or warming, are placed in the appropriate container when labeling is complete.

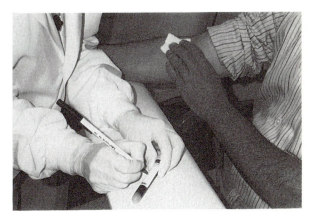

FIGURE 13–13. Labeling the tube.

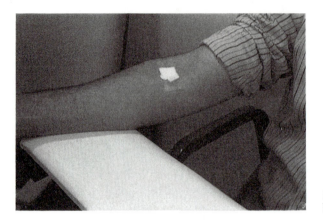

FIGURE 13–14. Patient's arm with bandage.

BANDAGING THE PATIENT'S ARM

Bleeding at the venipuncture site should stop within 5 minutes. Before applying the bandage the phlebotomist should examine the patient's arm to be sure the bleeding has stopped. For additional pressure, the adhesive bandage or tape is applied over a folded gauze square (Fig. 13–14). The patient should be instructed to remove the bandage within an hour and to avoid using the arm to carry heavy objects during that period.

LEAVING THE PATIENT

Prior to leaving the patient's room the phlebotomist disposes of all contaminated supplies such as alcohol pads and gauze in a biohazard container, removes gloves and disposes of them in the biohazard container, and washes the hands.

In the outpatient setting, patients can be excused when the arm is bandaged. If patients have been fasting and no more procedures are scheduled, they should be instructed to eat. Prior to calling the next patient the phlebotomist cleans up the area as described above.

In both the inpatient and outpatient settings, patients should be thanked for their cooperation.

COMPLETING THE VENIPUNCTURE PROCEDURE

The venipuncture procedure is complete when the specimen is delivered to the laboratory in satisfactory condition and all appropriate paperwork has been completed. These procedures will vary depending on institutional protocol and the types of specimens collected. The phlebotomist needs to be familiar with procedures such as stamping the time of specimen arrival in the laboratory on the requisition form or informing the nursing station that the procedure has been completed.

Delivering each specimen to the laboratory as soon as it is collected would not be efficient. However, this may be required for specimens requiring special handling and in STAT situations that are covered in the following chapters. When possible the phlebotomist should try to schedule patients so that a specimen requiring special handling is collected last.

SUMMARY OF VENIPUNCTURE TECHNIQUE WITH A VACUUM TUBE

1 Obtain and examine the requisition form.
2 Greet the patient.
3 Identify the patient.
4 Reassure the patient.
5 Position the patient.
6 Put on gloves.
7 Assemble equipment and supplies.
8 Apply the tourniquet.
9 Select the venipuncture site.
10 Release the tourniquet.
11 Cleanse the site.
12 Survey the supplies and equipment.
13 Reapply the tourniquet.
14 Confirm the venipuncture site.
15 Anchor the vein.
16 Insert the needle.
17 Mix the specimens as they are collected.
18 Remove the last tube from the holder.
19 Release the tourniquet.
20 Place sterile gauze over the needle.
21 Remove the needle and apply pressure.
22 Dispose of the needle.
23 Label the tubes.
24 Perform appropriate specimen handling.
25 Examine the patient's arm.
26 Bandage the patient's arm.
27 Thank the patient.
28 Dispose of used supplies.
29 Remove and dispose of gloves.
30 Wash hands.
31 Complete any required paperwork.
32 Deliver specimens to appropriate locations.

BIBLIOGRAPHY

National Committee for Clinical Laboratory Standards Approved Standard H3-A3: Procedures for Collection of Diagnostic Blood Specimens by Venipuncture. NCCLS, Villanova, PA, 1991.

Study Questions

1. List three reasons for requiring a requisition form prior to performing a venipuncture.

   a. _____

   b. _____

   c. _____

2. List five pieces of information that must be present on a requisition form.

   a. _____

   b. _____

   c. _____

   d. _____

   e. _____

3. List four pieces of information that must be present on a patient's ID band.

   a. _____

   b. _____

   c. _____

   d. _____

4. If no ID band is found on the patient's wrist, where should the phlebotomist look next?

   _____

5. An outpatient enters the drawing area. The phlebotomist asks "Are you Sandra Brown?" The patient answers "yes." The phlebotomist labels the tubes and performs the venipuncture. What is wrong with this situation?

   _____

   _____

6. The maximum length of time a tourniquet should be applied is

   _____ .

7. How does a properly applied tourniquet affect blood flow?

   _____

   _____

8. List the three major veins located in the antecubital fossa.

   a. _____

   b. _____

   c. _____

9. The preferred vein for venipuncture is the _____.

10. The vein located on the thumb side of the arm is the _____.

11. List three reasons for vein palpation.

    a. _____

    b. _____

    c. _____

12. List three reasons for allowing the alcohol to dry on a patient's arm prior to performing the venipuncture.

    a. _____

    b. _____

    c. _____

13. How does a phlebotomist prepare for the possibility of encountering a defective vacuum tube?

    _____

14. The cause of "rolling veins" is _____.

15. The angle of the needle during insertion is _____.

16. When should a specimen collected in a lavender top tube be mixed?

    _____

17. Place the following steps in the venipuncture technique in the correct order by numbering them 1 through 10.

    a. _____ Release the tourniquet

    b. _____ Identify the patient

    c. _____ Anchor the vein

    d. _____ Cleanse the site

    e. _____ Obtain a requisition form

    f. _____ Label the tubes

    g. _____ Bandage the puncture site

    h. _____ Insert the needle

    i. _____ Remove the needle and apply pressure

    j. _____ Select equipment

18. List five pieces of information that should be present on the specimen label.

    a. _____

    b. _____

    c. _____

    d. _____

    e. _____

19. What should phlebotomists do immediately after removing their gloves?

    _____

20. Determine if the following are acceptable or not acceptable when performing a venipuncture and explain your reason in one sentence.

    a. An outpatient with a sore back wishes to stand during the procedure.

       _____

       _____

    b. Assembling equipment prior to applying the tourniquet.

       _____

       _____

    c. Explaining the procedure to the patient.

       _____

       _____

    d. Requesting patients to pump their fists during sample collection.

       _____

       _____

    e. Palpating with the thumb.

       _____

       _____

    f. Cleansing the site in a circular motion from inside to outside.

       _____

       _____

    g. Bending the patient's elbow while applying pressure to the puncture site.

       _____

       _____

h. Bracing the hand holding the needle against the patient's arm during specimen collection.

_____

_____

21. State an error in routine venipuncture technique that may cause

a. A hematoma _____

b. Petechiae _____

Evaluation of Tourniquet Application and Vein Selection

Rating System
2 = Satisfactorily performed
1 = Needs improvement
0 = Incorrect/did not perform

_____ 1. Positions arm correctly for vein selection

_____ 2. Selects appropriate tourniquet application site

_____ 3. Places tourniquet in flat position behind arm

_____ 4. Smoothly positions hands when crossing and tucking tourniquet

_____ 5. Fastens tourniquet at appropriate tightness

_____ 6. Tourniquet is not folded into arm

_____ 7. Loop and loose end do not interfere with puncture site

_____ 8. Asks patient to clench fist

_____ 9. Selects antecubital area to palpate

_____ 10. Performs palpation using correct fingers

_____ 11. Palpates entire area or both arms if necessary

_____ 12. Checks depth and direction of veins

_____ 13. Removes tourniquet smoothly

_____ 14. Removes tourniquet in a timely manner

Total Points _____

Maximum Points = 28

COMMENTS:

Evaluation of Venipuncture Technique Using an Evacuated Tube

Rating System
2 = Satisfactorily performed
1 = Needs improvement
0 = Incorrect/did not perform

_____ 1. Examines requisition form

_____ 2. Greets patient, states procedure to be done

_____ 3. Identifies patient verbally

_____ 4. Examines patient's ID band

_____ 5. Compares requisition information with ID band

_____ 6. Puts on gloves

_____ 7. Selects correct tubes and equipment for procedure

_____ 8. Assembles and conveniently places equipment

_____ 9. Positions patient's arm

_____ 10. Applies tourniquet

_____ 11. Identifies vein by palpation

_____ 12. Releases tourniquet

_____ 13. Cleanses site and allows it to air dry

_____ 14. Reapplies tourniquet

_____ 15. Does not touch puncture site with unclean finger

_____ 16. Anchors vein below puncture site

_____ 17. Smoothly enters vein at appropriate angle with bevel up

_____ 18. Does not move needle when changing tubes

_____ 19. Collects tubes in correct order

_____ 20. Mixes anticoagulated tubes promptly

_____ 21. Fills tubes completely

_____ 22. Removes last tube collected from holder

_____ 23. Releases tourniquet

_____ 24. Covers puncture site with gauze

_____ 25. Removes the needle smoothly and applies pressure

_____ 26. Disposes of the needle in sharps container

_____ 27. Labels tubes

_____ 28. Examines puncture site

_____ 29. Applies bandage

_____ 30. Disposes of used supplies

_____ 31. Removes gloves and washes hands

_____ 32. Thanks patient

_____ 33. Converses appropriately with patient during procedure

Total Points _____

Maximum Points = 66

COMMENTS:

CHAPTER 14

Venipuncture Complications

Learning Objectives

Upon completion of this chapter, the reader will be able to:

1 Define the terms associated with venipuncture complications.
2 State the procedure for coordinating requisition forms, patient identification, and labeling of tubes for unidentified patients.
3 Discuss the procedures to follow when patients are asleep, not in their rooms, or being visited by a physician, member of the clergy, or friend.
4 Discuss the procedure to follow when a patient develops syncope during the venipuncture procedure.
5 State the policy regarding patients who refuse to have their blood drawn.
6 State the reasons why the tourniquet can only be applied for 1 minute.
7 List four methods used to locate veins that are not prominent.
8 List three conditions when it is not advisable to draw from veins in the legs or feet.
9 State reasons why blood should not be drawn from a hematoma, burned or scarred area, or an arm adjacent to a mastectomy.
10 State three methods for obtaining blood from a patient with an IV.
11 State the procedure to follow when drawing blood from a patient with a fistula.
12 Discuss cleansing of the venipuncture site prior to collecting a blood alcohol level.
13 Describe the venipuncture procedure using a syringe, including equipment examination, technique for exchanging syringes, transfer of blood to evacuated tubes, and disposal of the equipment.
14 Describe the venipuncture procedure using a butterfly, the technique involved, and disposal of equipment.
15 List six reasons why blood may not be immediately obtained from a venipuncture and the procedures to follow to obtain blood.
16 List 10 tests affected by hemolysis.
17 List seven venipuncture errors that may produce hemolysis.
18 List five causes of hematomas.
19 List five reasons for rejecting a specimen.

Terminology

Key Terms	Definition
Cannula	A tube which can be inserted into a cavity, for example, to form a temporary connection between an artery and a vein (used for dialysis)

Terminology
Continued

Key Terms	Definition
Catheter	Tube inserted into the body for injecting or withdrawing fluids
Edema	Accumulation of fluid in the tissues
Fistula	Permanent surgical connection between an artery and a vein (used for dialysis)
Heparin lock	Device inserted into a vein for administering medications and collecting blood
Indwelling line	Tube inserted into an artery or vein (primarily for administering fluids)
Lymphostasis	Stoppage of lymph flow
Occlusion	Obstruction of a lumen
Syncope	Fainting

Abbreviation	Definition
CVC	Central venous catheter

The venipuncture procedure discussed in Chapter 13 is what occurs in a routine situation; however, complications to the routine procedure can occur at any step. In this chapter the procedure is reviewed in the same order with emphasis on the complications that may be encountered.

REQUISITIONS

In the emergency room or other emergency situations the request for phlebotomy may be telephoned to the laboratory and the requisition picked up by the phlebotomist at the patient site. A requisition picked up in an emergency situation must still contain all pertinent information for patient identification. The patient ID number from the patient's wrist band may have to be written on the requisition form when a temporary identification system has been used.

GREETING THE PATIENT

Patients are frequently asleep and should be gently awakened and given time to become oriented prior to performing the venipuncture. Unconscious patients should be greeted in the same manner as conscious patients, because they may be capable of hearing and understanding even though they cannot respond. In this circumstance nursing personnel are often present and can assist with the patient, if necessary.

Physicians, members of the clergy, and visitors may be present when the phlebotomist enters the room. When the physician or clergy member is with the patient it is preferable to return at another time, unless the request is for a STAT or timed specimen. When this occurs the phlebotomist should explain the situation and request permission to perform the procedure at that time. Visitors should be greeted in the same manner as the patient and given the option to step outside. If they choose to stay, the phlebotomist should assess their possible reactions and may elect to pull the curtain around the bed. Visitors can sometimes be helpful in the case of pediatric or very apprehensive patients.

Patients are not always in the room when the phlebotomist arrives. The phlebotomist should attempt to locate the patient by checking with the nursing station, as the patient may be in the lounge or walking in the hall, or may have been taken to another department. If the specimen must be collected at a particular time, it may be possible to draw the patient in the area to which he or she has been taken. If this is not possible, the nursing station must be notified and the appropriate forms completed so that the test can be rescheduled. The requisition form is usually left at the nursing station.

PATIENT IDENTIFICATION

The phlebotomist will occasionally encounter a patient who has no ID band on either the wrist or the ankle. In this circumstance the phlebotomist must contact the nursing station and request that the patient be banded prior to the drawing of blood. The nurse's signature on the requisition form verifying identification should only be accepted in emergency situations and following strict hospital policy.

Unidentified patients are sometimes brought into the emergency room and a system must be in place to ensure they are correctly matched with their laboratory work. The American Association of Blood Banks requires that the patient be positively identified with a temporary but clear designation attached to the body. Some hospitals generate identification bands with an identification number and a tentative name, such as John Doe or Patient X. Commercial identification systems are particularly useful when blood transfusions are required. In these systems the identification band that is attached to the patient comes with matching identification stickers. The stickers are placed on the specimen tubes, requisition form, and any units of blood designated for the patient. Many hospitals use this type of system, in addition to the routine identification system, for all patients receiving transfusions.

PATIENT PREPARATION

It is not uncommon to encounter extremely apprehensive patients. Enlisting the help of the nurse who has been caring for the patient may help to calm the person's fears. It may also be necessary to ask for assistance from the nurse to hold the patient's arm steady during the procedure. Assistance from a nurse or parent is frequently required when working with children. Phlebotomists also may require nursing assistance when encountering patients in fixed positions, such as those in traction or body casts.

Apprehensive patients may be prone to fainting (**syncope**) and the phlebotomist should be alert to this possibility. It is sometimes possible to detect such patients during vein palpation, as their skin feels cold and damp. Keeping their minds off the procedure through conversation can be helpful. If a patient begins to faint during the procedure, remove the tourniquet and needle, and apply pressure to the venipuncture site. In the inpatient setting, notify the nursing station as soon as possible. In the outpatient area, make sure the patient is supported and that the patient lowers his or her head. Cold compresses applied to the forehead and back of the neck and ammonia inhalants will help to revive the patient. Outpatients who have been fasting for prolonged periods should be given something sweet to drink and required to remain in the area for 15 to 30 minutes. All incidents of syncope should be documented following hospital policy.

Phlebotomists must be alert for changes in a patient's condition and notify the nursing station. Such changes could include the presence of vomitus, urine, or feces; infiltrated or removed intravenous fluid lines; extreme breathing difficulty; and possibly a patient who has expired.

Changes in patient posture from an erect to a supine position will cause variations in some blood constituents, primarily substances that are not filtered by the kidney, such as cellular elements, plasma proteins, and compounds bound to plasma proteins. This is caused by the movement of water between the plasma and tissues when body position changes. Tests most noticeably affected are cell counts, protein, albumin, bilirubin, cholesterol, triglycerides, calcium, and enzymes. When inpatient and outpatient results are being compared, the physician may request that an outpatient lie down prior to specimen collection.

PATIENT REFUSAL   Some patients may refuse to have their blood drawn, and they have the right to do this. The phlebotomist can stress to the patient that the results are needed by the physician for treatment and discuss the problem with the nurse, who may be able to convince the patient to agree to have the test performed. If the patient continues to refuse, this should be written on the requisition form and the form should be left at the nursing station or the area stated in hospital policy.

EQUIPMENT ASSEMBLY

When positioning the needed equipment and supplies within easy reach, the phlebotomist should include extra vacuum tubes. It is not uncommon to find a vacuum tube that does not contain the proper amount of vacuum necessary to collect a full tube of blood. Accidentally pushing a tube past the indicator mark on the needle holder before the vein is entered will also result in loss of vacuum.

As discussed in Chapter 5, remember that only the necessary amount of equipment is brought into isolation rooms.

TOURNIQUET APPLICATION

As discussed in Chapter 12, a blood pressure cuff is sometimes used to locate veins that are difficult to find. The cuff should be inflated to a pressure below the systolic and above the diastolic blood pressure readings.

When dealing with patients with skin conditions, it may be necessary to place the tourniquet over the patient's gown or to cover the area with gauze prior to application. If possible another area should be selected for the venipuncture.

Application of the tourniquet for more than 1 minute will interfere with some test results. Tests most likely to be affected are those measuring large molecules, such as plasma proteins and lipids; or analytes affected by hemolysis, including potassium, lactic acid, and enzymes. Therefore, during multiple tube collections, it may be necessary to release the tourniquet before the last tube has been filled. Tourniquet application and fist clenching are not recommended when drawing specimens for lactic acid determinations.

Hemoconcentration and hemolysis can be prevented by releasing the tourniquet as soon as blood begins to flow into the first tube. However, difficulty filling additional tubes may be encountered and the tourniquet may have to be retightened or pressure applied to the area with the free hand to increase the amount of blood present in the vein.

SITE SELECTION

Not all patients have a median cubital, cephalic, or basilic vein that becomes immediately prominent when the tourniquet is applied. In fact, a high percentage of patients have veins that are not easily located and the phlebotomist may have to use a variety of techniques to locate a suitable puncture site. Many patients have prominent veins in one arm and not in the other; therefore, checking the patient's other arm should be the first thing done when a site is not easily located. Patients with veins that are difficult to locate often point out areas where they remember previous successful phlebotomies. Palpation of these areas may prove beneficial and is also good for patient relations.

Other techniques used by phlebotomists to enhance the prominence of veins include tapping the antecubital area with the index finger, massaging the arm upward from the wrist to the elbow, briefly hanging the arm down, and applying heat to the site. Remember that when performing these techniques, the tourniquet should not remain tied for more than 1 minute at a time.

If no palpable veins are found in the antecubital area, the wrist and hand should be examined. The tourniquet is retied on the forearm. Because the veins in these areas are smaller, it may be necessary to change equipment and use a smaller needle with a syringe or winged infusion set or a smaller vacuum tube.

Veins in the legs and feet are sometimes used as venipuncture sites. However, they should only be used with physician approval. Leg veins are more susceptible to infection and the formation of thrombi (clots), particularly in patients with diabetes, cardiac problems, and coagulation disorders.

Areas to Be Avoided

Veins that contain thrombi or have been subjected to numerous venipunctures often feel hard (sclerosed) and should be avoided as they may be blocked (**occluded**) and have impaired circulation.

The presence of a hematoma indicates that blood has accumulated in the tissue surrounding a vein. Puncturing into a hematoma is not only painful for the patient but will result in the collection of old, hemolyzed blood from the hematoma rather than circulating venous blood that is representative of the patient's current condition. If a vein containing a hematoma must be used, blood should be collected below the hematoma to ensure sampling of free flowing blood. Drawing from areas containing excess tissue fluid (**edema**) is also not recommended because the sample will be contaminated with tissue fluid.

Extensively burned and scarred areas, including tattoos, are more susceptible to infection; they also have decreased circulation and veins that are difficult to palpate.

Applying a tourniquet or drawing blood from an arm located on the same side of the body as a recent mastectomy can be harmful to the patient and produce erroneous test results. Removal of lymph nodes in the mastectomy procedure interferes with the flow of lymph fluid (**lymphostasis**) and increases the blood level of lymphocytes and waste products normally contained in the lymph fluid. The protective functions of the lymphatic system are also lost, so that the area becomes more prone to infection. Normal flow of lymph fluid usually returns in about 6 months; however, most patients remain hesitant to have blood drawn from the affected area and their wishes should be respected. In cases of a double mastectomy, the side associated with the oldest surgery should be used. The physician should be consulted if both procedures are recent.

Frequently the phlebotomist encounters patients receiving IV fluids in an arm vein. Whenever possible blood should then be drawn from the other arm. If an arm containing an IV drip must be used for specimen collection, the site selected must be below the IV insertion point and preferably in a different vein. The nurse should be asked to turn off the IV drip for at least 2 minutes and the first 5 mL of blood drawn must be discarded, as it may be contaminated with IV fluid. A new syringe is then used for the specimen collection. If a coagulation test is ordered, an additional 5 mL of blood should be drawn prior to collecting the coagulation test specimen because intravenous lines are frequently flushed with heparin. This additional blood can be used for other tests if they have been requested. When blood is collected from an arm containing an IV drip, this must be noted on the requisition form.

Using Central Venous Catheters

Blood also may be obtained from **indwelling lines** called central venous catheters (**CVCs**); however, this procedure must be performed by specially trained personnel, usually a member of the nursing staff, and physician authorization is required. Specific procedures must be followed for flushing the **catheters** with saline, and possibly heparin, when the blood collection is completed. Sterile technique procedures must be strictly adhered to when entering intravenous lines, as they provide a direct path for infectious organisms to enter the patient's blood stream.

Examples of CVCs include: Hickman and Groshong catheters that are surgically implanted; subcutaneous, jugular, and subclavian catheters; and more temporary devices such as Medi-Port and Port-a-Cath. **Heparin locks** are inserted to provide a means for administering frequently required medications and for obtaining blood specimens. They do not contain an IV line but techniques for using them for collecting blood specimens are similar to those for CVCs.

When intravenous fluids are being administered through the CVC, the flow should be stopped for 5 minutes prior to collecting the sample. Syringes larger than 20 mL should not be used, as the high negative pressure produced may collapse the catheter walls. At all times the first 5 mL of blood must be discarded and a new syringe must be used to collect the sample. Drawing coagulation tests from a venous catheter is not recommended, but if this is necessary, they should be collected after 20 mL of blood has been discarded or used for other tests.

The order of tube fill may vary slightly to accommodate the amount of blood that must be drawn prior to a coagulation test. As with other procedures, blood cultures are always collected first. If these are ordered, the draw will satisfy the additional discard needed for coagulation tests. Therefore the order of fill is:

1   Blood cultures
2   Anticoagulated tubes (light-blue, lavender, green, and gray)
3   Clotted tubes (red and serum separator tube [SST])

If blood cultures are not ordered, the coagulation tests (light-blue top tube) can be collected with a new syringe after the other specimens have been collected using the order shown above. Phlebotomists are frequently responsible for assisting the nurse who is collecting blood from the CVC and should understand these specimen collection requirements. The source of the specimen should be noted on the requisition form.

Patients receiving renal dialysis have a permanent surgical fusion of an artery and a vein called a **fistula** in one arm and this arm should be avoided for venipuncture due to the possibility of infection. The dialysis patient may also have a temporary connection between the artery and a vein formed by a **cannula** that contains a special T-tube connector with a diaphragm for drawing blood. Only specifically trained personnel are authorized to draw blood from a cannula.

CLEANSING THE SITE

Certain procedures, primarily blood cultures and arterial blood gases, require that the site be cleansed with a stronger antiseptic than isopropyl alcohol. The most frequently used solutions are povidone-iodine, or chlorhexidene gluconate for persons who are allergic to iodine.

Alcohol should not be used to cleanse the site prior to drawing a blood alcohol level. Thoroughly cleansing the site with soap and water will ensure the least amount of interference, and some institutions find iodine to be acceptable.

EXAMINATION OF PUNCTURE EQUIPMENT

When using a syringe the plunger is pulled back and pushed forward while the protective cap is still on the needle to ensure that it will move freely when the vein has been entered. The protective cap on the needle is then removed and the needle point is examined for imperfections.

PERFORMING THE VENIPUNCTURE

Although venipuncture is most frequently performed using an evacuated tube system, it may be necessary to use a syringe or butterfly apparatus to better control the pressure applied to the delicate veins found in pediatric and elderly patients, or when drawing from hand veins.

Using a Syringe

Except for a few minor differences, the procedure for drawing blood using a syringe is the same as when using an evacuated tube system. Blood is withdrawn from the vein by slowly pulling on the plunger of the syringe, using the hand that is free after anchoring of the vein is completed, as shown in Figure 14-1. When the vein is en-

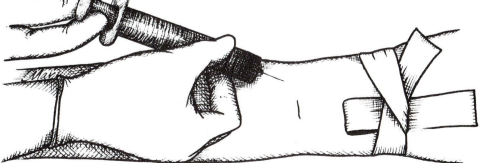

FIGURE 14–1. Venipuncture using a syringe.

tered, blood will appear in the hub of the needle and the plunger can then be pulled back at a speed that corresponds to the rate of blood flow into the syringe. Pulling the plunger back faster than blood is flowing may cause the walls of the vein to collapse (Fig. 14–3F) and can cause hemolysis. Again, it is important to anchor the hand holding the syringe firmly on the patient's arm so that the needle will not move when the plunger is pulled.

Ideally the size of the syringe used should correspond with the amount of blood needed; however, with small veins that easily collapse it may be necessary to fill two or more smaller syringes. This will require assistance, as blood from the filled syringe must be transferred to the appropriate tubes while the second syringe is being filled. Prior to exchanging syringes gauze must be placed on the patient's arm under the needle as blood will leak from the hub of the needle during the exchange.

As discussed in Chapter 12, blood is transferred from the syringe to evacuated tubes, following the prescribed order of fill, by puncturing the rubber tube stopper using a one-handed technique and allowing the blood to flow slowly into the tube. The entire assembly is then discarded into a sharps container.

Using a Butterfly

All routine venipuncture procedures utilized with evacuated tubes and syringes also apply to blood collection using a butterfly. By folding the plastic needle attachments upward while inserting the needle, the angle of insertion can be lowered to 10 to 15 degrees, thereby facilitating entry into small veins. Blood will appear in the tubing when the vein is entered. The needle can then be threaded securely into the vein and kept in place by holding the plastic wings against the patient's arm. Depending on the type of butterfly apparatus used, blood is collected into evacuated tubes or a syringe. To prevent hemolysis when using a small (23-gauge) needle, pediatric size vacuum tubes should be used.

When disposing of the butterfly apparatus use extreme care, as many accidental sticks result from unexpected movement of the tubing. Accidents can be prevented by placing the needle into a sharps container prior to removing the vacuum tube adaptor or the syringe and then allowing the tubing to fall into the container when they are removed. Use of an apparatus with automatic resheathing capability will also prevent problems. Do not manually push the apparatus into a full sharps container.

The venipuncture procedure using a butterfly is shown in Figure 14–2.

Complications

Not all venipunctures result in the immediate appearance of blood; however, in many instances this is only a temporary setback that can be corrected by slight movement of the needle. As shown in Figure 14–3B and C the bevel of the needle may be resting against the wall of the vein, and rotating the needle a quarter of a turn will allow blood to flow freely. Slowly advancing a needle that is not fully in a vein or pulling back a needle that has passed through a vein also may correct the problem (Fig. 14–3D and E). Gentle touching of the area around the needle with the cleansed gloved finger may determine the positions of the vein and the needle, and allow the needle to be slightly redirected. If the needle appears to be in the vein, a faulty vacuum tube may be the problem and a new tube should be used. The vein also may have collapsed (Fig. 14–3F) as a result of pressure from the vacuum tube, and use of a smaller vacuum tube may remedy the situation. If it does not, another puncture must be performed possibly using a syringe or butterfly. It is important for beginning phlebotomists to know these techniques, as they have a tendency to immediately remove the needle when blood does not appear. The patient must then be stuck again when it may not have been necessary.

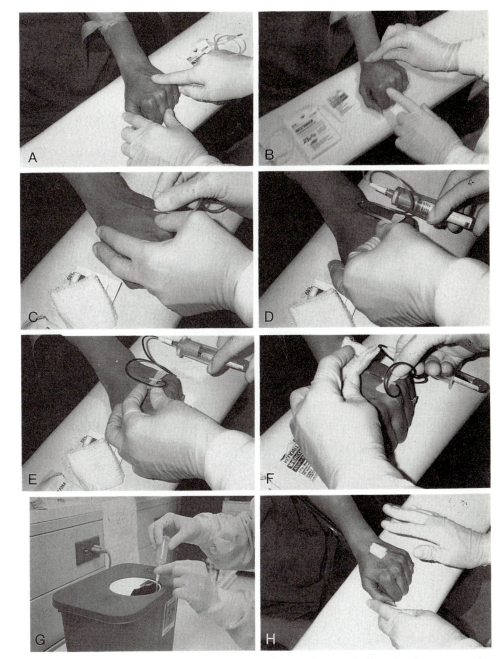

FIGURE 14–2. Venipuncture using a butterfly. *A*, Hand vein palpation. *B*, Cleansing the puncture site. *C*, Inserting the needle. *D*, Advancing an evacuated tube into the adapter. *E*, Blood flow through the butterly apparatus. *F*, Removing the needle. *G*, Disposing of the butterfly apparatus. *H*, Patient's hand with pressure bandage.

Movement of the needle should not include vigorous probing as this is not only painful to the patient but also enlarges the puncture site so that blood can leak into the tissues and form a hematoma.

When blood is not obtained from the initial venipuncture, the phlebotomist should select another site, either in the other arm or below the previous site, and re-

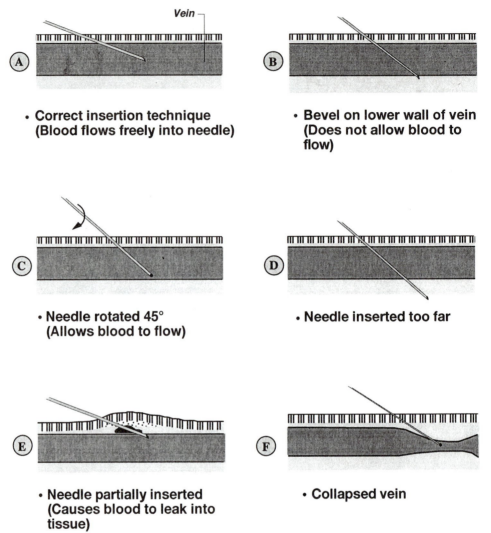

FIGURE 14–3. Possible reasons for failure to obtain blood.

peat the procedure. If the second puncture is not successful, another attempt should not be made by the same phlebotomist. Following hospital policy the phlebotomist should notify the nursing station and request that another phlebotomist perform the venipuncture.

Hemolyzed Specimens

Hemolysis is detected by the presence of pink or red plasma or serum. Rupture of the red blood cell membrane releases cellular contents into the serum or plasma and produces interference with many test results so that the specimen may need to be redrawn. Table 14–1 summarizes the major tests affected by hemolysis.

Errors in performance of the venipuncture account for the majority of hemolyzed specimens and include:

1 Using a needle with too small a diameter (above 23-gauge)
2 Using a small needle with a large vacuum tube
3 Using an improperly attached needle on a syringe so that frothing occurs as the blood enters the syringe

TABLE 14–1. **LABORATORY TESTS AFFECTED BY HEMOLYSIS**

Seriously Affected	Noticeably Affected	Slightly Affected
Potassium (K)	Serum iron (Fe)	Phosphorus (P)
Lactic dehydrogenase (LD)	Alanine aminotransferase	Total protein (TP)
Aspartate aminotransferase	(ALT)	Albumin
(AST)	Thyroxine (T4)	Magnesium (Mg)
Complete blood count (CBC)		Calcium (Ca)
		Acid phosphatase

4 Pulling the plunger of a syringe back too fast
5 Drawing blood from a hematoma
6 Vigorously mixing tubes
7 Forcing blood from a syringe into a vacuum tube
8 Failure to allow the blood to run down the side of a tube when using a syringe to fill the tube

REMOVAL OF THE NEEDLE

Improper technique when removing the needle is a frequent (although not the only) cause of a hematoma appearing on the patient's arm. Errors in technique that cause blood to leak or be forced into the surrounding tissue and produce hematomas include:

1 Failure to remove the tourniquet prior to removing the needle
2 Application of inadequate pressure to the site after removal of the needle
3 Excessive probing to obtain blood
4 Failure to insert the needle far enough into the vein
5 Inserting the needle through the vein
6 Bending the arm while applying pressure

Under normal conditions the elasticity of the vein walls prevents the leakage of blood around the needle during venipuncture. A decrease in the elasticity of the vein walls in older patients causes them to be more prone to developing hematomas. Using small bore needles and firmly anchoring the veins prior to needle insertion may prevent a hematoma in older patients.

DISPOSAL OF THE NEEDLE

There should be no deviations from the methods for needle disposal discussed in Chapter 12.

LABELING THE TUBES

Information contained on the labels of tubes from unidentified patients must follow the protocol used by the institution to provide a temporary but clear designation of the patient. When available, stickers from the patient's arm band should be attached to all specimens for the blood bank.

BANDAGING THE PATIENT'S ARM

Patients receiving anticoagulant medications or large amounts of aspirin, or patients with coagulation disorders may continue to bleed after pressure has been applied for 5 minutes. The phlebotomist should continue to apply pressure until the bleeding has stopped. The nurse should be notified in cases of excessive bleeding.

In the case of an accidental arterial puncture, which can usually be detected by the appearance of unusually red blood that spurts into the tube, the phlebotomist, not the patient, should apply pressure to the site for 10 minutes. The fact that the specimen is arterial blood should be recorded on the requisition form.

Some patients are allergic to adhesive bandages and it may be necessary to wrap gauze around the arm prior to applying the adhesive tape. Omitting the bandage in these patients and those with hairy arms is another option, particularly if it is requested by the patient. Bandages are not recommended for children under 2 years old, as they may put them in their mouths.

LEAVING THE PATIENT

Patients often request that the phlebotomist change the position of their bed or provide them with a drink of water. As this may not be in the best interest of the patient, the phlebotomist should tell the patient that she or he will inform the nurse of the request.

COMPLETING THE VENIPUNCTURE PROCEDURE

Specimens brought to the laboratory may be rejected if conditions are present that would compromise the validity of the test results.

Major reasons for specimen rejection are:

1 Unlabeled or mislabeled specimens
2 Inadequate volume
3 Collection in the wrong tube
4 Hemolysis
5 Clotted blood in an anticoagulant tube
6 Improper handling during transport, such as not chilling the specimen
7 Specimens without a requisition form
8 Obviously contaminated specimen containers

Phlebotomists should make sure that none of these conditions exist in the specimens they deliver to the laboratory.

BIBLIOGRAPHY

National Committee for Clinical Laboratory Standards Approved Standard H3-A3: Procedures for Collection of Diagnostic Blood Specimens by Venipuncture. NCCLS, Villanova, PA, 1991.

National Committee for Clinical Laboratory Standards Approved Guideline H18-A: Procedures for the Handling and Processing of Blood Specimens. NCCLS, Villanova, PA, 1990.

Read, DC, Viera, H, and Arkin, C: Effect of drawing blood specimens proximal to an in-place but discontinued intravenous solution. Am J Clin Pathol 90:702–706, 1988.

Statland, BE, and Per Winkle, MD: Preparing patients and specimens for laboratory testing. In Henry, JB (ed): Clinical Diagnosis and Management by Laboratory Methods. WB Saunders, Philadelphia, 1991.

Study Questions

1. How should a phlebotomist greet an unconscious patient?

   _____

   _____

2. What should the phlebotomist do when a physician is with the patient and the request is for a timed specimen?

   _____

   _____

3. If the phlebotomist cannot locate a patient, what procedure should be followed?

   _____

   _____

   _____

4. A phlebotomist encounters an inpatient without an ID band. When can the blood be drawn?

   _____

5. When should the needle be removed if the patient develops syncope?

   _____

6. True or False. A patient can refuse to have blood drawn.

7. Why should extra evacuated tubes be available when performing a venipuncture?

   _____

8. When a blood pressure cuff is used as a tourniquet, how will inflation of the cuff to a pressure above the patient's systolic pressure affect blood flow?

   _____

   _____

9. List four test results that are affected by prolonged tourniquet application.

   a. _____

   b. _____

   c. _____

   d. _____

10. If a vein is not easily located in the patient's dominant arm, what is the first thing the phlebotomist should do?

   _____

11. List four techniques to enhance the prominence of veins that are hard to find.

   a. _____

   b. _____

   c. _____

   d. _____

12. How does a vein that is occluded feel?

   _____

13. How does a mastectomy affect the adjacent blood supply?

   _____

   _____

14. Indicate if each of the following are acceptable or unacceptable venipuncture sites by placing an "A" or a "U" in front of the statement. Explain all "U" answers, using the words, contamination, infection, hemolysis, or decreased blood flow in the appropriate space.

                                                                    If "U"

   a. _____ Antecubital area above an IV drip that has
             been discontinued for 5 minutes   _____

   b. _____ The wrist below an antecubital hematoma   _____

   c. _____ Antecubital area containing a tattoo   _____

   d. _____ Vein surrounded by a hematoma   _____

   e. _____ Wrist below an IV drip that has been
             discontinued for 5 minutes   _____

   f. _____ Wrist containing scar tissue   _____

   g. _____ Arm with a fistula   _____

   h. _____ Right arm of a patient with a right
             mastectomy   _____

   i. _____ Veins on the back of the hand   _____

   j. _____ Vein that feels hard   _____

15. What precaution must be taken when coagulation tests are drawn from an indwelling line?

   _____

16. True or False. The phlebotomist can draw from the T-connection of a fistula.

17. List three site cleansing solutions other than isopropyl alcohol and state a reason for their use.

Solution	**Reason**
a. _____	_____
b. _____	_____
c. _____	_____

18. State two problems that may occur if the plunger of the syringe is pulled back too fast.

    a. _____

    b. _____

19. How can hemolysis be avoided when using a butterfly?

    _____

    _____

20. List three reasons why blood may not be obtained even though the needle is in the vein.

    a. _____

    b. _____

    c. _____

21. List two tests that are seriously affected by hemolysis. Do the same for tests that are noticeably and slightly affected.

Seriously	**Noticeably**	**Slightly**
a. _____	_____	_____
b. _____	_____	_____

22. List four causes of hematomas.

    a. _____

    b. _____

    c. _____

    d. _____

23. How can an accidental arterial puncture be detected and what should the phlebotomist do?

    _____

    _____

24. List six possible causes of specimen rejection and state a *specific* example of each.

a. _____

_____

b. _____

_____

c. _____

_____

d. _____

_____

e. _____

_____

f. _____

_____

Venipuncture Complications Exercise

1. An unidentified patient in the ER requires a transfusion. What precautions must the phlebotomist take?

   _____

   _____

   _____

2. The phlebotomist has a requisition to collect a chemistry profile and a PT. No blood is obtained from the left antecubital area. The phlebotomist then moves to the right antecubital area and obtains a full SST tube but cannot fill the light-blue tube. What should the phlebotomist do next?

   _____

   _____

3. A patient has an IV drip running in the left forearm. From the following sites, indicate your first choice with a "1," your second choice with a "2," and an unacceptable site with an "X."

   a. _____ The left wrist

   b. _____ The left antecubital area

   c. _____ The right antecubital area

4. A phlebotomist with a requisition for a PT, CBC, and glucose on a patient who is difficult to draw obtains 7 mL of blood using a syringe. Assuming the phlebotomist has a 2.7-mL light-blue top tube, a 3-mL lavender top tube, and a 3-mL red top tube, how should the blood be distributed?

   _____

   _____

   _____

5. The phlebotomist is assisting the nurse to collect a prothrombin time, CBC, and chemistry profile from an intravenous line.

   a. How many and what size syringes are needed and what is done with the blood collected in each?

   _____

   _____

   _____

   b. What should the phlebotomist write on the requisition form?

   _____

6. A phlebotomist needs to collect 20 mL of blood for serum chemistry tests and selects two 10-mL red top tubes. A successful puncture is performed; however, blood stops flowing when the first tube is only half full.

   a. Assuming the problem does not lie with the equipment, what is a possible reason for this?

   _____

   b. State two methods the phlebotomist could use to collect the required amount of blood.

   _____

   _____

7. When collecting a specimen from an elderly patient using routine evacuated tube equipment, the phlebotomist notices that the puncture site is beginning to swell.

   a. Why is this happening?

   _____

   b. What should the phlebotomist do?

   _____

   c. How can the specimen be collected?

   _____

   _____

8. While a CBC is being collected the patient develops syncope and the phlebotomist immediately removes the needle and lowers the patient's head. When the patient has recovered the phlebotomist labels the lavender top tube, which fortunately contains enough blood, and delivers it to the hematology section. Many results on this specimen are markedly lower than those on the patient's previous CBC.

   a. How could the quality of the specimen have caused this discrepancy?

   _____

   _____

   b. How could the venipuncture complication have contributed to this error?

   _____

   _____

   c. Could the phlebotomist have done anything differently? Explain your answer.

   _____

   _____

9. A nurse from the cardiac care unit reports that she is observing hematomas on the patients whenever Phlebotomist X is assigned to the floor. Considering the condition and treatment of the patients in this unit, what is the most probable error being made by Phlebotomist X? Explain your answer.

_____

_____

_____

10. A phlebotomist delivers a properly labeled specimen with sufficient volume collected in a red top tube to the chemistry section for a potassium determination. Fifteen minutes later the phlebotomist is asked to redraw the specimen.

a. Why did the chemistry section reject this specimen?

_____

b. What precautions should the phlebotomist take with the second specimen?

_____

_____

_____

Evaluation of Venipuncture Technique Using a Syringe

Rating System
2 = Satisfactorily performed
1 = Needs improvement
0 = Incorrect/did not perform

_____ 1. Examines requisition form

_____ 2. Greets patient, states procedure to be done

_____ 3. Identifies patient verbally

_____ 4. Examines patient's ID band

_____ 5. Compares requisition form with ID band

_____ 6. Puts on gloves

_____ 7. Selects tubes and equipment for procedure

_____ 8. Assembles and conveniently places equipment

_____ 9. Positions patient's arm

_____ 10. Applies tourniquet

_____ 11. Identifies vein by palpation

_____ 12. Releases tourniquet

_____ 13. Cleanses site and allows it to air dry

_____ 14. Reapplies tourniquet

_____ 15. Does not touch puncture site with unclean finger

_____ 16. Checks plunger movement

_____ 17. Anchors vein below puncture site

_____ 18. Smoothly enters vein at appropriate angle with bevel up

_____ 19. Does not move needle when plunger is retracted

_____ 20. Collects appropriate amount of blood

_____ 21. Releases tourniquet

_____ 22. Covers puncture site with gauze

_____ 23. Removes needle smoothly and applies pressure

_____ 24. Uses correct and safe technique to fill tubes

_____ 25. Fills tubes in correct order

_____ 26. Mixes anticoagulated tubes promptly

_____ 27. Disposes of needle and syringe in sharps container

_____ 28. Labels tubes

_____ 29. Examines puncture site

_____ 30. Applies bandage

_____ 31. Disposes of used supplies

_____ 32. Removes gloves and washes hands

_____ 33. Thanks patient

_____ 34. Converses appropriately with patient during procedure

Total Points _____

Maximum Points = 68

COMMENTS:

Evaluation of Venipuncture Technique Using a Butterfly

Rating System
2 = Satisfactorily performed
1 = Needs improvement
0 = Incorrect/did not perform

_____ 1. Examines requisition form

_____ 2. Greets patient, states procedure to be done

_____ 3. Identifies patient verbally

_____ 4. Examines patient's ID band

_____ 5. Compares requisition form with ID band

_____ 6. Puts on gloves

_____ 7. Selects tubes and equipment for procedure

_____ 8. Assembles and conveniently places equipment

_____ 9. Positions patient's hand

_____ 10. Applies tourniquet

_____ 11. Identifies vein by palpation

_____ 12. Releases tourniquet

_____ 13. Cleanses site and allows it to air dry

_____ 14. Reapplies tourniquet

_____ 15. Does not touch puncture site with unclean finger

_____ 16. Anchors vein below puncture site

_____ 17. Holds needle appropriately

_____ 18. Enters vein smoothly at appropriate angle with bevel up

_____ 19. Maintains needle securely in vein

_____ 20. Smoothly operates syringe or vacuum tube adapter

_____ 21. Fills tubes in the correct order

_____ 22. Mixes anticoagulated tubes promptly

_____ 23. Collects appropriate amount of blood

_____ 24. Releases tourniquet

_____ 25. Covers puncture site with gauze

_____ 26. Removes needle smoothly and applies pressure

_____ 27. Disposes of apparatus in sharps container

_____ 28. Labels tubes

_____ 29. Examines puncture site

_____ 30. Applies bandage

_____ 31. Disposes of used supplies

_____ 32. Removes gloves and washes hands

_____ 33. Thanks patient

_____ 34. Converses appropriately with patient during procedure

Total Points _____

Maximum Points = 68

COMMENTS:

CHAPTER 15 Special Venipuncture Collection

Learning Objectives

Upon completion of this chapter, the reader will be able to:

1 Define the terms and abbreviations associated with special venipuncture collection procedures.
2 State two reasons why fasting specimens are requested and name three tests affected by not fasting.
3 List four reasons for requesting timed specimens.
4 Explain the procedure for a 2-hour postprandial glucose test.
5 Correctly schedule specimen collections for a GTT.
6 Using an example, discuss diurnal variation of blood constituents.
7 State two reasons for therapeutic drug monitoring.
8 Differentiate between a trough and a peak level.
9 Discuss three timing sequences for the collection of blood cultures, reasons for selecting a particular timing sequence, and the number of specimens collected.
10 Describe the aseptic techniques required when collecting blood cultures.
11 Describe the procedure for collecting specimens for cold agglutinins.
12 List seven tests that must be chilled immediately after collection.
13 List five tests that are affected by exposure to light.
14 Define chain of custody.
15 List three tests frequently requested for forensic studies.

Terminology

Key Terms	Definition
Aseptic	Free of contamination by microorganisms
Basal state	Metabolic condition after 12 hours of fasting and lack of exercise
Chain of custody	Documentation of the collection and handling of forensic specimens
Diurnal	Variations occurring during the day
Fasting	Abstinence from food and liquids (except water) for a specified period
Forensic	Pertaining to legal proceedings
Lipemic	Pertaining to turbidity from lipids
Peak level	Specimen collected when a serum drug level is highest
Postprandial	After eating
Septicemia	Pathogenic microorganisms in the blood
Trough level	Specimen collected when a serum drug level is lowest

Terminology Continued	**Abbreviations**	**Definition**
	ARD	Antimicrobial removal device
	FUO	Fever of unknown origin
	pp	Postprandial
	TDM	Therapeutic drug monitoring

Certain laboratory tests require the phlebotomist to utilize techniques that are not part of the routine venipuncture procedure. These special techniques may involve patient preparation, timing of specimen collection, venipuncture techniques, and specimen handling. Phlebotomists must know when these techniques are required, how to perform them, and how specimen integrity is affected when they are not properly performed.

FASTING SPECIMENS

Normal values (reference ranges) for laboratory tests are determined using specimens from a normal, representative sample of volunteers who have usually been **fasting** and who have refrained from strenuous exercise for 12 hours (**basal state**). Not all tests are affected by fasting and exercise, as evidenced by the collection and testing of specimens throughout the day. Many diagnostic results can be obtained at any time. However, the best comparison of patients' results with the normal values can be made when the patients are in the basal state. This explains why phlebotomists begin their major hospital rounds very early in the morning and why the majority of outpatients arrive in the laboratory as soon as the drawing station opens.

Test results most critically affected in a nonfasting patient are glucose and triglyceride tests. When a fasting specimen is requested, it is the responsibility of the phlebotomist to determine if the patient has been fasting for the required length of time. If the patient has not, this must be reported to a supervisor or the nurse and noted on the requisition form.

Serum or plasma collected from patients shortly after a meal may appear cloudy (**lipemic**) due to the presence of fatty compounds. Lipemia will interfere with many test results.

TIMED SPECIMENS

Requisitions are frequently received requesting that blood be drawn at a specific time. Reasons for timed specimens include:

1 Measurement of the body's ability to metabolize a particular substance
2 Monitoring changes in a patient's condition (such as a steady decrease in hemoglobin)
3 Determining blood levels of medications
4 Measuring substances that exhibit **diurnal** variation (normal changes in blood levels at different times of the day)

Phlebotomists should arrange their schedules so as to be available at the specified time and should record the time of collection on the requisition and specimen tube.

The most frequently encountered timed specimens are discussed in this chapter. Other diagnostic procedures may also require timed specimens, and any request for a timed specimen should be strictly followed.

Two-Hour Postprandial Glucose

Comparison of a patient's fasting glucose level with the glucose level 2 hours after eating a meal or ingesting a measured amount of glucose is used to evaluate diabetes mellitus. Ideally the glucose level should return to the fasting level within 2 hours.

The phlebotomist must be able to explain the procedure to the patient, stressing the importance of eating a full meal and returning to the laboratory in time to have the blood drawn exactly 2 hours after the meal is completed.

Glucose Tolerance Test

The glucose tolerance test (GTT) is a procedure performed for the diagnosis of diabetes mellitus (hyperglycemia) and for evaluating persons with symptoms associated with low blood glucose (hypoglycemia). Phlebotomists are often responsible for the administration of this procedure, which includes patient instruction; administering the glucose solution; scheduling of samples; and the collection and organization of samples that consist of timed blood and urine collections. The procedure is scheduled for 3 hours to diagnose diabetes mellitus and 5 or 6 hours for evaluation of hypoglycemia.

GTT procedures should be scheduled to begin between 0700 and 0900 because glucose levels exhibit a diurnal variation. The phlebotomist draws a fasting glucose and requests the patient to collect a urine specimen. The fasting blood and urine specimens are tested prior to continuing the procedure to determine if the patient can be safely given a large amount of glucose. The phlebotomist then asks the patient to drink a standardized amount of flavored glucose solution within a period of 5 minutes. Timing for the remaining GTT specimens begins when the patient finishes drinking the glucose. Sample schedules are shown in Table 15–1. Notice that all timing is based on completion of the glucose drink.

The patient is given a copy of the schedule and instructed to remain fasting, drink water to facilitate urine collection, and return to the drawing station at the scheduled times.

Corresponding labels containing routinely required information and specimen order in the test sequence, such as 1-hour, 2-hour, and so on, are placed on the blood and urine specimens. Blood specimens that will not be tested until the end of the sequence should be collected in gray top tubes. Timing of specimen collection is criti-

TABLE 15–1. **SAMPLE GLUCOSE TOLERANCE TEST SCHEDULES**

Test Procedure	3-Hour Test	6-Hour Test
Fasting blood and urine	0700	0700
Patient finishes glucose	0800	0800
½-Hour specimen	0830	0830
1-Hour specimen	0900	0900
2-Hour specimen	1000	1000
3-Hour specimen	1100	1100
4-Hour specimen		1200
5-Hour specimen		1300
6-Hour specimen		1400

cal, as test results are related to the scheduled times; any discrepancies should be noted on the requisition. Consistency of venipuncture or dermal puncture must also be maintained, as glucose values differ between the two types of blood.

Some patients may not be able to tolerate the glucose solution, and if vomiting occurs, the time of the vomiting must be reported to a supervisor and a decision made concerning continuation of the test. Vomiting early in the procedure is considered to be most critical. Phlebotomists should also observe patients when they return for their scheduled sample collections for any changes in their condition, such as dizziness, that might indicate a reaction to the glucose and should report this to their supervisor.

Diurnal Variation

Substances primarily affected by diurnal variation are corticosteroids, hormones, serum iron, and glucose. Phlebotomists are often requested to draw specimens for these tests at specific times, usually corresponding to the peak diurnal level. Certain variations can be substantial. Plasma cortisol levels drawn between 0800 and 1000 will be twice as high as levels drawn at 1600, and serum iron levels drawn in the morning are one third higher than those drawn in the evening. Consequently, requests for plasma cortisol levels frequently specify that the test be drawn between 0800 and 1000, or at 1600. If the specimen cannot be collected at the specified time, the physician should be notified and the test rescheduled for the next day.

Therapeutic Drug Monitoring

The fact that medications affect all patients differently frequently results in the need to change dosages or medications. Some medications can reach toxic levels in patients who do not metabolize or excrete them within an expected time frame. Likewise there are patients who metabolize and excrete medications at an increased rate. To ensure patient safety and medication effectiveness the blood levels of many therapeutic drugs are monitored.

Examples of frequently monitored therapeutic drugs are digoxin, gentamycin, tobramycin, vancomycin, and theophylline. Random specimens are occasionally requested; however, the most beneficial levels are those drawn before the next dosage is given (**trough level**) and shortly after the medication is given (**peak level**). Trough levels are collected 30 minutes before the drug is to be given and represent the lowest level in the blood. Ideally trough levels should be tested prior to administering the next dose to ensure that the level is low enough for the patient to safely receive more medication. The time for collecting peak levels varies with the medication and the method of administration (intravenous, intramuscular, or oral). Information from drug manufacturers provides the recommended times for collection of peak levels. To ensure correct documentation of the peak and trough levels, requisitions and specimen tube labels should include the time and method of administration of the last dosage given, as well as the time that the specimen is drawn.

BLOOD CULTURES

One of the most difficult phlebotomy procedures is collection of blood cultures. This is because of the strict **aseptic** technique required and the need to collect multiple specimens in special containers. Blood cultures are requested on patients when symptoms of fever and chills indicate a possible infection of the blood by pathogenic microorganisms (**septicemia**). The patient's initial diagnosis is often fever of unknown origin (**FUO**).

Blood cultures are usually ordered STAT or as timed collections. Isolation of microorganisms from the blood is often difficult due to the small number of organisms needed to cause symptoms. Specimens are usually collected in sets of two or three drawn either 1 hour apart or just before the patient's temperature reaches its highest point (spike). If antibiotics are to be started immediately, the sets are drawn at the same time from different sites. The concentration of microorganisms will fluctuate and is often highest just before the patient's temperature spikes. This explains why collections may be ordered at 1-hour intervals or ordered STAT if a pattern has been observed in the patient's temperature chart. Specimens collected from multiple sites at the same time serve as a control for possible contamination and must be labeled as to the collection site, such as right arm antecubital vein, and their number in the series (#1, #2, or #3). A known skin contaminant must be cultured from at least two of the sites for it to be considered a possible pathogen.

Blood for culture may be drawn directly into bottles containing culture media; transferred to the bottles from a syringe; or drawn into sterile tubes containing anticoagulant and transferred to culture media in the laboratory. When transferring blood from a syringe to blood culture bottles, some laboratories require that a new needle be placed on the syringe for the transfer. Due to the increased risk of contact with contaminated needles, this practice has been discontinued in many institutions. Studies have shown little difference in contamination rates when needles are not changed. An anticoagulant must be present in the tube or media to prevent microorganisms from being trapped within a clot where they might be undetected; therefore, blood culture bottles must be mixed after the blood is added. The anticoagulant sodium polyanetholesulfonate (SPS) is used for blood cultures because it does not inhibit bacterial growth and may in fact enhance it by inhibiting the action of phagocytes, complement, and some antibiotics. Other anticoagulants should not be used. Some blood culture collection systems have antimicrobial removal devices (**ARDs**) containing resin that inactivates antibiotics. As shown in Figure 15–1, a variety of blood culture collection systems are available.

Venipuncture technique for collecting blood cultures follows routine procedure with the exception of the increased requirements for asepsis. Cleansing of the venipuncture site begins by vigorous scrubbing of the site with alcohol, starting in the center and progressing outward in concentric circles; this is followed by the application of 2% iodine or povidone-iodine in the same manner. The iodine must be allowed to dry for 1 minute. If the site must be retouched, the phlebotomist must cleanse the palpating finger in the same manner. The tops of the collection contain-

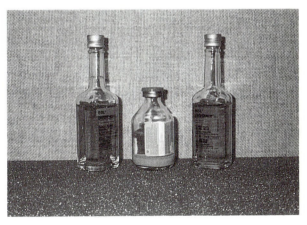

FIGURE 15–1. Blood culture collection systems.

ers are also cleansed with iodine at this time and then wiped with alcohol just prior to inoculation. To prevent irritation of the patient's arm, the iodine is removed with alcohol when the procedure is complete.

Two specimens are routinely collected for each blood culture set, one to be incubated aerobically and the other anaerobically. When a syringe is used, the anaerobic bottle should be inoculated first to prevent possible exposure to air.

Because the number of organisms present in the blood is often small, the amount of blood inoculated into each container is critical. There should be at least a 1:10 ratio of blood to media. Phlebotomists should follow the instructions for the system being used. Pediatric patients usually have a higher concentration of microorganisms so that a smaller volume of blood can be used.

SPECIAL SPECIMEN HANDLING PROCEDURES

Cold Agglutinins

Cold agglutinins are autoantibodies primarily produced by persons infected with *Mycoplasma pneumoniae* (atypical pneumonia). The autoantibodies react with red blood cells at temperatures below body temperature. Detection of a high titer of cold agglutinins in a patient's serum aids in the diagnosis of a *M. pneumoniae* infection.

Because the cold agglutinins in the serum attach to red blood cells when the blood cools to below body temperature, the specimen must be kept warm until the serum can be separated from the cells. Specimens are collected in tubes that have been warmed in an incubator at 37°C for 30 minutes and which contain no additives or gels that could interfere with the test. The phlebotomist can carry the warmed tube to the patient's room in a tightly closed fist, collect the specimen as quickly as possible, return the specimen to the laboratory in the same manner, and place it back in the incubator. Failure to keep a specimen warm prior to serum separation will produce falsely decreased test results.

Chilled Specimens

Specimens for arterial blood gases, ammonia, lactic acid, pyruvate, gastrin, ACTH, parathyroid hormone, and some coagulation studies must be chilled immediately after collection to prevent deterioration. For adequate chilling, the specimen must be placed in crushed ice or a mixture of ice and water at the bedside. It is important that these specimens be immediately returned to the laboratory for processing.

Specimens Sensitive to Light

Exposure to light will decrease the concentration of bilirubin, beta-carotene, vitamins A and B_6, and porphyrins. Specimens can be protected by wrapping the tubes in aluminum foil.

Legal (Forensic) Specimens

When drawing specimens for test results that may be used as evidence in legal proceedings, phlebotomists must use extreme care to follow the stated policies exactly. Documentation of specimen handling, called the **chain of custody**, is essential. It begins with patient identification and continues until testing is completed and results reported. Special forms are provided for this documentation and special containers and seals may be required (Fig. 15-2). For each person handling the speci-

AMERICAN MEDICAL LABORATORIES, INC.
14225 NEWBROOK DRIVE
CHANTILLY, VA 22021
(703) 802-6900

CHAIN-OF-CUSTODY FORM
Medical-Legal Specimen

Lab use only

INSTRUCTIONS FOR SUBMITTING SAMPLES

Section A – Specimen Collection: Fill out section A1 and an AML Request Form completely. Label all specimen containers with the patient name, date of collection and a peel-off label from the AML request form. Place dated and initialed security seals over the openings of the containers. If possible, have a witness sign. Have the patient (donor) sign Section A2, line 1 Received From line. The collector must also date and sign the form on the Received By line.

Section B – Specimen Transfers: When transferring specimens(s) the collector must sign line B1. Each person receiving specimen(s) must sign on the Received By line. Indicate job title, and date and time received. The condition of the specimen(s) should be noted by checking the appropriate box. The condition of the specimen(s) may be unacceptable for the following reasons: broken container or substantial leakage, torn seal(s), improper collection or storage for requested tests. Indicate under NOTE why the condition is unacceptable. The person that signs the Received By line is responsible for the security of the specimen(s) until the next person or secure area receives it. If the specimen(s) is being placed in a secure area, indicate location on the Received By line. Also indicate date and time.

A1. Patient Name _____ Age _____ Sex _____

    Client Name _____ Client Number _____

    Date _____ Time of Collection _____ AML Peel Off Sticker # _____

    Type and Number of Specimens _____

    Collection Witness Signature (if applicable) _____

A 2   Received From: (Patient or Authorized Signature) _____

      Received By (Collector) _____ Date/Time _____

B   1. Received From (Collector): _____ | Condition of Specimen
                                                         | Acceptable   ☐
      Received By _____ Title: _____ Date/Time _____ | Unacceptable ☐
                                                         | NOTES: _____

B   2. Received From: _____ | Condition of Specimen
                                            | Acceptable   ☐
      Received By _____ Title: _____ Date/Time _____ | Unacceptable ☐
                                            | NOTES: _____

B   3. Received From: _____ | Condition of Specimen
                                            | Acceptable   ☐
      Received By _____ Title: _____ Date/Time _____ | Unacceptable ☐
                                            | NOTES: _____

B   4. Received From: _____ | Condition of Specimen
                                            | Acceptable   ☐
      Received By _____ Title: _____ Date/Time _____ | Unacceptable ☐
                                            | NOTES: _____

B   5. Received From: _____ | Condition of Specimen
                                            | Acceptable   ☐
      Received By _____ Title: _____ Date/Time _____ | Unacceptable ☐
                                            | NOTES: _____

COC-FORM
9/94

FIGURE 15-2. Sample chain-of-custody form. (Courtesy of Janet Beatey, American Medical Laboratories Inc., Chantilly, VA.)

men, documentation must include the date, the time, and the identification of the handler. Patient identification and specimen collection should be done in the presence of a witness, frequently a law enforcement officer. Identification may include fingerprinting or heel-printing in paternity cases. Tests most frequently requested are alcohol and drug levels and DNA analysis.

As stated in the previous chapter, when collecting blood alcohol levels the site should be cleansed with soap and water or a nonalcoholic antiseptic solution. To prevent the escape of the volatile alcohol into the atmosphere, tubes should be completely filled and not left uncapped for longer than necessary.

BIBLIOGRAPHY

Lotspeich, CA: Specimen collection and processing. In Bishop, ML (ed): Clinical Chemistry: Principles, Procedures and Correlations. JB Lippincott, Philadelphia, 1985.

National Committee for Clinical Laboratory Standards Approved Standard H3-A3: Procedures for Collection of Diagnostic Blood Specimens by Venipuncture. NCCLS, Villanova, PA, 1991.

National Committee for Clinical Laboratory Standards Approved Guideline H18-A: Procedures for the Handling and Processing of Blood Specimens. NCCLS, Villanova, PA, 1990.

Statland, BE, and Per Winkle, MD. Preparing patients and specimens for laboratory testing. In Henry, JB (ed): Clinical Diagnosis and Management by Laboratory Methods. WB Saunders, Philadelphia, 1991.

Study Questions

1. Why are more phlebotomists utilized on the early morning shift?

   _____

2. A possible reason for a lipemic serum is _____.

3. At 0730 the phlebotomist receives requests for a cortisol level on Unit 4B, an FBS on Unit 4A, and a STAT crossmatch in the ER. In which order should the phlebotomist collect these specimens? Justify your answer.

   _____

   _____

   _____

4. Why should the fasting glucose specimens be tested prior to administering the glucose in a GTT?

   _____

   _____

5. Design a schedule for a 3-hour GTT assuming the patient has a fasting specimen drawn at 0715 and completes drinking the glucose at 0745.

   _____

   _____

   _____

   _____

   _____

6. True or False. A phlebotomist who cannot obtain the 1-hour sample in a GTT by venipuncture should immediately perform a capillary puncture.

7. When should trough and peak levels be drawn for TDM?

   _____

   _____

8. Which TDM level is used to determine if the medication should be administered? _____

9. Give two reasons why blood cultures are frequently ordered STAT.

   a. _____

   b. _____

10. The condition represented by a positive blood culture is called

   _____.

11. What is the purpose for inoculating two bottles of blood culture media each time a specimen is drawn? Which bottle is inoculated first?

_____

_____

12. The major source of false positive blood cultures is _____

_____.

13. True or False. A specimen for cold agglutinins will have a falsely decreased value if it is chilled immediately after collection. Why?

_____

_____

14. How will wrapping the collection tube in aluminum foil affect the results of a bilirubin test?

_____

15. How will the results of a serum gastrin test be affected if the specimen is held tightly in the phlebotomist's fist when being delivered to the laboratory?

_____

16. How is documentation of patient identification, specimen collection, and specimen handling performed when forensic studies are requested?

_____

_____

_____

Special Venipuncture Collection Exercise

1. An outpatient comes to the laboratory at 1300 with a requisition for a cardiac risk profile. Before collecting the specimen, what should the phlebotomist ask the patient?

   _____

2. Requisitions are received requesting that specimens for H & H be collected at 0800, 1200, 1600, and 2000 from a patient on a medical-surgical unit. Is there a reason for these requests and if so what is it?

   _____

   _____

3. An outpatient comes to the laboratory with a requisition for an FBS and a 2-hour pp glucose. What should the phlebotomist do?

   _____

   _____

   _____

4. A patient receiving a 3-hour GTT is unable to collect a urine specimen at the time of the 2-hour specimen and vomits 20 minutes before the 3-hour specimen is scheduled. What should the phlebotomist do?

   _____

   _____

   _____

5. At 0900 the phlebotomist arrives in a patient's room to collect a cortisol level. The patient is not in the room and the nurse reports that the patient is in the physical therapy department. What should the phlebotomist do?

   _____

   _____

6. Would it be unusual to receive requests to collect theophylline levels at 0800 and again at 1200? Explain your answer.

   _____

   _____

   _____

7. A phlebotomist is requested to draw three blood cultures within 30 minutes from a patient in the ER. Is this a reasonable request? Why or why not?

   _____

   _____

   _____

8. A phlebotomist collects two blood cultures in yellow top tubes and one in a lavender top tube and transfers each to bottles containing culture media. A known skin contaminant is cultured from two specimens.

   a. What errors in technique are indicated by this scenario?

   _____

   _____

   _____

   b. Why was one culture negative?

   _____

   _____

9. A phlebotomist collects a STAT ammonia level and is then paged to collect a cold agglutinin on the next floor and a CBC in the CCU. The phlebotomist sends the ammonia level to the laboratory in the pneumatic tube system; collects the cold agglutinin; goes to the CCU and draws the CBC; and delivers both specimens to the appropriate laboratory sections. How will the quality of these tests results be affected and why?

   _____

   _____

   _____

   _____

10. As an attorney for a defendant with a blood alcohol level above the legal limit, you are questioning the phlebotomist.

    a. State three questions you would ask the phlebotomist to try to discredit the laboratory result.

    _____

    _____

    _____

    b. How should a competent phlebotomist answer these questions?

    _____

    _____

    _____

Evaluation of Blood Culture Collection Technique

Rating System
2 = Satisfactorily performed
1 = Needs improvement
0 = Incorrect/did not perform

_____ 1. Examines requisition and identifies patient

_____ 2. Correctly assembles equipment

_____ 3. Applies tourniquet

_____ 4. Selects puncture site

_____ 5. Releases tourniquet

_____ 6. Cleanses site with alcohol

_____ 7. Cleanses site with iodine

_____ 8. Puts on gloves

_____ 9. Cleanses tops of blood culture containers

_____ 10. Reapplies tourniquet

_____ 11. Cleanses palpating finger if necessary

_____ 12. Performs venipuncture

_____ 13. Wipes tops of blood culture containers with alcohol

_____ 14. Changes syringe needles if this is required

_____ 15. Inoculates anaerobic container first

_____ 16. Dispenses correct amount of blood into containers

_____ 17. Mixes containers

_____ 18. Disposes of used equipment and supplies

_____ 19. Removes iodine from patient's arm

_____ 20. Bandages patient's arm

_____ 21. Correctly labels blood culture containers

_____ 22. Overall aseptic technique

Total Points _____

Maximum Points = 44

COMMENTS:

CHAPTER 16

Dermal Puncture

Learning Objectives

Upon completion of this chapter, the reader will be able to:

1 Define the terms associated with dermal puncture.
2 State the complications associated with puncture of the deep veins in infants.
3 List six reasons for performing dermal punctures on adults.
4 Describe the composition of capillary blood and name five test results that may differ between capillary and venous blood.
5 Discuss the types of skin puncture devices available.
6 Describe four types of microspecimen containers, as well as reasons for their use, method of collection, and advantages and disadvantages.
7 Discuss the purpose and methodology for puncture site warming.
8 Describe the acceptable sites for performing heel and finger punctures and the conditions when each is performed.
9 List four unacceptable areas for heel puncture.
10 State the complications produced by the presence of alcohol at the puncture site.
11 State the correct positioning of the lancet for dermal puncture.
12 Name the major cause of microspecimen contamination.
13 State the order of draw for dermal puncture specimens.
14 Describe the correct labeling of microspecimens.
15 Correctly perform dermal punctures on the heel and the finger.

Terminology

Key Terms	Definition
Calcaneus	Heel bone
Dermal	Pertaining to the skin
Ecchymoses	Hemorrhagic discoloration
Geriatric	Pertaining to old age
Microsample	A sample of less than 1 mL
Palmar	Pertaining to the palm of the hand
Plantar	Pertaining to the sole of the foot

Although venipuncture is the most frequently performed phlebotomy procedure, it is not appropriate in all circumstances. Current laboratory instrumentation and procedures make it possible to perform a majority of laboratory tests on **microsamples** of blood obtained by dermal puncture on both pediatric and adult patients.

In most institutions dermal puncture is the method of choice for collecting blood from infants and children under 2 years of age. Locating superficial veins large enough to accept even a small-gauge needle is difficult in these patients, and veins that are available may need to be reserved for intravenous therapy. Use of deep veins, such as the femoral, can be dangerous and may cause complications, including cardiac arrest; venous thrombosis; hemorrhage; damage to surrounding tissue and organs; infection; reflex arteriospasm, which can possibly result in gangrene; and injury caused by restraining the child. Drawing excessive amounts of blood from premature and small infants can rapidly cause anemia, as a 2-pound infant may have a total blood volume of only 150 mL.

In adults, dermal puncture may be required because of the inability to locate a suitable vein in:

1 Burned or scarred patients
2 Patients receiving chemotherapy who require frequent tests and whose veins must be reserved for therapy
3 Patients with thrombotic tendencies
4 **Geriatric** or other patients with very fragile veins
5 Persons performing home glucose monitoring

It may not be possible to obtain a satisfactory specimen by dermal puncture from patients who are severely dehydrated or who have poor peripheral circulation.

COMPOSITION OF CAPILLARY BLOOD

Blood collected by dermal puncture comes from the capillaries, arterioles, and venules; it is therefore a mixture of arterial and venous blood and may also contain small amounts of tissue fluid. Due to arterial pressure, the composition of this blood more closely resembles arterial rather than venous blood. Warming the site prior to specimen collection increases blood flow as much as sevenfold, thereby producing a specimen that is very close to the composition of arterial blood.

With the exception of arterial blood gases, very few chemical differences exist between arterial and venous blood. The concentration of glucose is higher in blood obtained by dermal puncture, and the concentrations of potassium, total protein, and calcium are lower. Therefore, when dermal punctures are performed, this should be noted on the requisition form. Alternating between dermal puncture and venipuncture should not be done when results are to be compared.

Hemolysis is more frequently seen in specimens collected by dermal puncture than in those collected by venipuncture. Excessive squeezing of the puncture site to obtain enough blood is often the cause. However, newborns in general have increased numbers of red blood cells and increased red cell fragility, which raises the possibility that hemolysis may occur even in properly collected samples. The presence of hemolysis may not be detected in specimens containing bilirubin, but it will interfere with not only the tests routinely affected by hemolysis but also with the frequently requested neonatal bilirubin determination.

DERMAL PUNCTURE EQUIPMENT

In addition to the previously discussed venipuncture equipment, a phlebotomy collection tray or drawing station should contain skin puncture devices, microsample collection containers, glass slides, and possibly a heel warmer for use in performing dermal punctures.

Skin Puncture Devices

As shown in Figure 16-1, a variety of skin puncture devices are commercially available, including manual and automatic lancets, with and without retractable blades. Many studies have been done comparing the various devices with respect to efficiency of collection, specimen hemolysis, and the formation of **ecchymoses** (bruising) at the collection site. No single method appears to be superior.

To prevent contact with bone, the depth of the puncture is critical and should not exceed 2.4 mm in a device used to perform heel sticks. There is concern that even this may be too deep. The puncture depth is controlled by the length of manual lancets, the spring release mechanism, and the use of platforms in automatic devices. Punctures should never be performed using an uncontrolled surgical blade. Some companies provide separate devices designed for heel sticks, finger sticks on children, and finger sticks on adults. The depth of the puncture can range from 0.85 mm in the Tenderfoot/Premi (Technidyne Corp., Edison, NJ) to 3.0 mm with the orange platform Autolet for adults (Ulster Scientific, New Paltz, NY).

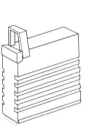

A

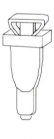

B

C

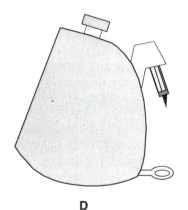

D

FIGURE 16-1. Skin puncture devices. *A*, Tenderfoot lancet. *B*, Blood lancet. *C*, Safety flow lancet. *D*, Autolet.

Phlebotomy Techniques

To produce adequate blood flow the depth of the puncture is actually much less important than the width of the incision. This is because the major vascular area of the skin is located at the dermal-subcutaneous junction, which in a newborn is only 0.35 to 1.6 mm below the skin (Fig. 16–2). Therefore, any of the commercial lancets will reach the blood vessels and the number of severed vessels depends on the incision width. Incision widths vary from needle stabs to 2.5 mm. Longer incisions should be avoided as they will produce unnecessary damage to the heel or finger.

Microspecimen Containers

Figure 16–3 illustrates some of the major specimen containers available for collection of microsamples, which include capillary tubes, micropipets, microcollection tubes, and micropipets with dilution systems. Some containers are designated for a specific test and others serve multiple purposes. The type of container chosen is usually related to laboratory preference, as advantages and disadvantages can be associated with each system.

Capillary Tubes

Capillary tubes are small glass tubes used to collect approximately 50 to 75 μL of blood for the primary purpose of performing a microhematocrit test. They are frequently referred to as microhematocrit tubes. The tubes are designed to fit into a hematocrit centrifuge and its corresponding hematocrit reader. Tubes are available plain or coated with ammonium heparin, and are color-coded, with a red band for heparinized tubes and a blue band for plain tubes. Heparinized tubes should be used for hematocrits collected by dermal puncture, and plain tubes are used when the test is being performed on previously anticoagulated blood. When sufficient blood has been collected, the end of the capillary tube that has not been used to collect the specimen is closed by embedding it in a clay sealant designated for use with the tubes.

Use of microhematocrit tubes to collect plasma or serum requires breaking the tube after centrifugation; extreme care must be used, as the fragile tubes may shatter or produce jagged edges that could puncture the person working with them. Likewise phlebotomists should use extreme care to prevent breakage when collecting specimens and sealing the tubes.

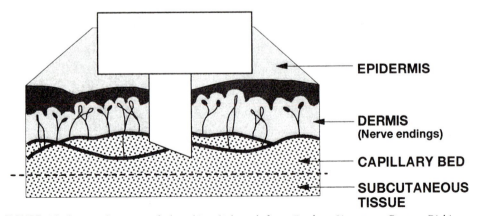

EPIDERMIS

DERMIS
(Nerve endings)

CAPILLARY BED

SUBCUTANEOUS
TISSUE

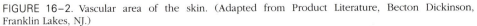

FIGURE 16–2. Vascular area of the skin. (Adapted from Product Literature, Becton Dickinson, Franklin Lakes, NJ.)

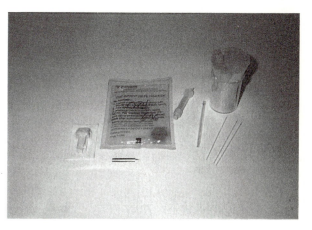

FIGURE 16–3. Microspecimen equipment.

Micropipets

Larger capillary tubes, called Caraway or Natelson pipets, are used when tests other than a microhematocrit are requested. The pipets have a tapered end for specimen collection and fill by capillary action. Pipet lengths vary from 75 mm for Caraway pipets to 150 mm for Natelson pipets. The capacity varies from 330 to 470 μL in Caraway pipets to 220 to 420 μL in Natelson pipets. Pipets are available plain or with ammonium heparin and are color-coded respectively with blue or red bands. After collection of the sample, the nontapered ends are sealed with specifically matched soft plastic caps or clay sealant.

For collection of serum or plasma, the tubes are centrifuged by carefully balancing them in cushioned centrifuge carriers. Serum or plasma can be removed by inserting a syringe needle into the tapered end and slowly drawing the specimen away from the red cells. Serum, plasma, or cells can also be collected by breaking the tube after centrifugation. This is done by scratching the tube with a file (scoring) just above the cell layer, holding the tube away from the body and carefully breaking it.

Microcollection Tubes

Plastic collection tubes such as the Microtainer (Becton Dickinson, Franklin Lakes, NJ) provide a larger collection volume and present no danger from broken glass. A variety of anticoagulants and additives, including separator gel, are available and the tubes are color-coded in the same way as vacuum tubes. As shown in Figure 16–3, the tubes are supplied with a capillary scoop collector top that is replaced by a color-coded plastic sealer top after the specimen is collected. Mixing of anticoagulated specimens is enhanced by the presence of small plastic beads in the collection tube. Microtainer tubes are designed to hold approximately 600 μL of blood, and separation is achieved by centrifugation in specifically designed centrifuges.

Micropipet and Dilution System

The Unopette System (Becton Dickinson, Franklin Lakes, NJ) is designed for tests that can be performed on diluted whole blood, primarily hematology tests. The system consists of a sealed plastic reservoir containing a measured amount of diluent, a calibrated glass capillary pipet in a plastic holder, and a plastic pipet shield. The amount and type of diluent and the size of the capillary pipet correspond to the specific test to be run. Pipets are designed to collect only the amount of blood for which they are calibrated.

The procedure for use of the Unopette System is shown in Figure 16–4A to C and includes:

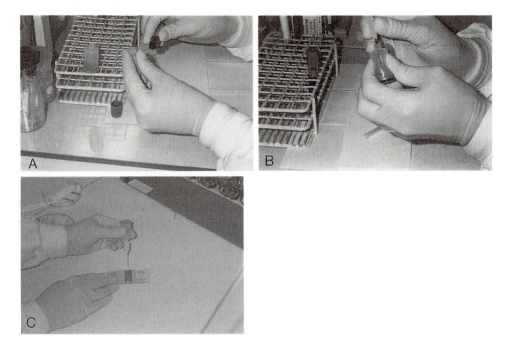

FIGURE 16–4. Unopette procedure. *A*, Filling the capillary pipet. *B*, Transferring blood to diluent. *C*, Loading diluted blood into a hemocytometer.

1 Puncturing the diaphragm of the reservoir with the point of the pipet shield
2 Filling the capillary pipet and wiping excess blood from the outside
3 Slightly squeezing the reservoir
4 Placing the index finger over the opening in the pipet holder and inserting the pipet into the reservoir
5 Releasing pressure on the reservoir and removing the finger from the holder opening to cause blood to be drawn into the diluent
6 Carefully rinsing the pipet by squeezing the reservoir without overflowing the pipet
7 Placing the index finger over the opening and inverting the reservoir to mix

Additional Dermal Puncture Supplies

Alcohol pads, sterile gauze, and sharps containers are required for the dermal puncture just as they are for the venipuncture. Blood smears used for the white blood cell differential and the examination of red blood cell morphology must be made during the dermal puncture procedure and require a supply of glass slides. Phlebotomists prepare these slides using the procedure discussed in Chapter 17.

As discussed previously, warming the puncture site increases blood flow to the area. This can be accomplished by using warm washcloths or towels, or a commercial heel warmer. A heel warmer is a packet containing sodium thiosulfate and glycerin that produces heat when the chemicals are mixed together by gentle squeezing of the packet. The packet should be wrapped in a towel and held away from the face during the initial activation. After heat is produced, the towel-covered packet is held against the puncture site for 3 to 5 minutes.

DERMAL PUNCTURE PROCEDURE

Many of the procedures associated with the venipuncture also apply to the dermal puncture; therefore major emphasis in this chapter will be on the techniques and complications that are unique to the dermal puncture.

Phlebotomist Preparation

Prior to performing a dermal puncture, the phlebotomist must have a requisition form containing the same information required for the venipuncture. When a specimen is collected by dermal puncture this must be noted on the requisition form because, as discussed above, the concentration of some analytes differs between venous and capillary blood.

Due to the variety of puncture devices and collection containers available for dermal puncture, phlebotomists should carefully examine the information on the requisition form to ensure that they have the appropriate equipment to collect all required specimens as well as the skin puncture device that corresponds to the age of the patient.

Phlebotomists frequently perform dermal punctures in the nursery and must observe its specified isolation procedures, such as the wearing of gowns and gloves, extensive handwashing, and carrying only the necessary equipment to the patient area. At all times equipment should be kept out of reach of the patient.

Patient Identification and Preparation

Patients for dermal puncture must be identified using the same procedures used for venipuncture (requisition form, verbal identification, and ID band). In the nursery an identification band *must* be present on the infant and not just on the bassinet. Verbal identification of pediatric outpatients may have to be obtained from the parents.

Approaching pediatric patients can be difficult, and the phlebotomist must present a friendly, confident appearance while explaining the procedure to the child and the parents. Do not say the procedure will not hurt, and explain the necessity of remaining very still.

Parents should be given the choice of staying with the child or leaving the room. If they choose to stay they may be asked to assist in holding and comforting the child. Very agitated children may need to have their legs and free hand restrained. This can be accomplished by a parent or coworker, or by confining the child in a blanket or commercially available papoose-style wrap. If a restraint is used, parental consent must be obtained and documented in the patient's medical record.

When necessary the finger or heel from which the sample is to be taken may be warmed. This is most commonly required for patients with very cold fingers, for heel sticks to collect multiple samples, and for the collection of capillary blood gases. Warming is performed by moistening a towel with warm water (40°C), or by activating a commercial heel warmer and covering the site for 3 to 5 minutes.

Site Selection

As mentioned in the discussion of skin puncture devices, a primary danger in dermal puncture is accidental contact with the bone followed by infection (osteomyelitis). This can be avoided by selection of puncture sites that provide sufficient distance between the skin and the bone. The primary dermal puncture sites are the heel and the distal segments of the third and fourth fingers. The plantar surface of the large toe is also acceptable. Performing dermal punctures on earlobes is usually not recommended. The choice of a puncture area is based on the age and size of the patient.

Areas selected for dermal puncture should not be callused, scarred, bruised, edematous, or infected. Punctures should *never* be made through previous puncture sites as this can easily introduce microorganisms into the puncture and allow them to reach the bone.

Heel Puncture Sites

The heel is used for dermal punctures on infants less than 1 year of age because it contains more tissue than the fingers and has not yet become callused from walking.

Acceptable areas for heel puncture are shown in Figure 16-5 and are described as the medial and lateral areas of the **plantar** (bottom) surface of the heel. Notice that these areas can be determined by drawing imaginary lines extending back from the middle of the large toe and from between the fourth and fifth toes. It is in these areas that the distance between the skin and the **calcaneus** (heel bone) is greatest. The short distance between the back (posterior curvature) of the heel and the calcaneus (Fig. 16-5) is the reason why this area is never acceptable for heel puncture.

Punctures should not be performed in other areas of the foot, and particularly not in the arch, where they may cause damage to nerves and tendons. In larger infants the plantar surface of the large toe may be used.

Finger Puncture Sites

Finger punctures are performed on adults and children over 1 year of age. Fingers of infants less than 1 year old may not contain enough tissue to prevent contact with the bone.

The fleshy areas located near the center of the third and fourth fingers on the **palmar** side are the sites of choice for finger puncture (Fig. 16-6). Because the tip and sides of the finger contain only about half the tissue mass of the central area, the possibility of bone injury is increased in these areas. Problems associated with use of

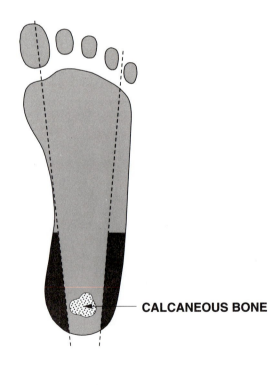

CALCANEOUS BONE

■ PUNCTURE ZONE

FIGURE 16-5. Acceptable heel puncture sites.

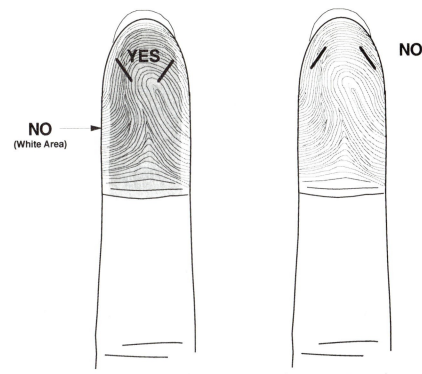

FIGURE 16–6. Acceptable finger puncture sites and correct puncture angle.

the other fingers include possible calluses on the thumb, increased nerve endings in the index finger, and decreased tissue in the fifth finger. Patients who routinely perform home glucose monitoring may request a specific finger and their wishes should be accommodated.

Summary of Dermal Puncture Site Selection

1 Use the medial and lateral areas of the plantar surface of the heel.
2 Use the central fleshy area of the third or fourth fingers.
3 Do not use the back of the heel.
4 Do not use the arch of the foot.
5 Do not puncture through old sites.
6 Do not use areas with visible damage.

Cleansing the Site

The selected site is cleansed with 70% isopropyl alcohol, using a circular motion. The alcohol should be allowed to dry on the skin for antiseptic action and the residue may be removed with a sterile gauze to prevent interference with certain tests. Failure to allow the alcohol to dry will:

1 Cause a stinging sensation for the patient
2 Contaminate the specimen
3 Hemolyze red blood cells
4 Prevent formation of a rounded blood drop because blood will mix with the alcohol and run down the finger

Use of povidone-iodine is not recommended for dermal punctures, as specimen contamination may elevate some test results, including bilirubin, phosphorus, and uric acid.

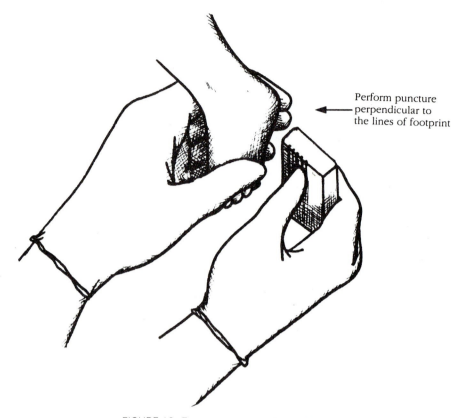

Perform puncture perpendicular to the lines of footprint

FIGURE 16–7. Correct position for heel puncture.

Performing the Puncture

While the puncture is performed, the heel or finger should be well supported and held firmly, without squeezing the puncture area. Massaging the area before the puncture may increase blood flow to the area. The heel is held between the thumb and index finger of the nondominant hand, with the index finger held over the heel and the thumb below the heel (Fig. 16-7). The finger is held between the thumb and index finger with the palmar surface facing up.

Punctures performed with a manual lancet should be made with one continuous motion and automatic devices should be placed firmly on the puncture site. Be sure the device chosen for the puncture corresponds to the size of the patient. As shown in Figure 16-6, the blade of the lancet should be aligned to cut across (perpendicular to) the grooves of the finger or heel print. This will aid in the formation of a rounded drop as the blood will not have a tendency to run into the grooves.

After completing the puncture the lancet should be placed in an appropriate sharps container. A new puncture device must be used if an additional puncture is required.

Specimen Collection

Prior to beginning the blood collection the first drop of blood must be wiped away with a sterile gauze. This will prevent contamination of the specimen with residual alcohol and tissue fluid released during the puncture. When collecting microspecimens it is important to understand that even a minute amount of contamination can severely affect the sample quality. Therefore blood should be freely flowing from the puncture site as a result of firm pressure and should not be obtained by milking of the surrounding tissue, which will release tissue fluid. The most satisfactory blood flow is obtained by alternately applying and releasing pressure to the area. Tightly squeezing the area with no relaxation cuts off blood flow to the puncture site.

Because collection containers fill by capillary action, the collection tip can be lightly touched to the drop of blood and the blood will be drawn into the container. Collection devices should not touch the puncture site and should not be scraped over the skin, as this will produce specimen contamination and hemolysis. Fingers are positioned slightly downward but with the palmar surface facing down during the collection procedure (Fig. 16 – 8).

To prevent the introduction of air bubbles, capillary tubes and micropipets are held horizontally while being filled. The presence of air bubbles limits the amount of blood that can be collected per tube and will interfere with blood gas determinations and tests performed with Unopettes. When the tubes are filled they are sealed with sealant clay or designated plastic caps.

Microcollection tubes are slanted down during the collection, and blood is allowed to run through the capillary collection scoop and down the side of the tube. Gently tapping the bottom of the tube may be necessary to force blood to the bottom. When a tube is filled, the scoop is removed and the color-coded top attached. Tubes with anticoagulants should be inverted 8 to 10 times.

Order of Draw

The order of draw for collecting multiple specimens from a dermal puncture is important because of the tendency of platelets to accumulate at the site of a wound. Therefore, tests for the evaluation of platelets, such as the blood smear, platelet count and CBC, must be collected first. The blood smear should be made first, followed by the Unopette Platelet System or the lavender top Microtainer, and then the specimens for other tests.

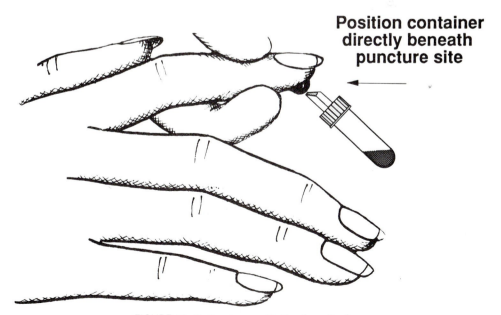

Position container directly beneath puncture site

FIGURE 16–8. Specimen collection from the finger.

When sufficient blood has been collected, pressure is applied to the puncture site with a sterile gauze. The finger or heel is elevated and pressure is applied until the bleeding stops.

Bandages are not used for children under 2 years old because they may remove them, place them in their mouths, and possibly aspirate them. Adhesive may also cause irritation to sensitive skin.

Labeling the Specimen

Microsamples must be labeled with the same information required for venipuncture specimens. Labels can be wrapped around microcollection tubes or groups of capillary pipets. For transport, capillary pipets are then placed in a large tube, because the outside of the capillary pipets may be contaminated with blood. This procedure also helps to prevent breakage.

Completion of the Procedure

The dermal puncture procedure is completed in the same manner as the venipuncture; this includes disposing of all used materials in appropriate containers, removing gloves, washing hands, and thanking the patient and the parents for their cooperation.

All special handling procedures associated with venipuncture specimens also apply to microspecimens. Microspecimens are frequently ordered STAT.

To prevent excessive removal of blood from small infants, many nurseries have a log sheet for documenting the amount of blood collected each time a procedure is requested. The phlebotomist should record the amount of blood collected on the log sheet prior to leaving the area.

If the phlebotomist fails to collect a sufficient amount of blood after performing two punctures, the nursing station should be notified and another phlebotomist should be asked to complete the procedure.

Summary of Dermal Puncture Technique

1   Obtain and examine the requisition form.
2   Assemble equipment and supplies.
3   Greet the patient and the parents.
4   Identify the patient.
5   Position the patient and the parents.
6   Put on gloves.
7   Organize equipment and supplies.
8   Select the puncture site.
9   Warm the puncture site if necessary.
10   Cleanse and dry the puncture site.
11   Perform the puncture.
12   Wipe away the first drop of blood.
13   Make blood smears if requested.
14   Collect the hematology specimen and then other specimens.
15   Mix the specimens if necessary.
16   Apply pressure.
17   Dispose of the puncture device.
18   Label the specimens.
19   Perform appropriate specimen handling.
20   Thank the patient and parents.
21   Dispose of used supplies.
22   Remove and dispose of gloves.
23   Wash hands.

24 Complete any required paperwork.

25 Deliver specimens to the appropriate locations.

BIBLIOGRAPHY

National Committee for Clinical Laboratory Standards Approved Standard H4-A3: Procedures for the Collection of Diagnostic Blood Specimens by Skin Puncture. NCCLS, Villanova, PA, 1991.

National Committee for Clinical Laboratory Standards Approved Guideline H14-A2: Devices for the Collection of Skin Puncture Blood Specimens. NCCLS, Villanova, PA, 1990.

Study Questions

1. List six possible complications associated with femoral puncture in infants.

   a. _____

   b. _____

   c. _____

   d. _____

   e. _____

   f. _____

2. Daily collection of 3 mL of blood from a premature infant may produce

   _____.

3. Why are dermal punctures often performed on (a) patients receiving chemotherapy, (b) geriatric patients, and (c) diabetic patients?

   a. _____

   b. _____

   c. _____

4. State a major concern when collecting a specimen for potassium and bilirubin by dermal puncture.

   _____

5. Describe the composition of capillary blood.

   _____

   _____

6. Can dermal puncture and venipuncture collections be alternated on a patient receiving 4-hour H & H tests? Why?

   _____

   _____

7. The maximum length of a puncture device used on the heel is

   _____.

8. True or False. Surgical blades should be used when collecting more than 100 μL of blood.

9. The location of the major vascular area of the skin is _____ .

10. Which is more important for producing adequate blood flow, the width or depth of the puncture? _____

11. Collection of a microhematocrit by dermal puncture is performed using a tube that is color-coded (red) (blue). Circle one.

Dermal Puncture Exercise

1. A phlebotomist must collect a CBC and a glucose from a diabetic patient with casts on both arms. How could these tests be collected?

_____

_____

2. The phlebotomy supervisor notices that many of the specimens collected by the nurses on the pediatric unit must be collected again because they are hemolyzed. What should the supervisor stress when presenting a continuing education inservice to the nurses?

_____

_____

_____

3. Is it necessary for phlebotomists to have both heparinized and nonheparinized microhematocrit tubes in the collection tray? Why or why not?

_____

_____

4. A manual platelet count is requested on a patient receiving chemotherapy. What would be the most efficient method for collecting this specimen?

_____

5. A very agitated 2-year-old needing a CBC is carried into the outpatient drawing area by his equally agitated mother. How should the phlebotomist handle this situation?

_____

_____

_____

6. A phlebotomy student is having difficulty obtaining rounded drops when performing dermal punctures. What part of the student's technique should the instructor check?

_____

_____

7. After failing to collect a sufficient amount of blood from two dermal punctures, the phlebotomist asks a coworker to complete the collection. What additional technique could the second phlebotomist perform to obtain sufficient blood flow?

_____

8. A phlebotomist delivers a lavender top Microtainer to hematology and two red top Microtainers to chemistry. The hematology supervisor is concerned because the platelet count is much lower than the previous day's count and all other CBC parameters match the previous values. Could the phlebotomy technique have caused this? Why or why not?

_____

_____

9. While selecting a site for a heel puncture, the phlebotomist notices that a previous puncture has been performed on the back of the heel. What should the phlebotomist do?

_____

10. A phlebotomist enters the nursery, performs the specified isolation procedures, checks the infant's name on the bassinet, selects an area on the plantar surface of the heel, cleanses the area with iodine, collects and labels the specimen, and bandages the heel. What is wrong with this scenario?

_____

_____

_____

_____

Evaluation of a Microtainer Collection by Heel Stick

Rating System
2 = Satisfactorily performed
1 = Needs improvement
0 = Incorrect/did not perform

_____ 1. Places collection tray in designated area

_____ 2. Checks requisition and selects necessary equipment

_____ 3. Washes hands, puts on gown

_____ 4. Assembles equipment and carries it to patient

_____ 5. Identifies patient using ID band

_____ 6. Puts on gloves

_____ 7. Warms heel

_____ 8. Selects appropriate puncture site

_____ 9. Cleanses puncture site with alcohol and allows it to air dry

_____ 10. Does not contaminate puncture device

_____ 11. Performs puncture smoothly

_____ 12. Wipes away first drop of blood

_____ 13. Collects rounded drops into lavender Microtainer without scraping

_____ 14. Does not milk site

_____ 15. Collects adequate amount of blood

_____ 16. Mixes Microtainer

_____ 17. Cleanses site and applies pressure until bleeding stops

_____ 18. Removes all collection equipment from area

_____ 19. Disposes of puncture device in sharps container

_____ 20. Disposes of used supplies

_____ 21. Labels tube

_____ 22. Removes gloves and washes hands

_____ 23. Removes and disposes of gown

_____ 24. Completes nursery log sheet

Total Points _____

Maximum Points = 48

COMMENTS:

Evaluation of Finger Stick on an Adult Patient

Rating System
2 = Satisfactorily performed
1 = Needs improvement
0 = Incorrect/did not perform

_____ 1. Greets patient and explains procedure

_____ 2. Examines requisition form

_____ 3. Asks patient to state full name

_____ 4. Compares requisition and patient's statement

_____ 5. Organizes and assembles equipment

_____ 6. Selects appropriate finger

_____ 7. Warms finger if necessary

_____ 8. Puts on gloves

_____ 9. Gently massages finger

_____ 10. Cleanses site with alcohol and allows to air dry

_____ 11. Does not contaminate puncture device

_____ 12. Smoothly performs puncture across fingerprint

_____ 13. Wipes away first drop of blood

_____ 14. Collects two microhematocrit tubes without air bubbles

_____ 15. Seals tubes

_____ 16. Cleanses site and asks patient to apply pressure

_____ 17. Labels tubes

_____ 18. Examines site and applies bandage

_____ 19. Thanks patient

_____ 20. Disposes of puncture device in sharps container

_____ 21. Disposes of used supplies

_____ 22. Removes gloves

_____ 23. Washes hands

Total Points _____

Maximum Points = 46

COMMENTS:

Evaluation of Unopette Collection on a 2-Year-Old Child

Rating System
2 = Satisfactorily performed
1 = Needs improvement
0 = Incorrect/did not perform

_____ 1. Greets patient and parent

_____ 2. Examines requisition

_____ 3. Identifies patient using correct verbal ID procedure

_____ 4. Explains procedure to patient and parent

_____ 5. Determines if parent needs/wants to hold patient

_____ 6. Puts on gloves

_____ 7. Organizes equipment

_____ 8. Punctures reservoir diaphragm

_____ 9. Gently massages finger

_____ 10. Cleanses site with alcohol and allows to air dry

_____ 11. Does not contaminate puncture device

_____ 12. Smoothly performs puncture across fingerprint

_____ 13. Wipes away first drop of blood

_____ 14. Removes pipet shield

_____ 15. Completely fills pipet with no air bubbles

_____ 16. Wipes blood from outside of pipet without drawing blood out of the pipet

_____ 17. Places index finger over opening in overflow chamber

_____ 18. Squeezes reservoir

_____ 19. Places pipet firmly into reservoir

_____ 20. Removes index finger and releases reservoir

_____ 21. Rinses pipet by squeezing reservoir

_____ 22. Does not force fluid out of overflow chamber

_____ 23. Places shield on overflow chamber

_____ 24. Mixes container

_____ 25. Cleanses site and applies pressure until bleeding stops

_____ 26. Applies bandage

_____ 27. Labels Unopette

_____ 28. Disposes of puncture device in sharps container

_____ 29. Disposes of used supplies

_____ 30. Thanks patient and parent

_____ 31. Removes gloves and washes hands

Total Points _____

Maximum Points = 62

COMMENTS:

CHAPTER 17

Special Dermal Puncture

Learning Objectives

Upon completion of this chapter, the reader will be able to:

1. Define the terms and abbreviations associated with special dermal puncture procedures.
2. Discuss the necessary precautions for collecting high-quality specimens for neonatal bilirubin tests.
3. Describe the appearance of an acceptable blood smear.
4. List six possible errors in technique that cause unacceptable blood smears.
5. Prepare an acceptable blood smear using the instructions provided.
6. State the purpose of the bleeding time and three reasons why it may be prolonged.
7. Discuss the standardization of the bleeding time since its introduction by Duke and errors in technique that affect test results.
8. Correctly perform a bleeding time following the instructions provided in the text or by the manufacturer of the incision device.
9. Briefly discuss why and how neonatal filter paper screening tests are collected.
10. Discuss the performance of ancillary blood glucose testing including puncture technique and other procedures that must be performed.
11. Perform an ancillary blood glucose test following the manufacturers instructions for the instrument provided.

Terminology

Key Terms	Definition
Feathered edge	Area of the blood smear where the microscopic examination is performed
Panic value	Laboratory test result critical to patient survival
Phenylalanine	Naturally occurring amino acid
Phenylketonuria	Presence of abnormal phenylalanine metabolites in the urine
Plasmodium	Genus of malaria parasites
Platelet plug	Initial blockage of a vascular puncture by platelets
Volar	Pertaining to the palm side of the forearm

Abbreviations	Definition
ABGT	Ancillary blood glucose test
BT	Bleeding time
HDN	Hemolytic disease of the newborn
PKU	Phenylketonuria

Several of the special collection techniques discussed in Chapter 15 also apply to specimens collected by dermal puncture. These include:

1 Collecting of fasting specimens
2 Performing glucose tolerance tests
3 Collecting timed specimens for postprandial glucose (It is recommended that sodium fluoride be used when collecting neonatal glucose tests as the normally high red blood cell count increases glycolysis.)
4 Therapeutic drug monitoring
5 Specimens affected by diurnal variation
6 Specimens that must be warmed or chilled during transport
7 Forensic specimens

Procedures primarily associated with dermal punctures are:

1 The collection of neonatal bilirubins
2 Preparation of blood smears
3 Bleeding time test
4 Collection of neonatal filter paper screening tests
5 Ancillary (bedside) glucose testing

COLLECTION OF NEONATAL BILIRUBINS

One of the most frequently performed tests on newborns measures bilirubin levels, and specimens for this determination are often collected at timed intervals over several days. Bilirubin is a very light-sensitive chemical and is rapidly destroyed when exposed to light.

Increased serum bilirubin in newborns may be caused by the presence of hemolytic disease of the newborn (**HDN**) or it may simply be due to the fact that the liver of newborns (particularly premature infants) is often not developed enough to process the bilirubin produced from the normal breakdown of red blood cells. Bilirubin test results are critical to infant survival and mental health because the blood-brain barrier is not fully developed in neonates, a condition that allows bilirubin to accumulate in the brain and cause permanent or lethal damage. Bilirubin levels reaching 18.0 mg/dL or rising at a rate of 0.5 mg/dL per hour indicate the need for an exchange transfusion.

Phlebotomy technique is critical to the determination of accurate bilirubin results, and specimens must be protected from excess light during and after the collection. Infants that appear jaundiced are frequently placed under an ultraviolet light (bili light) to lower the level of circulating bilirubin. This light must be turned off during specimen collection. Amber-colored Microtainer tubes are available for collecting bilirubins, or if multiple capillary pipets are used, the filled tubes should be shielded from light. Hemolysis must be avoided; it will falsely lower bilirubin results in some procedures and must be corrected for in others. Also, specimens must be collected at the specified time so that the rate of bilirubin increase can be determined.

PREPARATION OF BLOOD SMEARS

Blood smears are needed for the microscopic examination of blood cells that is performed for the differential part of the CBC, for special staining procedures, and for the reticulocyte count. Phlebotomists must make smears when one of these tests is ordered and a dermal puncture is performed. When specimens are collected by venipuncture the smear is usually made in the laboratory from the EDTA tube, and some laboratories have automated instruments for smear preparation. Performing smears at the bedside following a venipuncture may sometimes be necessary to ensure a fresh smear. However, this can be dangerous, as blood must be forced from the needle onto the slide and the needle cannot be disposed of until the smear has been made. Also blood smears must be considered infectious until they have been fixed with alcohol in the laboratory, and gloves must be worn when handling them. Carrying numerous smears in a crowded collection tray can cause contamination of equipment and ungloved hands.

Learning to prepare an acceptable blood smear requires considerable practice and can be a source of frustration for beginning phlebotomists; however, once the technique is mastered, it is seldom that an acceptable smear is not achieved on the first attempt. The technique for preparing a blood smear is described here and illustrated in Figure 17–1 and Figure 17–2.

1 Obtain three clean glass slides and perform the dermal puncture in the manner discussed in Chapter 16. Be sure to wipe away the first drop of blood.
2 Place the second drop of blood in the center of a glass slide approximately 0.5 to 1 inch from the end, or just below the frosted end, by lightly touching the drop with the slide. The drop should be 1 to 2 mm in diameter.
3 Immediately place the slide in one of the positions shown in Figure 17–2. Choose the one that works best for you.
4 Place a second slide (spreader slide) with a clean smooth edge in front of the drop at a 25- to 30-degree angle inclined over the blood.
5 Draw the spreader slide back to the edge of the drop of blood, allowing the blood to spread across the end.
6 When blood is evenly distributed across the spreader slide, lightly push the spreader slide forward with a continuous movement all the way past the end of the smear slide. Be sure to maintain the 25- to 30-degree angle and not to apply pressure to the spreader slide.
7 Place the slide in an area where it can dry undisturbed and repeat the procedure for the second smear.
8 Smears collected on slides with frosted ends are labeled by writing the patient information on the frosted area with a pencil. Labels containing the appropriate information are attached to the thick end of smear slides that do not have frosted ends.

A properly prepared blood smear has a smooth film of blood that covers approximately one half to two thirds of the slide, does not contain ridges or holes, and has a lightly **feathered edge** without streaks. The microscopic examination is performed in the area of the feathered edge because here the cells have been spread

BLOOD SMEAR PREP

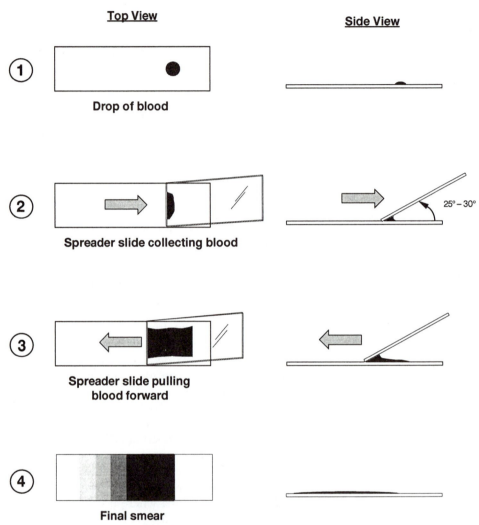

FIGURE 17–1. Preparation of a blood smear.

into a single layer. An uneven smear indicates that the cells are not evenly distributed; therefore, test results will not be truly representative of the patient's blood. Errors in technique that result in an unacceptable specimen are summarized in Table 17–1.

BLOOD SMEARS FOR MALARIA

The parasites (*Plasmodium* species) that cause malaria invade the red blood cells and their presence is detected by microscopic examination of thick and thin blood

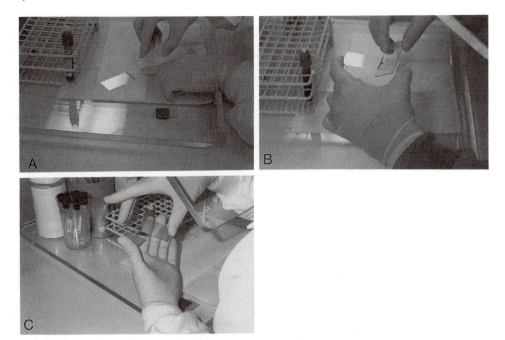

FIGURE 17–2. Examples of slide positioning for blood smear preparation.

smears. Patients with malaria exhibit periodic episodes of fever and chills related to the multiplication of the parasites within the red blood cells. Therefore, specimen collection is frequently requested on a STAT or timed basis similar to that of blood cultures. Smears may be prepared from EDTA anticoagulated blood, or at the bedside following dermal puncture.

Thin smears (two or three) are prepared in the manner previously described. Thick smears are made by placing a large drop of blood in the center of a glass slide and then using the corner of another glass slide to spread the blood into a circle about the size of a dime. The smear must be allowed to dry for at least 2 hours prior to staining. Thick smears concentrate the specimen for detection of the parasites, and thin smears are then examined for parasitic morphology and identification.

TABLE 17–1. **EFFECT OF TECHNICAL ERRORS ON BLOOD SMEARS**

Discrepancy	Possible Cause
Uneven distribution of blood (ridges)	Pressure on the spreader slide
	Movement of the spreader slide not continuous
Holes in the smear	Dirty slide
No feathered edge	Spreader slide not pushed the entire length of the smear slide
Streaks in the feathered edge	Chipped or dirty spreader slide
	Spreader slide not placed flush against the smear slide
	Pulling the spreader slide into the drop of blood so that the blood is pushed instead of pulled
Smear too thick and long	Drop of blood is too big
	Angle of spreader slide is greater than 30°
Smear too thin and short	Drop of blood is too small
	Angle of spreader slide is less than 25°

BLEEDING TIME

The bleeding time (**BT**) is performed to measure the time required for platelets to form a plug strong enough to stop bleeding from an incision. The length of the bleeding time is increased when the platelet count is low, in platelet disorders that affect the ability of the platelets to stick to each other and for the incision to form a plug, and in persons taking medications that contain aspirin. Test results can also be affected by the type and condition of the patient's skin, vascularity, temperature, and the phlebotomist's technique. Therefore the bleeding time is considered a screening test, and abnormal results are followed by additional testing. Bleeding times are frequently ordered as part of a presurgical workup.

Measurement of the bleeding time was first introduced by Duke in 1910 and was performed by timing the length of bleeding from a lancet puncture of the ear-lobe. The Duke method is not as well standardized as current methods; however, it may occasionally be requested in special situations.

Standardization of the bleeding time began in 1941 when Ivy modified the Duke method by performing the incision on the **volar** surface of the forearm and inflating a blood pressure cuff to 40 mm Hg to control blood flow to the area. These modifications are still a part of the bleeding time procedure. In 1969 Mielke introduced a plastic template, used with a surgical blade rather than a lancet, to control the length and depth of the incision. Automated disposable incision devices, such as the Simplate-R and Simplate-IIR (Organon Teknika Corp, Durham, NC) and Surgicutt (International Technidyne, Edison, NJ), that produce standardized incisions of 1 mm in depth and 5 mm in length have now replaced the original template method.

Steps in performing the bleeding time using an automated device are:

1 Identify the patient following routine protocol.
2 Explain the procedure to the patient, including the possibility of leaving a small scar, and obtain information about any prescribed or over-the-counter medications, particularly aspirin, that may have been taken in the last 7 to 10 days. Many medications contain salicylate (aspirin); therefore, the contents of any medication mentioned by the patient should be checked prior to performing the test, and if salicylate has been taken the physician should be notified.
3 Place the patient's arm on a steady surface with the volar surface facing up.
4 Select an area, approximately 5 cm below the antecubital crease and in the middle of the arm, that is free of surface veins, scars, bruises, and edema.
5 Cleanse the area with alcohol and allow it to dry.
6 Place a blood pressure cuff on the upper arm.
7 Remove the incision device from its package and release the safety lock, being careful not to touch the blade area.
8 Inflate the blood pressure cuff to 40 mm Hg. This pressure must be maintained throughout the procedure.
9 Place the incision device firmly, but without making an indentation, on the arm and position it so that the incision will be horizontal (parallel to the antecubital crease) (Fig. 17–3). In adults, horizontal incisions are slightly more sensitive to hemorrhagic disorders and are less likely to leave a scar, whereas in newborns a vertical incision is preferable for the same reasons.
10 Depress the trigger and simultaneously start a stopwatch and then remove the incision device.
11 After 30 seconds remove the blood that has accumulated on the incision by gently "wicking" it onto a circle of Whatman No. 1 filter paper or Surgicutt

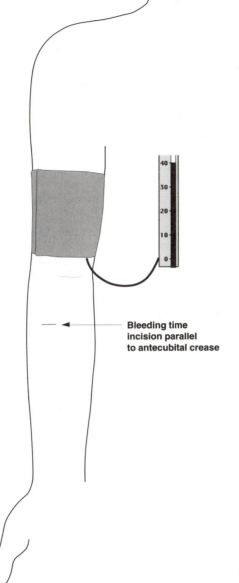

Bleeding time incision parallel to antecubital crease

FIGURE 17–3. Template bleeding time procedure.

Bleeding Time Blotting Paper (International Technidyne, Edison, NJ) (Fig. 17–4). Do not touch the incision as this will disturb formation of the **platelet plug** and prolong the bleeding time.

12 Continue to remove blood from the incision in the manner described every 30 seconds until the bleeding stops.

13 Record the time on the stopwatch to the nearest 30 seconds.

14 Deflate and remove the blood pressure cuff.

15 Clean the patient's arm, apply a butterfly bandage to tightly hold the edges of the incision together, and cover this with a regular bandage. Instruct the patient to leave the bandages on for 24 hours.

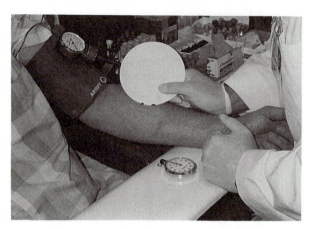

FIGURE 17-4. Wicking of blood during the bleeding time procedure.

16 Depending on the method and device used, normal bleeding times range from 2 to 10 minutes. The test can be discontinued after 20 minutes and reported as greater than 20 minutes.

NEONATAL SCREENING

Screening of newborns for 50 inherited metabolic disorders can currently be performed from blood collected by heel stick and placed on specially designed filter paper. Most states have laws requiring the screening of newborns for the presence of the most prevalent disorders: **phenylketonuria (PKU)**, which is caused by the lack of the enzyme needed to metabolize **phenylalanine**, and hypothyroidism. Both disorders produce severe mental retardation, but this can be avoided by changes in diet and the use of medication if they are detected within the first few weeks of life. Routine screening is not usually performed for other disorders, but they may be requested when symptoms or family history indicates a need or when state law requires a more extensive battery of neonatal tests.

The filter paper blood screening test for PKU utilizes bacterial growth to determine the presence or absence of phenylalanine in the blood. The blood-impregnated filter paper disks are placed on culture media containing bacteria and the media is then observed for bacterial growth, as shown in Figure 17-5. Hypothyroidism is detected by performing immunochemical analysis of the dried blood.

It can be understood from this brief explanation of the bacterial testing procedure that correct collection of the blood specimen is critical for accurate test results. Special collection kits consisting of a patient information form attached to specifically designed filter paper that has been preprinted with an appropriate number of 0.5-inch-diameter circles are used. The filter paper and the ink must be biologically inactive and approved by the Food and Drug Administration. The phlebotomist must be careful not to touch or contaminate the area inside the circles or to touch the dried blood spots.

The heel stick is performed in the routine manner and the first drop of blood is wiped away. A large drop of blood is then applied directly into a filter paper circle. To obtain an even layer of blood only one drop should be used to fill a circle. Blood is applied to only one side of the filter paper and there must be enough to soak

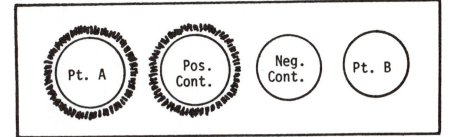

FIGURE 17–5. Sample bacterial inhibition test. (From Strasinger, SK: Urinalysis and Body Fluids, ed. 3. FA Davis, Philadelphia, 1994, p. 119, with permission.)

through the paper and be visible on the other side. As shown in Figure 17–6, if a circle is not evenly or completely filled a new circle and a larger drop of blood should be used. The collected specimen must be allowed to air dry in a suspended horizontal position, at room temperature, and away from direct sunlight. To prevent cross-contamination, specimens should not be stacked during or after the drying process.

Collection of blood in heparinized capillary pipets and then immediate transfer to the filter paper circles is an acceptable but not recommended technique. Each circle requires 100 μL of blood, which must be added without scratching or denting the filter paper with the capillary tip.

The dorsal hand vein collection technique is also acceptable for filter paper collections. This technique can be used to collect specimens from a superficial hand vein directly into appropriate microspecimen containers. A short, 21- to 23-gauge needle with a clear hub is inserted into the vein and blood drips from the hub of the needle into the collection container. Use of this technique requires additional training and is an institutional decision, as saving all veins for IV therapy may be preferred.

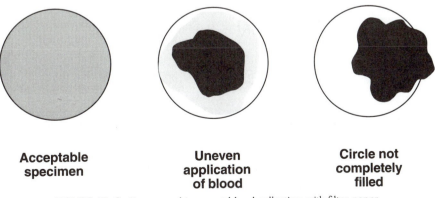

Acceptable specimen   **Uneven application of blood**   **Circle not completely filled**

FIGURE 17–6. Correct and incorrect blood collection with filter paper.

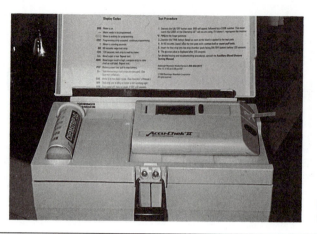

FIGURE 17–7. Instrument used to perform bedside glucose testing.

ANCILLARY (BEDSIDE) BLOOD GLUCOSE TEST

The development of small, handheld instruments capable of measuring blood glucose levels from a drop of blood applied to a paper reagent strip (Fig. 17–7) allows glucose levels to be measured at the bedside by phlebotomists, other medical staff, and even the patients themselves.

Institutional protocol specifies which personnel may perform bedside testing, and these persons must receive training and demonstrate proficiency prior to performing patient tests. Many slightly different types of glucose analyzers are available and the specific manufacturers' instructions must be followed. The phlebotomist must also know about possible sources of test error, understand and perform appropriate maintenance and quality control of the instrument and quality control of the reagent strips, as well as document all actions taken.

The dermal puncture is performed according to routine procedure; however, currently some manufacturers do not recommend wiping away the first drop of blood. The appropriate area of the reagent strip is covered with blood by lightly touching it to a large hanging drop of blood. Care must be taken not to contaminate the testing area by rubbing it against the patient's skin or touching the pad prior to collection. Reagent strips must be stored in tightly closed containers and should not be used if they appear discolored or are past their expiration date.

Test results appear on the analyzer screen and are recorded in the appropriate place by the phlebotomist. The phlebotomist must be aware of values that the institution has determined to be critically high or low (**panic values**) and immediately report them to the nursing staff or physician.

BIBLIOGRAPHY

Brown, BA: Hematology: Principles and Procedures, ed. 6. Lea & Febiger, Philadelphia, 1992.

Buchanan, GR, and Holtkamp, CA: A comparative study of variables affecting the bleeding time using two disposable devices. Am J Clin Pathol, 9(1), 1989.

Clagg, ME: Venous sample collection from neonates using dorsal hand veins. Lab Med, April, 1989.

Henry, JB: Clinical Diagnosis and Management by Laboratory Methods. WB Saunders, Philadelphia, 1991.

Koepke, JA: Bleeding time test (Tips on Technology). Medical Laboratory Observer, 25(7), 1993.

National Committee for Clinical Laboratory Standards Tentative Guideline C30-T: Ancillary (Bedside) Blood Glucose Testing in Acute and Chronic Care Facilities. NCCLS, Villanova, PA, 1991.

National Committee for Clinical Laboratory Standards Approved Standard LA4-A2: Blood Collection on Filter Paper for Neonatal Screening Programs. NCCLS, Villanova, PA, 1992.

Study Questions

1. The color code for a Microtainer used to collect a glucose from a newborn should be ———————— .

2. List two reasons for elevated neonatal bilirubins.

   a. ————————————————————————————————

   b. ————————————————————————————————

3. Why are neonatal bilirubins frequently ordered as timed tests?

   ————————————————————————————————————

   ————————————————————————————————————

4. A neonatal bilirubin collected at 0600 is 10.0 mg/dL, the specimen collected at 1800 reads 12.0 mg/dL, and the specimen collected the next morning at 0600 has a value of 5.0 mg/dL.

   a. State an error in phlebotomy technique that could cause the last result.

   ————————————————————————————————————

   b. State a specimen characteristic that could cause the last result.

   ————————————————————————————————————

5. Name two tests that require a blood smear.

   a. ————————————————————————————————

   b. ————————————————————————————————

6. True or False. Unfixed blood smears are a biologic hazard.

7. The proper angle of the spreader slide when preparing a blood smear is ———————————————————— .

8. If the angle of the spreader slide is too large, the blood smear will be too ———————————— and ———————————— .

9. What is the purpose of the feathered edge on a blood smear?

   ————————————————————————————————————

   ————————————————————————————————————

10. A chipped spreader slide will cause ———————————————————— .

11. Why is a blood smear containing ridges or holes considered unacceptable?

   ————————————————————————————————————

   ————————————————————————————————————

12. What laboratory error could occur if only thin smears are prepared for a malaria test?

   ————————————————————————————————————

13. A prolonged bleeding time may be caused by

    a. _____

    b. _____

    c. _____

14. State the basic principle of the bleeding time.

    _____

    _____

    _____

15. True or False. To obtain an accurate bleeding time result, the patient must be given aspirin prior to having the test performed.

16. State the standardizations added to the Duke bleeding time by:

    a. Ivy _____

    b. Mielke _____

17. What is the purpose of "wicking?"

    _____

    _____

18. In adults the bleeding time incision is made (horizontal) (vertical) to the antecubital crease. (Circle one) Why?

    _____

    _____

19. The normal bleeding time is approximately _____ .

20. Name two disorders in which neonatal filter paper tests are frequently used for screening.

    a. _____

    b. _____

21. How should blood collected on a filter paper disk appear?

    _____

    _____

22. State a reason why collecting blood for filter paper testing with a capillary pipet or from a dorsal hand vein may not be recommended.

    a. Capillary pipet _____

    b. Dorsal hand vein _____

23. List seven topics that should be included in an ancillary blood glucose testing training program.

    a. _____

    b. _____

    c. _____

    d. _____

    e. _____

    f. _____

    g. _____

24. State two reasons for discarding a blood glucose reagent strip and obtaining another one.

    a. _____

    b. _____

25. When should ABGT test results be immediately reported to a physician or nurse?

    _____

Special Dermal Puncture Exercise

1. The phlebotomy supervisor is asked to present an inservice to the nurses who collect neonatal bilirubins on the night shift. Specimens are not hemolyzed; however, test results are consistently lower than those of tests collected on the morning and evening shifts.
   What should the supervisor stress?

   _____

2. A phlebotomist collects three Caraway micropipets for a bilirubin, labels a large tube, places the sealed tubes into it and leaves the tube on the counter in chemistry while everyone is at lunch. The chemistry supervisor rejects the specimen.
   Why? How could this have been avoided?

   _____

   _____

   _____

3. In what circumstance might a phlebotomist deliver a blood smear without a feathered edge to the hematology section?

   _____

4. Bleeding times performed by a new employee are consistently prolonged. What part of the employee's technique should the supervisor observe most closely? Why?

   _____

   _____

   _____

5. A phlebotomist performs a bleeding time on an outpatient using correct technique and the result is prolonged. The next day the physician sends the patient back to the laboratory for a repeat test. The phlebotomy supervisor prepares to perform the test, but after talking to the patient stops and calls the physicians' office. The test is canceled.
   What had the first phlebotomist failed to do?

   _____

6. A phlebotomist with requisitions for two bleeding times is gone for 2 hours and returns with results of 40 minutes and 45 minutes. The phlebotomy supervisor tells the phlebotomist to reread the bleeding time procedure in the procedure manual. Why?

   _____

   _____

7. A phlebotomist with a requisition for a bleeding time identifies the patient, checks on medications, selects and chooses an appropriate site, inflates the blood pressure cuff to halfway between the systolic and diastolic pressure, performs the puncture, wipes away the first drop, starts the stopwatch, blots the area with gauze every 30 seconds until the bleeding stops, records the time, and completes the procedure.
   What is wrong with this scenario?

   _____

   _____

   _____

   _____

8. How could failure to wipe away the first drop of blood affect the results of a filter paper PKU?

   _____

   _____

9. A phlebotomist has requisitions for a blood smear and a bleeding time. Can this be accomplished with one puncture? Why or why not?

   _____

   _____

10. A phlebotomist performs a bedside glucose test using correct technique and reports a critically low value. A repeat test by another phlebotomist is normal.
    What did the first phlebotomist fail to do prior to performing the test?

    _____

Evaluation of Blood Smear Preparation

Rating System
2 = Satisfactorily performed
1 = Needs improvement
0 = Incorrect/did not perform

_____ 1. Obtains requisition form

_____ 2. Obtains three clean glass slides

_____ 3. Identifies patient

_____ 4. Puts on gloves

_____ 5. Selects and cleanses an appropriate site and allows it to air dry

_____ 6. Performs puncture

_____ 7. Wipes away first drop

_____ 8. Puts correct size drop on appropriate area of slide

_____ 9. Positions slide

_____ 10. Places spreader slide at correct angle

_____ 11. Pulls spreader slide back to blood drop

_____ 12. Allows blood to spread across spreader slide

_____ 13. Pushes spreader slide evenly forward

_____ 14. Places smear to dry

_____ 15. Collects second smear using correct technique

_____ 16. Labels smears

_____ 17. Smear has feathered edge with no streaks

_____ 18. Blood is evenly distributed

_____ 19. Smear does not have holes

_____ 20. Smear is not too long or too thick

_____ 21. Smear is not too short or too thin

_____ 22. Disposes of equipment and supplies

_____ 23. Removes gloves and washes hands

Total Points _____

Maximum Points = 46

COMMENTS:

NAME _____

Evaluation of Bleeding Time Technique

Rating System
2 = Satisfactorily performed
1 = Needs improvement
0 = Incorrect/did not perform

_____ 1. Obtains requisition form

_____ 2. Identifies patient

_____ 3. Explains procedure to patient

_____ 4. Asks patient about medications

_____ 5. Assembles equipment

_____ 6. Puts on gloves

_____ 7. Positions patient's arm

_____ 8. Selects appropriate site

_____ 9. Cleanses site and allows it to air dry

_____ 10. Puts blood pressure cuff on upper arm

_____ 11. Opens and does not contaminate puncture device

_____ 12. Inflates blood pressure cuff to 40 mm Hg

_____ 13. Correctly aligns puncture device on patient's arm

_____ 14. Simultaneously punctures and starts stopwatch

_____ 15. Quickly removes puncture device

_____ 16. Correctly wicks blood after 30 seconds

_____ 17. Continues wicking every 30 seconds

_____ 18. Recognizes endpoint and discontinues timing

_____ 19. Records stopwatch time

_____ 20. Deflates and removes blood pressure cuff

_____ 21. Cleans patient's arm

_____ 22. Applies butterfly bandage

_____ 23. Applies regular bandage

_____ 24. Instructs patient when to remove bandages

_____ 25. Disposes of equipment and supplies

_____ 26. Removes gloves and washes hands

Total Points _____

Maximum Points = 52

COMMENTS:

NAME _____

Evaluation of Neonatal Filter Paper Collection

Rating System
2 = Satisfactorily performed
1 = Needs improvement
0 = Incorrect/did not perform

_____ 1. Obtains requisition

_____ 2. Performs nursery isolation procedures

_____ 3. Assembles equipment

_____ 4. Identifies patient

_____ 5. Puts on gloves

_____ 6. Selects appropriate heel site

_____ 7. Cleanses site and allows it to air dry

_____ 8. Performs the puncture

_____ 9. Wipes away first blood drop

_____ 10. Evenly fills a circle

_____ 11. Fills all required circles correctly

_____ 12. Does not touch inside of circles or blood spots

_____ 13. Places filter paper in appropriate transport position

_____ 14. Applies pressure until bleeding stops

_____ 15. Disposes of equipment and supplies

_____ 16. Correctly completes all required paperwork

_____ 17. Removes gown and gloves

_____ 18. Washes hands

Total Points _____

Maximum Points = 36

COMMENTS:

Evaluation of Bedside Glucose Testing

Rating System
2 = Satisfactorily performed
1 = Needs improvement
0 = Incorrect/did not perform

_____ 1. Obtains requisition form

_____ 2. Performs instrument quality control

_____ 3. Checks expiration date of reagent strips

_____ 4. Identifies patient

_____ 5. Explains procedure to patient

_____ 6. Assembles equipment and supplies

_____ 7. Puts on gloves

_____ 8. Selects and prepares appropriate site

_____ 9. Removes reagent strip from container and closes container

_____ 10. Does not contaminate reagent strip

_____ 11. Performs puncture

_____ 12. Wipes away first blood drop

_____ 13. Fills appropriate area of reagent strip

_____ 14. Does not touch reagent strip to patient's skin

_____ 15. Correctly operates instrument

_____ 16. Correctly handles and processes reagent strip

_____ 17. Asks patient to apply pressure to site

_____ 18. Records glucose result

_____ 19. Inspects and cleanses site

_____ 20. Applies bandage

_____ 21. Disposes of equipment and supplies

_____ 22. Cleans instrument

_____ 23. Removes gloves and washes hands

_____ 24. States examples of low and high panic values

Total Points _____

Maximum Points = 48

COMMENTS:

CHAPTER 18 Arterial Blood Collection

Learning Objectives

Upon completion of this chapter, the reader will be able to:

1 Define the terms and abbreviations associated with arterial blood collection.
2 Define arterial blood gases and describe their diagnostic function.
3 List the equipment and materials needed to perform arterial punctures and discuss preparation of materials.
4 Define "steady state" and list additional patient information that must be collected when performing blood gas determinations.
5 State four factors that are considered when selecting a site for arterial puncture and name the preferred site.
6 Perform and state the purpose of the Modified Allen Test.
7 Describe the steps in the performance of an arterial puncture.
8 State six technical errors associated with arterial puncture and their effect on the specimen.
9 Discuss six complications of arterial puncture, including their effect on the patient and the precautions taken to avoid them.
10 Describe the collection of capillary blood gases including sources of technical error.

Terminology

Key Terms	Definition
Arteriospasm	Spontaneous constriction of an artery
Blanch	Turn pale
Collateral circulation	Additional vessels supplying circulation to a particular area
Local anesthetic	Substance that paralyses nerve endings in the area of injection
Luer tip	Part of a syringe that attaches to the needle
Magnetic "flea"	Small metal filing
Partial pressure	Concentration of a gas within a particular site
Respiration rate	Number of breaths per minute
Steady state	A 30-minute period of controlled stable oxygen consumption and no physical exercise
Streptokinase	Clot lysis activator
Thrombolytic therapy	Administration of medication to enhance clot lysis
Urokinase	Clot lysis activator
Ventilation device	Apparatus to control the amount of oxygen inhaled

Terminology
Continued

Abbreviations	Definition
ABGs	Arterial blood gases
CBGs	Capillary blood gases
Pco_2	Partial pressure of carbon dioxide
pH	Negative log of the hydrogen ion concentration (less than 7 is acid and above 7 is alkaline)
Po_2	Partial pressure of oxygen
RDS	Respiratory distress syndrome
t-PA	Tissue plasminogen activator

The composition of arterial blood is uniform throughout the body, whereas the composition of venous blood varies as it picks up waste products from different areas of the body. However, because arterial punctures are more uncomfortable and dangerous for the patient and more difficult to perform, laboratories have established normal values for most laboratory tests based on venous blood. Arterial blood is needed for the assessment of blood gases and may also be requested for the measurement of ammonia and lactic acid.

Performing arterial punctures is not a primary duty for phlebotomists, and all institutions require specialized training for personnel who perform them. Training must include learning about the complications associated with arterial puncture, precautions to be taken for patient safety, and specimen handling procedures to prevent alteration of the test results. Personnel trained to perform arterial punctures include physicians, nurses, medical technologists, and respiratory therapists. In many institutions collecting and testing of arterial blood gases (**ABGs**) has become the responsibility of the respiratory therapy department. In institutions where the laboratory performs the testing, phlebotomists may be required to perform the puncture, or to assist the person performing the puncture by preparing and delivering the specimen to the laboratory following special procedures.

To provide phlebotomists with a thorough understanding of arterial punctures, whether or not they are required to perform them, this chapter will cover the equipment, patient preparation, puncture technique, specimen handling, and complications of the procedure. Collection of capillary blood gases (**CBGs**), a procedure routinely performed by phlebotomists, is also covered.

ARTERIAL BLOOD GASES

Testing of ABGs measures the ability of the lungs to exchange oxygen and carbon dioxide by determining the **partial pressure** of oxygen (**Po_2**) and carbon dioxide (**Pco_2**) present in the arterial blood, and the **pH** of the blood. Under normal conditions arterial blood will have a higher Po_2 than Pco_2, because oxygen enters the arterial blood flowing through the lungs and carbon dioxide released from the tissues accumulates in the venous blood. Conditions requiring the measurement of blood gases include chronic obstructive pulmonary disease (COPD), cardiac and respiratory failures, severe shock, lung cancer, diabetic coma, coronary bypass, open heart surgery, and respiratory distress syndrome (**RDS**) in premature infants. Patients requiring blood gas determinations are often critically ill.

ARTERIAL PUNCTURE EQUIPMENT

Arterial blood is collected and transported in specially prepared syringes. Specimens can be introduced directly into blood gas analyzers from the collection syringe as shown in Figure 18-1. This is necessary to protect the specimen from contact with room air. Syringes for the collection of blood gas samples are made of glass or specifically designed gas-impermeable plastic and are fitted with plungers that will move spontaneously due to the arterial pressure rather than requiring manual aspiration. They should be no larger than the volume of specimen required, usually 1 to 3 mL.

The anticoagulant used for blood gases is sodium heparin, which must be present in the syringe when the specimen is collected. Plastic syringes containing the appropriate amount of dried heparin can be purchased, or the syringe can be prepared with liquid heparin just prior to performing the procedure. To heparinize a syringe:

1 Obtain a vial of sodium heparin with a concentration of 1000 IU/mL.
2 Attach a 20-gauge needle to the collection syringe.
3 Cleanse the top of the heparin vial with alcohol.
4 Draw 0.5 to 1.0 mL of heparin into the syringe.
5 Pull the plunger back to expose the area of the syringe that will be in contact with the blood and rotate the syringe so that the entire surface has been heparinized.
6 Remove the 20-gauge needle and replace it with the needle to be used for performing the puncture (usually a 21- to 23-gauge needle with a length of ⅝ to 1½ inches).
7 Hold the syringe with the needle pointing up and expel the air; then point the needle down, expel the excess heparin, and carefully recap the needle.

By expelling the heparin with the needle pointing downward, the space in the needle that would normally contain air contains heparin, so that air cannot be introduced into the specimen. It is important to expel the excess heparin from the syringe barrel because the presence of excess heparin will lower the pH value.

A tightly fitting cap must be available to place on the **Luer tip** of the collection syringe after the needle has been removed. It is also desirable to have a small rubber or plastic block to stick the needle into immediately after it is withdrawn from the patient. This prevents air contamination while the patient is being cared for and until the phlebotomist is free to apply the Luer cap.

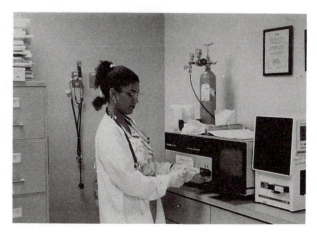

FIGURE 18-1. Technician performing arterial blood gas determination.

A container of crushed ice, or ice and water, is required for maintaining specimen integrity until it can be tested. The container must be large enough to cover the entire blood specimen with the ice and water.

Some institutions administer a **local anesthetic** prior to performing arterial punctures. This requires a 1-mL hypodermic syringe with a 25- or 26-gauge needle containing 0.5 mL of an anesthetic such as lidocaine.

Materials for care of the puncture site include povidone-iodine or chlorhexidene for cleansing the site, alcohol pads to remove the iodine after the procedure is complete, gauze pads to apply pressure to the site, and bandages.

As shown in Figure 18–2 ABG kits containing site care materials, a preheparinized syringe and needle, and syringe caps are available. Materials used for specimen labeling must be waterproof.

ARTERIAL PUNCTURE PROCEDURE

As discussed previously for the venipuncture and the dermal puncture, when an arterial puncture is performed, a requisition containing appropriate information is required, patients must be properly identified, and specimens must be labeled with required information.

Phlebotomist Preparation

After carefully examining the requisition form the phlebotomist must collect all the required equipment, and heparinize the collection syringe (if necessary), and prepare the syringe to administer the local anesthetic. All equipment must be conveniently accessible when the puncture is being performed.

Additional patient information concerning the conditions under which the specimen was obtained must be provided either on the requisition form or a designated ABG form. This includes:

1 Time of collection
2 Patient's temperature
3 Patient's **respiration rate**
4 Amount of oxygen the patient is receiving, specified either as room air or the concentration shown on the oxygen monitor, and the type of **ventilation device** in use
5 Patient activity, such as comatose, agitated, or anesthetized

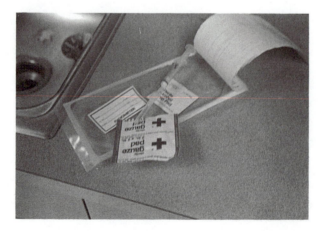

FIGURE 18–2. Arterial blood collection kit.

The patient should have been receiving the specified amount of oxygen and have refrained from exercise for at least 30 minutes prior to obtaining the sample. This is referred to as a **"steady state."**

Patient Preparation

Patients are often apprehensive about arterial punctures and considerable time and care must be taken to reassure them, as an agitated patient will not be in a steady state. Telling the patient that a local anesthetic will be administered after the site has been selected may aid in relaxing an apprehensive patient.

Site Selection

Arterial punctures can be hazardous, a situation that limits the number of acceptable sites. To be acceptable as a puncture site, an artery must be:

1 Large enough to accept at least a 23-gauge needle
2 Located near the skin surface so that deep puncture is not required
3 In an area where injury to surrounding tissues will not be critical
4 Located in an area where other arteries are present to supply blood (**collateral circulation**) in case the punctured artery is damaged

The radial artery located on the thumb side of the wrist and sometimes the brachial artery located near the basilic vein in the antecubital area are the only sites used by phlebotomists. Physicians and specially trained personnel must collect specimens from sites such as the femoral artery, umbilical and scalp veins in infants, and the foot artery (dorsal pedis) in adults. These are also the only personnel authorized to insert and collect specimens from arterial cannulas.

Although it is smaller than the brachial artery, the radial artery is the arterial puncture site of choice because:

1 The ulnar artery can provide collateral circulation to the hand.
2 It lies close to the surface of the wrist and is easily accessible.
3 It can be easily compressed against the wrist ligaments, so that pressure can be applied more effectively on the puncture site after removal of the needle and there is less chance of a hematoma.

In spite of its large size and the presence of adequate collateral circulation, the brachial artery is not routinely used; this is due to its depth, its location near the basilic vein and median nerve, and the fact that it lies in soft tissue that does not provide adequate support for postpuncture pressure.

Modified Allen Test

Prior to performing a radial artery puncture it is essential to determine that the ulnar artery is capable of providing collateral circulation to the hand. Failure to do this could result in loss of the hand or its function.

The Modified Allen Test (Fig. 18–3) is performed as follows:

1 Extend the patient's wrist over a rolled towel and ask the patient to form a fist.
2 Locate the pulses of the radial and ulnar arteries on the palmar surface of the wrist by palpating with the second and third fingers, not the thumb, which has a pulse.
3 Compress both arteries and, while they are occluded, have the patient open and close the fist several times until the palm turns pale (**blanches**).
4 Release pressure on the *ulnar artery only* and watch to see that color returns to the palm. This should occur within 5 seconds if the ulnar artery is functioning.

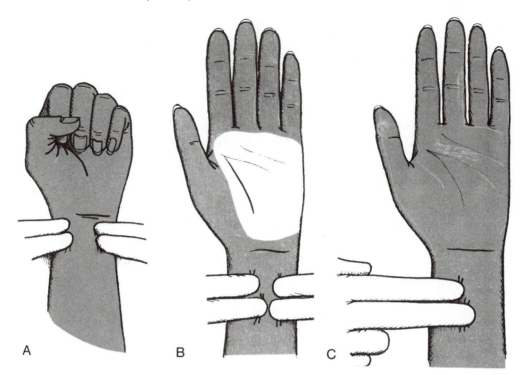

FIGURE 18–3. Modified Allen Test procedure. *A*, Apply pressure to the radial and ulnar arteries while the patient opens and closes the fist. *B*, While applying pressure, look for blanching of the palm. *C*, Release pressure only on the ulnar artery; if color returns to the palm, the test result is positive.

5 If color does not appear (negative Modified Allen Test), the radial artery must not be used. If the Modified Allen Test is positive, proceed with the procedure by palpating the radial artery to determine its depth, direction, and size.

Preparing the Site

The risk of infection is higher in arterial punctures than venipunctures. Therefore, the puncture site is cleansed with alcohol followed by povidone-iodine or chlorhexidene and the area is allowed to air dry. The gloved palpating fingers are cleansed in the same manner.

A local anesthetic may be administered at this time. This is done by injecting a small amount of anesthetic just under the skin, or into the surrounding tissue if the artery is deep. Before injecting the anesthetic, gently pull back on the plunger and check for the appearance of blood, which would indicate that a blood vessel rather than tissue has been entered. Should this happen a new anesthetic syringe must be prepared and a slightly different injection site must be chosen. Allow 2 minutes for the anesthetic to take effect, and if the patient is apprehensive allow him or her to relax for 5 minutes.

Performing the Puncture

Just prior to performing the puncture the artery is relocated with the cleansed finger of the nondominant hand. The finger is placed directly over the area where the needle should enter the artery — not where the needle enters the skin.

The heparinized syringe is held like a dart in the dominant hand and the needle is inserted about 5 to 10 mm below the palpating finger at a 45- to 60-degree angle with the bevel up (Fig. 18–4). The needle is slowly advanced into the artery until

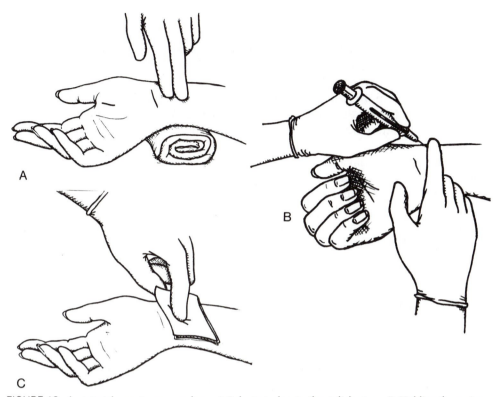

FIGURE 18–4. Arterial puncture procedure. *A*, Palpate to locate the radial artery. *B*, Holding the syringe like a dart, make the puncture at a 45- to 60-degree angle. *C*, Apply firm pressure to the puncture site for 5 minutes.

blood appears in the needle hub. At this time arterial pressure should cause blood to pump into the syringe. If blood does not appear, the needle may be slightly redirected but must remain under the skin. Blood that does not pulse into the syringe and appears dark rather than bright red may be venous blood and should not be used.

When enough blood has been collected, remove the needle and apply firm pressure to the site with a gauze pad. The phlebotomist, not the patient, must apply firm pressure for a minimum of 5 minutes. Arterial punctures are often performed on patients receiving anticoagulant therapy (coumadin or heparin) or **thrombolytic therapy** (tissue plasminogen activator [**t-PA**], **streptokinase**, or **urokinase**). Application of pressure for longer than 5 minutes may be necessary for patients receiving this type of therapy.

With the hand holding the syringe, immediately expel any air that has entered the specimen and stick the end of the needle into the rubber or plastic block to prevent additional exposure to air. Rotate the syringe to mix the anticoagulant with the entire specimen and place the specimen in ice until both hands are free to continue processing the specimen.

After 5 minutes check the patient's arm and, if bleeding has stopped, discontinue the pressure and remove the iodine with alcohol.

Completion of the Procedure

When both hands are free, the syringe is removed from the ice, the needle is discarded in an appropriate container, and the Luer cap is applied to the hub of the syringe. The specimen is labeled and returned to the ice bath.

After pressure has been removed for 2 minutes, the patient's arm is rechecked to be sure a hematoma is not forming, in which case additional pressure is required.

The radial artery is checked for a pulse below the puncture site and the nurse is notified if a pulse cannot be located.

A pressure bandage is applied if no complications are discovered.

In the same manner as discussed with previous phlebotomy procedures, prior to leaving the room the phlebotomist disposes of used materials in appropriate containers, removes gloves and washes hands, and thanks the patient.

Summary of Steps in the Arterial Puncture

1   Obtain a requisition form.
2   Collect equipment.
3   Greet and identify the patient.
4   Explain the procedure and reassure the patient.
5   Obtain metabolic and oxygen therapy information and ensure a steady state.
6   Organize equipment, heparinize the collection syringe, and prepare the anesthetic syringe.
7   Support and hyperextend the patient's wrist.
8   Perform the Modified Allen Test.
9   Put on gloves.
10   Locate and palpate the radial artery.
11   Cleanse the site and the palpating finger.
12   Administer the anesthetic if necessary and wait 2 minutes.
13   Place a cleansed gloved finger over the arterial puncture site.
14   Insert needle, bevel up at a 45- to 60-degree angle 10 to 15 mm below the palpating finger.
15   Allow syringe to fill.
16   Remove needle and apply pressure.
17   Expel any air bubbles from the syringe.
18   Stick needle into rubber block.
19   Roll syringe to mix.
20   Place syringe in ice bath.
21   Maintain pressure on puncture site for 5 minutes.
22   Examine puncture site and remove pressure if bleeding has stopped.
23   Remove needle from syringe and replace with Luer cap.
24   Dispose of needle.
25   Label specimen and return to ice bath.
26   Reexamine puncture site for hematoma formation.
27   Check for a radial pulse below the puncture site.
28   Apply a pressure bandage.
29   Dispose of used materials.
30   Remove gloves and wash hands.
31   Thank the patient.
32   Immediately deliver specimen to the laboratory.

SPECIMEN HANDLING

Arterial specimens are maintained in ice and delivered to the laboratory immediately after collection. Many errors in technique can produce erroneous results. These are summarized in Table 18–1.

TABLE 18–1. **EFFECT OF TECHNICAL ERRORS ON ABG RESULTS**

Technical Error	Effect
Air bubbles present	Atmospheric oxygen enters the specimen and carbon dioxide from the specimen enters the air bubbles
Improper cooling	Blood cells in the specimen continue their metabolism, utilizing oxygen and producing carbon dioxide and acids that lower the pH
Too much heparin	pH is lowered
Too little heparin/inadequate mixing	Clots that interfere with the analyzer are present
Venous rather than arterial sample	Falsely decreased P_{O_2} and increased P_{CO_2}
Improper plastic syringe	Atmospheric and specimen gases diffuse through the plastic

ARTERIAL PUNCTURE COMPLICATIONS

As mentioned previously, the arterial puncture is more dangerous for the patient than the venipuncture. Possible complications include hematoma formation, arteriospasm, thrombosis, hemorrhage, infection, and nerve damage.

Hematomas are more common following arterial puncture because the increased pressure forces blood into the surrounding tissue. Failure of the phlebotomist to maintain pressure for at least 5 minutes and to check the site, use of arteries located in soft tissues where pressure is difficult to apply, and the decrease in elasticity in the arteries of older persons are frequent causes of hematomas.

An **arteriospasm** is a spontaneous, usually temporary, constriction of an artery in response to a sensation such as pain. Closure of the artery prohibits collection of the specimen and prevents oxygen from reaching the tissues, so that tissue destruction and possible gangrene result. This is why the presence of collateral circulation is essential when performing arterial punctures.

Formation of a clot (thrombus) on the inside wall of an artery or vein in response to a puncture hole can produce occlusion of the vessel, particularly if the thrombus continues to grow due to irritation, such as that which may be caused by the continued presence of a cannula. Collateral circulation again becomes important.

Patients with coagulation disorders or receiving anticoagulant or thrombolytic therapy have an increased risk of bleeding following arterial puncture. Puncture of a large artery, such as the femoral, using a large-gauge needle can produce considerable hemorrhaging in these patients.

Failure to adequately cleanse the arterial puncture site, resulting in the introduction of microorganisms into the arterial circulation is more likely to cause infection than if microorganisms are introduced into the venous circulation. In the arterial circulation the organisms are easily carried into many areas of the body without coming in contact with the protective capabilities of the lymphatic system, which runs in close proximity to the venous circulation.

The possibility of nerve damage is greater with arterial puncture due to the need to puncture deeper into the tissue to reach the artery, thereby increasing the possibility of encountering a nerve. As mentioned previously, the brachial artery is located very near the median nerve.

Considering these possible complications it is easy to understand why phlebotomists should only perform arterial punctures after receiving specialized training and when the requisition form indicates an arterial puncture. They should never perform an arterial puncture just because they have been unsuccessful with the venipuncture.

CAPILLARY BLOOD GASES

Performing deep arterial punctures in newborns and young children is usually not recommended; therefore, unless blood can be obtained from umbilical or scalp arteries, blood gases are performed on capillary blood. As discussed in Chapter 6 capillary blood is actually a mixture of venous and arterial blood, with a higher concentration of arterial blood.

Specimens are collected in heparinized blood gas pipets designed to correspond with the volume and sampling requirements of the blood gas analyzer being used. Plugs or sealant clay are needed for both ends of the pipets and a **magnetic "flea"** and circular magnet are used to mix the specimen.

After warming the site to 40°C to 42°C for 5 to 10 minutes to increase the flow of arterial blood, blood is collected using the technique described in Chapter 16. Pipets must be completely filled and must not contain air bubbles. When the pipet is full, one end is immediately sealed, the magnetic flea is inserted into the open end, the round magnet is slipped over the tube and the other end is sealed. The blood is mixed by moving the magnet up and down the tube several times. The tubes are labeled, placed horizontally in an ice bath, and immediately transported to the laboratory.

BIBLIOGRAPHY

Bishop, ML: Clinical Chemistry: Principles, Procedures and Correlations. JB Lippincott, Philadelphia, 1992.

National Committee for Clinical Laboratory Standards Approved Standard H11-A2: Percutaneous Collection of Arterial Blood for Laboratory Analysis. NCCLS, Villanova, PA, 1992.

Shapiro, BA, et al: Clinical Application of Blood Gases. Year Book Medical Publishers, Chicago, 1982.

Study Questions

1. List and define the components of a blood gas analysis.

   _____

   _____

   _____

2. Name three hospital units that frequently order blood gases.

   a. _____

   b. _____

   c. _____

3. Name a hospital department other than the clinical laboratory that may be responsible for collecting and analyzing blood gases.

   _____

4. Why are specimens for ABGs not transferred into anticoagulant tubes after collection?

   _____

5. What special property must be present in plastic syringes used to collect blood gases?

   _____

6. The anticoagulant used for ABGs is _____ .

7. When preparing a syringe for collecting ABGs, why is the needle pointed downward when expelling the anticoagulant?

   _____

   _____

8. List five items of patient information required when collecting ABGs that are not required for routine venipuncture.

   a. _____

   b. _____

   c. _____

   d. _____

   e. _____

9. Why is the presence of collateral circulation important when selecting an arterial puncture site?

   _____

   _____

10. List three reasons why the radial artery is the artery of choice for arterial puncture.

    a. _____

    b. _____

    c. _____

11. List three reasons why the brachial artery is not the artery of choice for arterial punctures.

    a. _____

    b. _____

    c. _____

12. Place the following steps performed in the Modified Allen Test in the correct order, using the numbers 1 to 6.

    a. _____ Patient opens and closes fist several times

    b. _____ Patient opens hand

    c. _____ Ulnar artery is released

    d. _____ Pressure is applied to radial and ulnar arteries

    e. _____ Patient's palm is observed for blanching

    f. _____ Patient's palm is observed for color

13. True or False. When a negative Modified Allen Test is encountered, blood should be collected from the ulnar rather than the radial artery.

14. If a local anesthetic is used in arterial blood collection, when and where is it administered?

    _____

    _____

15. What is the angle of needle insertion for arterial punctures, and why does it differ from the angle used for venipunctures?

    _____

    _____

16. State whether the Po_2 and Pco_2 results will be falsely decreased or increased as a result of the following technical errors.

	Po_2	Pco_2
a. Improper cooling	_____	_____
b. Presence of air bubbles	_____	_____
c. Collection of venous blood	_____	_____

17. State two technical errors that will falsely lower the pH.

    a. _____

    b. _____

18. Match the following complications of arterial puncture with the most possible cause or effect. Complications may be used more than once.

    Cause/Effect

    a. _____ Presence of an arterial cannula

    b. _____ Pressure applied to the site for 2 minutes

    c. _____ Patient receiving t-PA

    d. _____ Gangrene of the fingers

    e. _____ Use of the brachial artery

    f. _____ Failure to cleanse the palpating finger

    g. _____ Inability to obtain a radial pulse after the puncture

    Complication

    1. Hematoma

    2. Arteriospasm

    3. Thrombosis

    4. Hemorrhage

    5. Infection

19. Name two pieces of equipment used when collecting capillary blood gases that are not used with other dermal or arterial punctures. What is their purpose?

    Equipment   **Purpose**

    a. _____   _____

    b. _____   _____

20. Why must the site for collection of capillary blood gases be warmed prior to specimen collection?

    _____

Arterial Puncture Exercise

1. Arterial blood gases are requested on a patient who has just been transported back to the room from radiology and reconnected to the bedside ventilator. When should the phlebotomist collect the specimen? Why?

   _____

   _____

2. How would failure to stick the needle into a rubber block and rotate the specimen immediately after collection affect the specimen?

   _____

   _____

3. When performing an arterial puncture the phlebotomist notices that the blood is not pulsating into the syringe.

   a. What other observation should the phlebotomist make?

   _____

   b. Should the phlebotomist be concerned?

   _____

   c. Why or why not?

   _____

4. When performing a venipuncture in the antecubital area, the phlebotomist notices that the blood is pulsating into the evacuated tube.

   a. What other observation should the phlebotomist make?

   _____

   b. What blood vessel may have been punctured?

   _____

   c. What additional precautions should the phlebotomist take to protect the patient?

   _____

5. A phlebotomist has difficulty collecting a capillary blood gas specimen from a very agitated pediatric patient. After 30 minutes the phlebotomist is able to mix two partially filled tubes and place them on ice.

a. State four errors in this scenario.

_____

_____

_____

_____

b. What course of action should be taken?

_____

Evaluation of Modified Allen Test Performance

Rating System

2 = Satisfactorily performed
1 = Needs improvement
0 = Incorrect/did not perform

_____ 1. Explains procedure to patient

_____ 2. Extends patient's wrist

_____ 3. Asks patient to make a fist

_____ 4. Locates radial and ulnar arteries using appropriate fingers

_____ 5. Compresses both arteries

_____ 6. Asks patient to open and close fist several times

_____ 7. Looks for blanching of patient's palm

_____ 8. Tells patient to leave hand open

_____ 9. Releases pressure on the ulnar artery only

_____ 10. Observes color of patient's palm

_____ 11. States if the test is positive or negative

_____ 12. Explains the significance of the test result

Total Points _____

Maximum Points = 24

COMMENTS:

NAME _____

Evaluation of Arterial Puncture Technique

Rating System

2 = Satisfactorily performed
1 = Needs improvement
0 = Incorrect/did not perform

_____ 1. Obtains requisition form

_____ 2. Assembles equipment

_____ 3. Identifies patient

_____ 4. Explains procedure to the patient

_____ 5. Determines that patient is in a steady state

_____ 6. Obtains metabolic and oxygen therapy information

_____ 7. Organizes equipment

_____ 8. Heparinizes collection syringe

_____ 9. Prepares anesthetic syringe

_____ 10. Supports and hyperextends the patient's wrist

_____ 11. Performs and interprets the Modified Allen Test

_____ 12. Puts on gloves

_____ 13. Locates and palpates the radial artery

_____ 14. Cleanses the site with alcohol; allows it to air dry

_____ 15. Cleanses the site with iodine; allows it to air dry

_____ 16. Cleanses palpating finger

_____ 17. Administers local anesthetic and waits 2 minutes

_____ 18. Places palpating finger over puncture site

_____ 19. Inserts needle, bevel up, at a 45- to 60-degree angle

_____ 20. Inserts needle 10 to 15 mm below palpating finger

_____ 21. Allows syringe to fill by arterial pressure

_____ 22. Removes needle and applies pressure

_____ 23. Consistently maintains pressure on site for 5 minutes

_____ 24. Expels air bubbles from syringe

_____ 25. Sticks needle into rubber block

_____ 26. Rolls syringe to mix

_____ 27. Places syringe in ice bath

_____ 28. Examines puncture site after 5 minutes

_____ 29. Replaces syringe needle with Luer cap

_____ 30. Disposes of needle

_____ 31. Labels specimen

_____ 32. Reexamines patient's arm

_____ 33. Checks for a radial pulse

_____ 34. Removes iodine and applies pressure bandage

_____ 35. Disposes of used supplies

_____ 36. Removes gloves and washes hands

_____ 37. Thanks patient

_____ 38. Immediately delivers iced specimen to the laboratory

Total Points _____

Maximum Points = 76

COMMENTS:

NAME _____

Evaluation of Capillary Blood Gas Collection

Rating System

2 = Satisfactorily performed
1 = Needs improvement
0 = Incorrect/did not perform

_____ 1. Obtains requisition

_____ 2. Performs nursery isolation procedures

_____ 3. Identifies patient

_____ 4. Begins 5-minute heel warming

_____ 5. Assembles equipment

_____ 6. Puts on gloves

_____ 7. Selects appropriate heel site

_____ 8. Cleanses site and allows it to air dry

_____ 9. Performs puncture

_____ 10. Wipes away first drop of blood

_____ 11. Fills Natelson tube without bubbles

_____ 12. Seals one end of Natelson tube

_____ 13. Adds magnetic "flea" and magnet

_____ 14. Seals second end of tube

_____ 15. Mixes specimen

_____ 16. Applies pressure to site until bleeding stops

_____ 17. Labels tube

_____ 18. Places tube on ice

_____ 19. Disposes of equipment and supplies

_____ 20. Removes gown and gloves

_____ 21. Washes hands

_____ 22. Immediately transports iced specimen to laboratory

Total Points _____

Maximum Points = 44

COMMENTS:

CHAPTER 19

Additional Duties of the Phlebotomist

Learning Objectives

Upon completion of this chapter, the reader will be able to:

1 Define the terms and abbreviations associated with the additional duties of the phlebotomist.
2 Provide patients with instructions and containers for the collection of random, first morning, midstream clean-catch, and 24-hour urine specimens.
3 Provide patients with instructions and containers for the collection of random and timed fecal specimens.
4 Provide patients with instructions and containers for the collection of semen specimens.
5 Correctly collect a throat culture.
6 Discuss the major components and concerns of the blood donor selection process.
7 Compare and contrast the blood donor collection process and the routine venipuncture.
8 Briefly describe the purpose of and the collection procedure for sweat electrolytes, including the precautions to protect specimen integrity.
9 Describe the distribution of tubes for cerebrospinal fluid analysis.
10 Discuss the responsibilities of a phlebotomist when accepting a specimen for transport to a laboratory section.
11 State four rules for safe operation of a centrifuge.
12 Define basic terms associated with computers.
13 State three routine phlebotomy duties that can involve a phlebotomist in the use of a LIMS.

Terminology

Key Terms	Definition
Accessioning	Assigning of specific identification numbers and distribution of specimens
Aliquot	Portion of a sample
Autologous donation	Donation of a unit of blood designated to be available to the donor during surgery
Hardware	Solid components of a computer system
Hemostat	Surgical clamp
Iontophoresis	Electrical stimulation of soluble salt ions used in the collection of sweat electrolyte specimens
Mnemonics	Memory-aiding abbreviations
Modem	Computer-telephone connection

Terminology
Continued

Key Terms	Definition
Pilocarpine	Sweat-inducing chemical
Software	Computer applications programs
Therapeutic phlebotomy	Collection of a unit of blood performed as a patient treatment
Unit of blood	405 to 495 mL of blood collected with 63 mL of anticoagulant

Abbreviations	Definition
AABB	American Association of Blood Banks
CPU	Central processing unit
CRT	Cathode ray tube
FDA	Food and Drug Administration
g	Gravitational force
LIMS (LIS)	Laboratory information management system
RAM	Random access memory
RCF	Relative centrifugal force
ROM	Read only memory
rpm	Revolutions per minute
VDT	Video display terminal

Although collection of quality blood specimens is the primary duty of phlebotomists, they are frequently assigned other responsibilities related to specimen collection and handling. These additional duties may include:

1 Providing instructions and materials to patients for the collection of urine, fecal, and semen specimens
2 Collecting throat cultures
3 Transporting and receiving nonblood specimens
4 Preparing specimens for delivery to laboratory sections or shipment to reference laboratories
5 Interviewing blood donors
6 Performing donor blood collections and therapeutic phlebotomies
7 Performing sweat electrolyte collections
8 Entering and retrieving patient information and charges with the computer

The extent to which phlebotomists are assigned these duties varies greatly among laboratories, as do the protocols for performing them. This chapter is intended to provide phlebotomists with basic information associated with these additional functions.

PATIENT INSTRUCTION

Because they are located in the central processing or **accessioning** area of the laboratory where patient contact is most frequent, phlebotomists often provide instructions to patients and may receive calls from physicians' office personnel requesting instructions. Instructions may be given verbally, using guidelines stated in the laboratory procedure manual, or may be handed to the patient in written form. The phlebotomist should be prepared to answer questions regarding the instructions. Depending on the test requested, patients may be collecting the specimen while at the laboratory or collecting the specimen at home and returning it to the laboratory. The facilities for specimen collection should be at a location convenient to the laboratory.

Urine Specimen Collection

Frequently collected urine specimens include random, first morning, midstream clean-catch, and 24-hour (timed) specimens. Phlebotomists should explain to patients that the composition of urine changes quickly and specimens should be delivered promptly to the laboratory, or refrigerated.

Random specimens are collected from patients in the laboratory in disposable containers. They are used primarily for routine urinalysis.

A first morning specimen is the specimen of choice for urinalysis because it is more concentrated and may be used to confirm results obtained from random specimens. Patients are provided with a container and instructed to collect the specimen immediately after arising and return it to the laboratory within 1 hour.

Midstream clean-catch specimens are used for urine cultures. Patients are provided with sterile containers and antiseptic materials for cleansing the genitalia. Sterile soapy gauze pads followed by gauze pads soaked in sterile water are recommended for women, and mild antiseptic towelettes followed by sterile water-soaked gauze pads for men. Women should be instructed to spread the labia and cleanse from front to back. The tip of the penis is cleansed for men; the cleansing should include retraction of the foreskin if the man is uncircumcised. Patients are instructed to begin voiding into the toilet, then collect the specimen without touching the inside of the container, and finish voiding into the toilet. Midstream clean-catch specimens are collected at the laboratory and delivered immediately to the microbiology section.

Timed or 24-hour specimens require larger containers that may contain a preservative specific for a particular substance to be quantitatively measured (Fig. 19-1). To obtain an accurate timed specimen it is necessary for the patient to begin and end the collection period with an empty bladder.

> *Example:* Day 1 — 0700: Patient voids and *discards* urine, then collects all urine for 24 hours
>
> Day 2 — 0700: Patient voids, and *adds* this urine to the previously collected urine

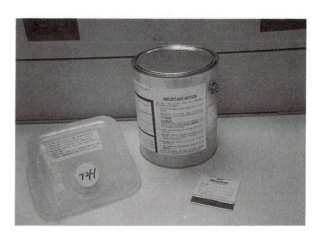

FIGURE 19–1. Containers for urine and fecal specimens.

Fecal Specimen Collection

The laboratory provides patients with several types of containers for collection of fecal specimens. Random specimens used for cultures, ova and parasites, microscopic examination for cells, fats and fibers, and detection of blood are collected in cardboard containers with wax-coated interiors or plastic containers. Large paint-can style containers are used for collection of 72-hour specimens for fecal fats (Fig. 19–1). Mailing kits containing reagent-impregnated filter paper are provided to screen for the presence of occult (hidden) blood.

Patients should be instructed to return the specimen to the laboratory as soon as possible and to avoid contaminating the specimen with urine or toilet water. It may be necessary to collect the specimen in a large container such as a bedpan and then transfer it to the laboratory container.

Semen Specimen Collection

Patients presenting requisitions for semen analysis should be instructed to abstain from sexual activity for 3 days prior to collecting the specimen. Ideally the specimen should then be collected at the laboratory in a sterile container. The specimen must not be collected in a condom, as these frequently contain spermicidal agents.

If the specimen is collected at home, it must be kept warm and delivered to the laboratory within 1 hour. When accepting a semen specimen, it is essential that the phlebotomist record the time of specimen collection, not specimen receipt, on the requisition form because certain parameters of the semen analysis are based on specimen life span.

Figure 19–2 shows an example of laboratory instructions given to patients with requisitions for semen analysis.

THE FAUQUIER HOSPITAL LABORATORY

COMPLETE SEMEN ANALYSIS COLLECTION

The laboratory hours for semen analysis are 8:00 AM to 2:00 PM, Monday through Friday. Please call extension 501/502 (347-2550) to set up an appointment.

The following are guidelines for proper specimen collection. Please instruct patient to:

1. Collect specimen after 3 days of abstinence.

2. Collect semen into a sterile **plastic** container (condom specimens are unacceptable)—keep warm (body temperature) during transport.

3. Bring specimen immediately to laboratory (within half an hour of collection) and then go to Outpatient Registration.

Semen should be analyzed within one hour after collection.

•••

POSTVASECTOMY SPECIMENS

Collect semen in plastic container, it does **not** require special handling. Deliver to laboratory anytime after collection—Monday through Friday between 8:00 AM and 4:00 PM.

FIGURE 19–2. Sample patient instructions. [Courtesy of Anita Sutherland, MT(ASCP), The Fauquier Hospital, Warrenton, VA.]

COLLECTION OF THROAT CULTURES

In some institutions, the duties of the phlebotomist may include collection of throat cultures from outpatients, often children. They are performed primarily for the detection of a streptococcal infection, "strep throat." Specimens may be collected for the purpose of performing a culture or a rapid immunologic Group A Strep test.

Materials needed include a tongue depressor, collection swab in a sterile tube containing transport media, such as a Becton Dickinson (Franklin Lakes, NJ) Culturette, and possibly a flashlight.

To obtain the specimen (Fig. 19–3):

1 Have the patient tilt the head back and open the mouth wide.
2 Gently depress the tongue with the tongue depressor.
3 Being careful not to touch the cheeks, tongue, or lips, swab the area in the back of the throat, including the tonsils and any inflamed or ulcerated areas.
4 Return the swab to the holder tube and crush the ampule of transport media, making sure the released media is in contact with the swab.
5 Label the specimen and deliver it to the microbiology section.

BLOOD DONOR COLLECTION

Phlebotomists may be assigned to work in the blood donor collection station as a part of their routine duties or they may obtain employment in a donor station. In the donor station, units of blood are collected for the purpose of providing the blood bank with a supply of blood and blood components for transfusions. A **unit of blood** consists of 405 to 495 mL of blood mixed with 63 mL of anticoagulant. Experienced phlebotomists are needed to perform donor unit collections. Blood donor collections are performed following guidelines established by the American Association of Blood Banks (**AABB**) and the Food and Drug Administration (**FDA**) for donor selection and unit collection and processing.

Donor Selection

Persons volunteering to donate blood must be interviewed and tested to ensure that the donation will not be physically harmful to them, as well as to determine that their blood is unlikely to cause an adverse condition in the recipient. Donor units are always tested with all available tests for blood-borne pathogens; however, exclusion of donors with possible exposure to these pathogens provides additional protection for the recipient.

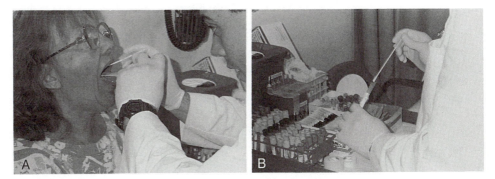

FIGURE 19–3. Throat culture collection. *A*, Swabbing the back of the throat. *B*, Returning the swab to its sterile container.

Donor registration requires identification (including name, address, telephone number, date of birth, social security number, sex) and date of last donation (at least 8 weeks is required between donations). This information is needed in case the donor must be contacted at a later time. Donors must also sign a consent form permitting the laboratory to draw the blood and test it for blood-borne pathogens.

Donors should be 17 years of age or older, weigh at least 110 pounds, and have a temperature of 99.5°F or lower, blood pressure no higher than 180/100 mm Hg, and a hemoglobin level of 12.5 g/dL or higher. The donor should also appear to be in good health.

Donors are asked an extensive list of questions regarding their previous medical history, medications currently being taken, and their social habits particularly related to blood-borne pathogen exposure. Persons performing this interview must be certain that all questions are fully understood by the donor and that the donor understands the importance of a truthful answer to the future health of the recipient. It is also required that all donors be given a private opportunity to indicate that after the unit is collected it should not be used for transfusion. This can be done by providing the donor with a choice between two bar codes to attach to the unit. The unit can then be scanned for acceptability during processing.

Donor Collection

Units of blood are collected into sterile, closed systems consisting of one or more plastic bags connected to tubing and a sterile needle. Large-bore needles, usually 16- to 18-gauge, are used for collection of donor units, both to prevent hemolysis and to facilitate collection of the large amount of blood. Some systems utilize special thin-walled needles that provide a larger bore without increasing the diameter of the needle, so that there is less discomfort for the donor. The plastic bags fill by gravity and must be located below the collection site. They are frequently placed in an automatic mixing device that is also designed to stop when the unit reaches a weight that is consistent with the appropriate volume of blood. **Hemostats** may be applied to the tubing to start and stop the flow of blood into the bag.

A large vein, usually located in the antecubital area, is necessary to accommodate the large needle and supply the required amount of blood. Aseptic site preparation is essential to prevent introduction of microorganisms into the unit of blood. Cleansing is a two-step process, beginning with a soap or dilute iodine scrub and followed by application of more concentrated iodine or chlorhexidene that is allowed to dry for 30 seconds.

Venipuncture is performed in the usual manner, and when blood appears in the tubing, the needle is securely taped to the donor's arm. Donors are encouraged to open and close their fists during the collection to speed the flow of blood. In contrast to routine venipuncture, hemoconcentration is acceptable in donor blood. After removal of the needle, donors are instructed to elevate the arm and apply firm pressure to the puncture site. The phlebotomist completes any required procedures such as transferring blood from the tubing into tubes for testing and discards the needle. Labels corresponding to those on the unit collection bag must be attached to all additional tubes.

Donors should not be left alone during the collection period and should be carefully observed for dizziness or nausea during and after the collection is completed. They are usually offered fruit juice and a snack before they leave the donor station.

Patients scheduled for elective surgery may choose to donate units of their own blood to be transfused back to them during their surgery if blood is needed. This is referred to as an **autologous donation** and has become a common procedure due to the concern about transmission of blood-borne pathogens. Patients may donate as often as every 72 hours, providing they have their physician's approval and a hemoglobin level of at least 11.0 g/dL.

Phlebotomists may also perform a procedure called a **therapeutic phlebotomy**. In this procedure a unit of blood that will not be used for transfusion is collected from patients with conditions causing overproduction of red blood cells (polycythemia) or iron (hemochromatosis). Patients requiring therapeutic phlebotomy are not as healthy as routine blood donors and should be carefully monitored during the collection period. Frequently, therapeutic phlebotomy is performed in a designated area of the laboratory or in a hospital unit and not in the donor station.

Due to the requirements of additional personnel, equipment, documentation of compliance with the regulations imposed by the AABB and the FDA and the legal responsibilities, not all hospitals have donor stations. However most hospitals do collect autologous donations and perform therapeutic phlebotomy.

COLLECTION OF SWEAT ELECTROLYTES

Measurement of the sweat electrolytes, sodium and chloride, is performed to confirm the diagnosis of cystic fibrosis, a genetic disorder of the mucous-secreting glands. Because cystic fibrosis involves multiple organs, many clinical symptoms can lead the physician to suspect its presence. Symptoms usually appear early in life; therefore, sweat electrolytes are frequently collected from infants.

Specimen collection is time-consuming and must be performed under very controlled conditions to ensure that the small amount of sample collected is not altered by contamination or evaporation.

Patients are induced to sweat using a technique called pilocarpine **iontophoresis**, which is illustrated in Figure 19–4. **Pilocarpine**, a sweat-inducing chemical, is applied to an area of the forearm or leg that has been previously cleansed with deionized water. The pilocarpine is then iontophoresed into the skin by the application of a mild electrical current provided by a device designed for pilocarpine iontophoresis. Following iontophoresis the area exposed to the pilocarpine is again thoroughly cleansed with deionized water and dried.

Several methods are available for collection of sweat for electrolyte analysis, including the use of preweighed gauze or filter paper pads or coil collectors. The collection apparatus is placed on the stimulated area, covered securely with plastic, if the collection material is gauze or filter paper, and allowed to remain for a specified length of time, usually 30 minutes.

Regardless of the collection method used, it is essential that:

1 The collection apparatus is handled only with sterile forceps or powder-free gloves and not contaminated by use of the fingers.
2 The collection apparatus is tightly sealed during the collection period to prevent evaporation of the collected sweat.
3 The collected sweat is tightly sealed during transportation to the laboratory to prevent evaporation.

Phlebotomists may be required to perform sweat electrolyte collections or to assist personnel from the chemistry section with the collection. If the collection of sweat electrolytes is one of the phlebotomist's duties, the phlebotomist is usu-

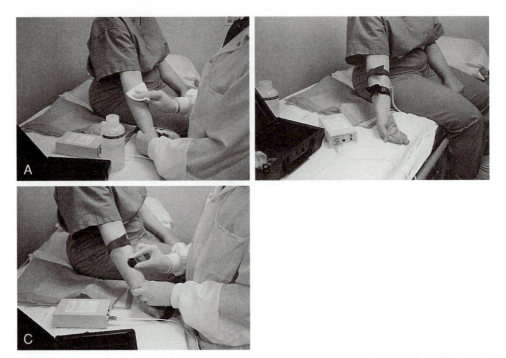

FIGURE 19–4. Sweat collection by means of pilocarpine iontophoresis. *A,* Cleansing the collection site with distilled water. *B,* Performing iontophoresis sweat stimulation. *C,* Applying the sweat collection container.

ally required to notify the chemistry section when a collection is requested and to obtain collection materials (which may have to be preweighed) from the department.

RECEIVING AND TRANSPORTING SPECIMENS

Phlebotomists encounter a variety of specimens other than those they personally collect. When collecting blood in the hospital units they are often asked to transport specimens back to the laboratory. Many inpatient and outpatient specimens are delivered to the central processing area, and phlebotomists must be knowledgeable about any special handling requirements, the laboratory sections that analyze the specimens, and the laboratory policy for accepting specimens. A procedure manual detailing specimen requirements should be present in the central processing area.

In addition to urine, fecal, and semen specimens, common specimens received in the laboratory that are not collected by phlebotomists include cerebrospinal, synovial, pleural, pericardial, peritoneal (ascitic), and amniotic fluids; and tissue specimens.

Cerebrospinal fluid is delivered in tubes usually numbered 1 through 3, representing the order in which the specimen was collected. Tube No. 1 is designated for chemistry, tube No. 2 for microbiology, and tube No. 3 for hematology.

Specimens such as synovial (joint), pleural (chest), pericardial (heart), and peritoneal (abdominal) fluids are frequently collected in evacuated tubes corresponding to those used for similar tests performed on blood. Specimens with a large quantity of fluid designated for cytology may also be received.

Amniotic fluid collected from the fetal sac may be tested for the presence of bilirubin, to monitor hemolytic disease of the newborn, and lipids, to determine fetal lung maturity; or it may be examined by the cytogenetics section for the presence of abnormal chromosomes. Specimens for bilirubin analysis must be protected from light in the same manner as blood specimens, and specimens for cytogenetic analysis should be delivered immediately for processing to preserve the limited number of cells present.

Tissue specimens are routinely received in a preservative solution and are processed by the histology section. Specimens that are not preserved must be immediately delivered to the histology section.

When delivering specimens to laboratory sections, phlebotomists should be sure to alert the technical personnel about the specimen. If specimens are delivered to sections when no personnel are present, as may be the case on evening and night shifts, the phlebotomist must be aware of specimen preservation requirements. This information should be available in the procedure manual or may be posted in the section; it will vary with the type of specimen and the section to which it is delivered. For example, cerebrospinal fluid (CSF) specimens are refrigerated in hematology and left at room temperature in microbiology.

Specimens accepted by phlebotomists, either on the units or in the laboratory, must be accompanied by a requisition form containing appropriate information and must have a label containing information that correlates with the requisition form. Specimens in containers that are visibly contaminated should not be accepted.

SPECIMEN PROCESSING, ACCESSIONING, AND SHIPPING

In some laboratories, particularly in large hospitals, phlebotomists may be involved in centrifuging, **aliquoting**, and assigning accession numbers or bar codes to specimens prior to their delivery to the laboratory sections. They may also process and package specimens sent to reference laboratories.

Universal precautions must be strictly followed when processing all specimens (Fig. 19–5). In accordance with Occupational Safety and Health Administration

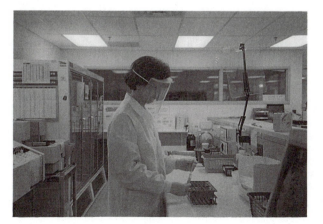

FIGURE 19–5. Blood specimen processing.

(OSHA) regulations, protective apparel must include gloves, fluid-resistant lab coats that are completely closed, and face shields with protective sides. Specimens must never be centrifuged in uncapped tubes.

Specimen processing involving centrifugation and aliquoting is primarily associated with laboratory tests performed on plasma and serum. Plasma is obtained by centrifugation of anticoagulated blood, and serum is similarly obtained from clotted blood. To prevent contamination of plasma and serum by cellular constituents, it is recommended that specimens be separated within 2 hours. Anticoagulated specimens can be centrifuged immediately after collection, and the plasma removed. Specimens collected without anticoagulant must be fully clotted prior to centrifugation. Clotting time can vary from 15 minutes, when clot activators are present, to an hour, for specimens from patients receiving anticoagulant therapy. Loosening clots from the side of the tube (rimming) prior to centrifugation is not recommended as it may cause hemolysis.

In the accessioning area there are a number of types of centrifuges available, including table models, floor models, and refrigerated models. The relative centrifugal force (**RCF**) of a centrifuge is expressed as gravity (**g**) and is determined by the radius of the rotor head and the speed of rotation (revolutions per minute [**rpm**]). Most laboratory specimens are centrifuged at 850 to 1000 g for 10 minutes. Improper use of the centrifuge can be dangerous, and the following rules of operation must be observed:

1   Tubes placed in the cups of the rotor head must be equally balanced. This is accomplished by placing tubes of equal size and volume directly across from each other. Failure to do this will cause the centrifuge to vibrate and possibly break the tubes. A final check for balancing should be made just prior to closing the centrifuge lid (Fig. 19-6).

2   A centrifuge should never be operated until the top has been firmly fastened down, and the top should never be opened until the rotor head has come to a complete stop. Should a tube break during centrifugation, pieces of glass and biohazardous aerosols will be sprayed from a centrifuge that is not covered.

3   Do not walk away from a centrifuge until it has reached its designated rotational speed without evidence of excessive vibration.

4   If a tube breaks in the centrifuge, the cup containing the broken glass must be completely emptied into a sharps container and disinfected. The inside of the

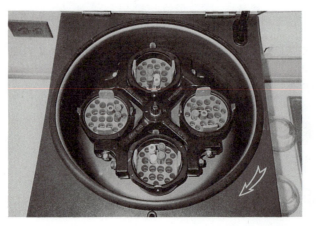

FIGURE 19-6. A properly balanced centrifuge.

centrifuge must also be cleaned of broken glass and disinfected. Puncture-resistant gloves should be worn for the cleanup.

Separation of serum and plasma from the cellular elements and specimen aliquoting require careful attention to detail so that specimens are placed in properly labeled tubes. Care must also be taken to prevent the formation of aerosols when stoppers are removed from evacuated tubes. Specimens should not be poured from one tube to another. As discussed in Chapter 12, stoppers should be covered with gauze and twisted rather than "popped" off. Use of evacuated tubes with barrier gels provides immediate separation. A variety of transfer systems is available. All systems are designed to prevent the formation of aerosols and to provide minimum contact with the specimen by laboratory personnel. Some automated instruments are equipped to sample directly from the sealed tube.

When preparing specimens for transport to reference laboratories information provided by the reference laboratory regarding specimen stability, type of specimen, and volume required must be consulted. Many laboratories contract with a particular reference laboratory that may pick up specimens on a daily basis or provide specific packaging materials. Persons preparing specimens for shipping must be sure to include all necessary labels and requisition forms in the package.

Specimens requiring refrigeration can be shipped in Styrofoam containers with refrigerant packs of ice enclosed in a leakproof bag. Specimens that must remain frozen are packaged in containers with dry ice.

USE OF THE LABORATORY COMPUTER

In recent years computers have become an essential part of the laboratory. Phlebotomists are in contact with the laboratory computer through the generation of requisitions and specimen labels, registration of outpatients, and the receipt of specimens from hospital units. They should understand the basic components of computer systems, be able to enter and retrieve data, be willing to learn new applications as the laboratory computer system expands, and realize that computers are intended to increase the efficiency and accuracy of patient care.

Most people currently have some experience using micro or personal computers in school, the workplace, or at home. The differences between these computers and laboratory computers are primarily the amount of information that can be processed, the speed of processing, and the ability to transfer information to other computers. Therefore the actual computer operated by a phlebotomist will appear no different than a familiar school or home model, although it may be connected to a higher powered minicomputer or mainframe computer for transfer and storage of data. Data can be transferred among the laboratory sections or other hospital departments and by computer-telephone connections (**modems**) to outside agencies such as physicians' offices.

A knowledge of basic computer terminology needed to effectively operate the computer begins with the terms hardware and software. As its name implies, **hardware** refers to the solid components of the computer, including the central processing unit (**CPU**), workstation, printer, and storage disks. The CPU contains the power supply, integrating circuits, processing chips, and random access memory (**RAM**) chips. RAM determines the amount of data that can be newly entered into or retrieved from the CPU during operation. The data must be saved prior to shutting off the computer. The workstation consists of the keyboard for data input and the monitor that displays the entered data. The monitor may be referred to as the **CRT** (cathode ray tube) or the **VDT** (video display terminal); however, these terms are becoming obsolete. The printer provides output of data, and many types that vary in speed and quality of print are available. Depending on the computer system, data may be stored on removable "floppy disks," hard disks, or in central computer system storage devices.

The term **software** refers to the instructions provided to the computer and consists of an operating system that is specific for the particular brand of computer because of the read only memory (**ROM**) installed by the manufacturer. The application programs such as word processing, spreadsheets, and data management must be compatible with the hardware that is being used.

Many application programs for laboratory use are currently available and the decision to use a particular program is determined by the requirements of the laboratory. These laboratory information management systems (**LIMS**) may be used only by the laboratory or may be integrated into a hospitalwide computer system. Companies that provide LIMS work closely with the laboratory staff to adapt the system to correspond with particular laboratory operations.

Phlebotomists first come in contact with a LIMS through the receipt of computer-generated requisitions and specimen labels. They must learn to recognize the information provided, to be sure that it corresponds with the required information discussed in Chapter 13, and to compare this information with the information on the specimen labels. Many computer-generated requisitions also provide the phlebotomist with the number and type of tubes to be collected.

Phlebotomists required to input or retrieve data with the computer are assigned a password that allows them to use the computer. The purpose of the password is to provide computer security so that patient data will only be available to authorized personnel. Phlebotomists should understand that any computer transaction performed when their password has been used to enter the computer can be traced back to them; therefore, the password should not be given to other persons.

Data are frequently entered or retrieved with computers through the use of codes, which can be numeric (1 = retrieve information) or memory-aiding abbreviations (**mnemonics**), such as typing *RI* to retrieve information. The method will vary with the system in use. Another method of data entry is the use of bar codes, from which information can be scanned into the computer by a specially designed light source (this method has been used in retail stores for many years). The black and white stripes of varying width on a bar code correspond to letters and numbers, and are grouped together to represent patient names, identification numbers, and laboratory tests. Use of bar code systems decreases the possibility of laboratory error due to clerical mistakes.

Additional computer duties for phlebotomists may include generation of collection lists and schedules, posting of patient charges, computing monthly phlebotomy workloads, and retrieving information for personnel in physicians' offices (Fig. 19-7). Because of the variety of laboratory information systems available, the major learning requirement of a technically trained phlebotomist (or other laboratory worker) when entering a new job is usually the use of the computer system. This can only increase as laboratories expand their computer applications.

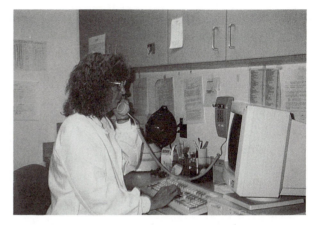

FIGURE 19–7. A phlebotomist using a laboratory computer.

BIBLIOGRAPHY

Henry, JB: Clinical Diagnosis and Management by Laboratory Methods. WB Saunders, Philadelphia, 1991.

National Committee for Clinical Laboratory Standards Approved Standard C34-A; Sweat Collections and Quantitative Analysis. NCCLS, Villanova, PA, 1994.

Quinley, ED: Immunohematology Principals and Practice. JB Lippincott, Philadelphia, 1993.

Strasinger, SK: Urinalysis and Body Fluids, ed. 3. FA Davis, Philadelphia, 1994.

Study Questions

1. If a urine specimen cannot be delivered to the laboratory within 1 hour, how should the specimen be stored?

   _____

2. State the specific type of specimen a patient should be instructed to collect for the following tests.

   a. Urine culture   _____

   b. Quantitative fecal fat   _____

   c. Routine urinalysis   _____

   d. Ova and parasites   _____

   e. Follow-up urinalysis   _____

   f. Quantitative urine creatinine _____

3. Name a specimen and test that patients can mail to the laboratory.

   _____

4. Why should a patient begin and end a timed urine collection period with an empty bladder?

   _____

   _____

5. True or False. A patient delivers a semen specimen to the laboratory in a condom for fertility studies. He should be given a sterile container and told to collect another specimen in 3 days. Explain your answer.

   _____

   _____

6. What information (other than patient ID) must be placed on the requisition that accompanies a semen specimen?

   _____

7. Describe the areas that should be swabbed when collecting a throat culture.

   _____

   _____

8. Name three areas that should be avoided when collecting a throat culture.

   a. _____

   b. _____

   c. _____

9. State the purpose of:

    a. An autologous donation

    _____

    _____

    b. A therapeutic phlebotomy

    _____

    _____

10. State the reason for the following parts of the donor selection process.

    a. Identification information _____

    _____

    b. Physical examination _____

    _____

    c. Medical and social history _____

    _____

11. Place a "Q" for qualify or a "D" for disqualify in front of the following results of a donor selection process.

    a. _____ Weight: 220 pounds

    b. _____ Hemoglobin: 11.0 g/dL

    c. _____ Rehabilitated heroin user

    d. _____ Blood pressure: 160/90 mm Hg

    e. _____ Hepatitis 5 years ago

12. Why do the following procedures in the collection of donor blood differ from those of routine venipuncture?

    a. Cleansing the site

    _____

    _____

    b. Needle gauge

    _____

    _____

    c. Clenching and unclenching of donor's fist

    _____

    _____

13. Sweat electrolytes are collected to confirm the diagnosis of

_____ .

14. List three collection errors that could produce falsely elevated sweat electrolytes.

    a. _____

    b. _____

    c. _____

15. The name of the technique used for collection of sweat electrolytes is

    _____.

16. While you are alone in the central processing area, a patient presents you with a requisition for an unfamiliar test. Where can you obtain information for the collection of this specimen?

    _____

17. Cerebrospinal fluid specimens labeled No. 1, No. 2, and No. 3 are delivered to the laboratory. What section should they be delivered to?

    a. No. 1 _____

    b. No. 2 _____

    c. No. 3 _____

18. Match the following specimens with the area of the body from which they were collected.

Specimen	**Body Area**
a. _____ Ascitic fluid	1. Heart
b. _____ Synovial fluid	2. Lymph node
c. _____ Pericardial fluid	3. Joint
d. _____ Pleural fluid	4. Abdomen
	5. Chest

19. State a special handling requirement for amniotic fluid to be tested for HDN.

    _____

20. List three reasons why a specimen delivered to the central processing area would be unacceptable.

    a. _____

    b. _____

    c. _____

21. What protective apparel must be worn when processing blood specimens?

    _____

    _____

    _____

22. True or False. Specimens collected in light-blue top tubes must be allowed to sit for 30 minutes prior to centrifugation. Explain your answer.

_____

_____

23. List two factors that determine the RCF of a centrifuge.

    a. _____

    b. _____

24. State three causes of aerosol production when processing specimens.

    a. _____

    b. _____

    c. _____

25. Given the following tubes and spaces in a centrifuge rotor head, show how you would balance the centrifuge by placing the numbers of the appropriate tubes in the space on the rotor head.

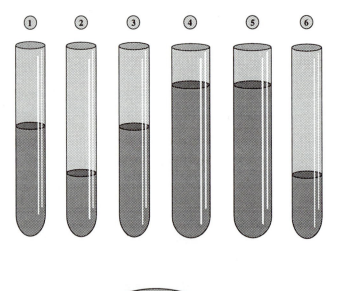

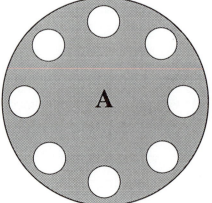

26. Match the following terms or statements with the appropriate computer component.

Term/Statement	Component
a. _____ Application program	1. CPU
b. _____ Floppy disk	2. Workstation
c. _____ RAM	3. Printer
d. _____ LIMS	4. Storage device
e. _____ Output device	5. Software
f. _____ Input device	
g. _____ Power supply	
h. _____ Keyboard	
i. _____ CRT	
j. _____ Hard disk	

27. A phlebotomist is counseled by the supervisor because two computer entry errors on the previous day were traced back to the phlebotomist. The phlebotomist states that he or she did not use the computer on that day. Explain how this could occur and how it could be avoided.

_____

_____

28. How does the use of bar codes contribute to laboratory accuracy?

_____

_____

29. How can a LIMS be adapted to aid a phlebotomist in the collection of appropriate specimens?

_____

_____

30.

```
TRAINING, PATIENT
45Y M   0323/PT
01/26   0324/PTT
BLUE
```

Should a specimen with the above label be accepted for testing? Why or why not?

_____

_____

CHAPTER 20 Quality Phlebotomy

Learning Objectives

Upon completion of this chapter, the reader will be able to:

1 Define the terms and abbreviations associated with quality phlebotomy.
2 Discuss the interactions of QC, QA, CQI, and TQM, and their differences.
3 List five methods used to document a quality assurance program in the phlebotomy department.
4 List the information contained in a procedure manual and describe how the manual is used by the phlebotomist.
5 Discuss the role of variables in the development of a quality assurance program.
6 State the purpose of a floor book and the information it contains.
7 List nine types of records that can be used to monitor the quality of specimen ordering.
8 Discuss the role of delta checks in laboratory quality assurance.
9 Describe methods used for quality control of phlebotomy equipment.
10 State possible errors that may occur through the use of outdated or defective vacuum tubes.
11 Name tests that may be affected by the following patient variables: diet, posture, exercise, stress, alcohol, tobacco, and diurnal variation.
12 List the tests affected by prolonged tourniquet application.
13 List five puncture sites to be avoided to prevent specimen contamination and five sites that may cause patient injury.
14 Discuss four tests that can be affected by improper site cleansing.
15 State four errors in phlebotomy puncture and specimen collection technique that affect specimen quality.
16 Discuss methods of specimen transport and name the tests most affected by excessive vibration.
17 Describe the quality control of specimen processing equipment.
18 Discuss methods to prevent specimen alteration during processing.
19 Discuss the role of the phlebotomist in the various areas of medical TQM.

Terminology

Key Terms	Definition
Continuous quality improvement	Institutional program focusing on customer expectations
Delta check	Comparison of a patient's current results with previous results
Documentation	Written evidence
Floor book (laboratory reference manual)	Document providing laboratory information to other areas of the hospital

Terminology
Continued

Key Terms	Definition
Lot	Group of products manufactured at the same time under the same conditions
Pneumatic tube system	Air-driven transport system
Procedure manual	Detailed documentation of procedures and methods used in performing tests
Quality assurance	Methods used to guarantee quality patient care
Quality control	Methods used to monitor the quality of procedures
Tachometer	Instrument for measuring speed
Total quality management	Institutional policy to provide customer satisfaction
Turn-around-time	Amount of time between the request for a test and the reporting of results
Variable/indicator	Measurable condition used to evaluate quality of service

Abbreviations	Definition
CQI	Continuous quality improvement
QA	Quality assurance
QC	Quality control
TAT	Turn-around-time
TQM	Total quality management

Throughout the previous chapters many of the aspects of providing quality patient care have been discussed in relation to phlebotomy techniques. These procedures provide the **quality control (QC)** needed to ensure that acceptable standards are being met while the procedures are being performed. This QC is a part of the laboratory's overall program of quality assurance. In this last chapter it is appropriate to review these quality control procedures, combine them with additional information, and discuss their interactions in laboratory quality assurance and the institutional processes of total quality management and continuous quality improvement. The actions of the phlebotomist in these programs are critical to their success.

QUALITY ASSURANCE

Quality assurance (QA) is the program through which the laboratory guarantees quality patient care by providing accurate and reliable test results in an appropriate and timely manner. The Joint Commission on Accreditation of Healthcare Organizations requires a planned systematic process for the monitoring and evaluation of the quality and appropriateness of patient care services and the resolving of identified problems. The phlebotomy department is a central part of the laboratory quality assurance program due to its close contact with patients and other hospital personnel. The quality of laboratory testing is strictly dependent on the quality of the specimens received.

Documentation of a quality assurance program requires:

1   Written policies and procedures covering all aspects of service

2   Evidence of compliance with standards of good practice and achievement of expected outcomes

3   Collection of data (metrics) to monitor and evaluate the program

4   Evidence of work being performed efficiently and in the best interests of the patient

5   Actions taken to resolve problems

In the phlebotomy department documentation is provided in a variety of ways. These include a detailed procedure manual present in the department, **floor books (laboratory reference manuals)** provided to the nursing units, identification of variable factors associated with the performance of phlebotomists, policies developed to provide guidelines to control and monitor these variables, and continuing education records for all members of the department.

Procedure Manual

Periodic review, in order to gain a thorough knowledge of the phlebotomy department procedure manual, is of major importance to quality performance in phlebotomy. The manual is present in the department at all times and phlebotomists should not hesitate to refer to it when unfamiliar requests are encountered. It is the responsibility of the phlebotomy supervisor to enter all policy and procedure changes into the manual, notify personnel of the changes, and document an annual review of the entire manual.

For each test or procedure performed, the procedure manual provides the principle and purpose, specimen type and method of collection, equipment and supplies needed, standards and controls, step-by-step procedure, specific procedure notes, limitations and variables of the method, corrective actions, method validation, normal values, and references. The procedure manual documents the intention of the laboratory to comply with the standards of good practice to achieve expected outcomes.

Variables/ Indicators

Identification of variables, sometimes referred to as indicators, provides the basis for the development of the procedures and policies of the department. Variables can be divided into three groups: preanalytical, analytical, and postanalytical. Phlebotomists are primarily involved with preanalytical variables, which include the ordering, collection, transportation, and processing of specimens. Their actions in these areas affect the quality of the analytical results obtained in the various laboratory sections. They continue to be involved in the postanalytical phase because the timeliness of collection affects the amount of time required to report the test results. Their duties may also include delivery of reports to the units and retrieval of results from the computer. Major emphasis in this discussion will be placed on the application of quality assurance to preanalytical variables.

Ordering of Tests

This is a joint effort between the phlebotomy department and the personnel on the hospital units who generate the requests for laboratory tests. The laboratory must facilitate test ordering by providing a floor book (laboratory reference manual). Information contained in the floor book includes:

1   Laboratory schedules for collection of routine specimens (Fig. 20-1). These may be called "sweeps" and are scheduled to correspond with the primary times that patient specimens are requested. Examples of scheduled sweeps are the early morning, when patients are in a basal state, and late morning and afternoon, when physicians have completed their patient visits. Unit personnel need to understand that whenever possible issuing test requisitions to the laboratory

THE FAUQUIER HOSPITAL
SPECIMEN PROCESSING DEPARTMENT

COLLECTION TIMES

I Routine blood tests will be collected by the laboratory personnel at the following times:
AM collection 0530–0730
Routine daily draws 1000
                   1300
                   1600
                   1900
                   2100

II Routine orders for tests placed after 2200 hours will be collected with the 0530 AM draw.

III The laboratory will operate in a STAT mode from the hours of 2200 to 0700 due to reduced staffing on the overnight shift.

IV Floor collected specimens, i.e., urine, body fluids, CSF, sputums, etc., should be delivered to the laboratory as soon as possible for prompt processing.

V **STAT** tests will be collected within 10 minutes of receipt of order in the laboratory.
ASAP tests will be collected as soon as possible or within 30 minutes of receipt of order in the laboratory.
NOW testing is not recognized by the laboratory.

FIGURE 20–1. Sample of a laboratory collection schedule. [Courtesy of Anita Sutherland, MT(ASCP), The Fauquier Hospital, Warrenton, VA.]

at these times increases not only the efficiency of the phlebotomy department but also the entire laboratory, because tests can then be performed in batches.

2 A list of laboratory tests including the type of specimen required, specimen handling procedures, normal values, and any pertinent patient preparation or scheduling requirements. Personnel may be referred to additional instructions provided separately in the floor book. As shown in Figure 20-2, instructions can also be included on computer-generated requisitions. The appearance of "clean-catch" under the heading of special instructions prompts personnel col-

```
********************** FLOOR COLLECTED REQUISITION  ************************

==========================================================================
Pt# 279377          TRAINING, PATIENT #1          Room-Bed: 9999-99
==========================================================================

DR: VON ELTEN, S.                      Current Date-Time:  01/26/94-12:27
                                       BY: LRAS

Test: CULTURE, URINE  **        Order# 0318        PRIORITY [ R ]

Sp Inst: CLEAN CATCH


        Start Date-Time  01/26/94        Stop Date-Time: 01/26/94
                         12:27                           12:27

SOURCE OF SPECIMEN: _____


COLLECTED BY: _____  DATE: _____ TIME: _____


********  THIS REQUEST MUST ACCOMPANY THE SPECIMEN TO THE LABORATORY  ********
```

FIGURE 20-2. Sample requisition with special instructions. [Courtesy of Anita Sutherland, MT(ASCP), The Fauquier Hospital, Warrenton, VA.]

lecting the specimen to check the floor book for additional information.

3   Any changes or additions to laboratory policies affecting personnel in the unit should be promptly added to the floor book and all personnel should be notified of the changes.

As discussed in previous chapters, requisition forms must contain the required patient information and request the tests actually ordered by the physician. Errors in requisitioning include generation of duplicate requisitions and the missing of tests, either by the person transferring the physician's orders to the requisition or by the phlebotomist when organizing or reading the requisitions. The discovery of a missed test by personnel on the unit frequently causes a routine test to be ordered STAT, and a test overlooked by the phlebotomist may cause the patient to undergo a second, unnecessary venipuncture.

Monitoring of specimen ordering can include records of:

1   The number of incomplete requisitions
2   The number of duplicate requisitions
3   The number of missed tests
4   Delays in the collection of timed tests
5   The number of STAT requests by hospital location
6   The time between test requests and collection
7   The number of unit collected specimens rejected
8   **Turn-around-time** (**TAT**) (the amount of time between the ordering of a test and the reporting of the test results)
9   Physician complaints

Evaluation of these records may then be used to determine the need for additions or changes to the floor book; for inservice continuing education presentations to personnel ordering tests in order to reduce the number of errors or decrease the number of STAT requests; for additional phlebotomists or changes in staffing schedules to provide faster specimen collection; and for additional training of phlebotomists who are missing tests or inefficiently collecting specimens.

A sample corrective action procedure is shown in Figure 20 – 3.

SPECIMEN COLLECTION

Variables affecting specimen quality are present at all stages of venipuncture, dermal puncture, arterial puncture, and special collection procedures. Their presence forms the basis for the techniques discussed in previous chapters, and their importance is reemphasized in this section.

Patient Identification

Failure to properly identify a patient is the most serious error in phlebotomy and can result in injury or death to the patient. Identification of errors may be made in the laboratory, before the patient is harmed, through an analytical quality assurance procedure known as the **delta check**. A delta check is a comparison between a patient's previous test results and the current results. Variation of results outside of established parameters alerts laboratory personnel to the possibility of an error. Documentation of errors in patient identification will result in suspension and dismissal.

Phlebotomy Equipment

Assuring the sterility of needles and puncture devices and the stability of evacuated tubes, anticoagulants, and additives is essential to patient safety and specimen quality.

Disposable needles and puncture devices are individually packaged in tightly

THE FAUQUIER HOSPITAL
SPECIMEN PROCESSING DEPARTMENT

TDM FLOW SHEET

In response to problems documenting the times blood was drawn for trough/peak levels to monitor therapeutic drugs, the TDM Flow Sheet has been implemented.

The Flow Sheet will be started by the phlebotomist drawing the trough level and be sent to the pharmacy after the peak level.

Procedure:

1. TDM Flow Sheets are kept in the specimen processing area.

2. A label with patient's information is placed on the Flow Sheet in the appropriate area.

3. Phlebotomist will date the sheet and initial/time when the trough has been drawn.

4. The Flow Sheet is left with the patient's nurse for completion of medication information.

5. The phlebotomist initials/times again when the peak is drawn.

6. The TDM Flow Sheet is returned to the laboratory and placed in the pharmacy box for collection by the pharmacy.

Return to pharmacy box

TDM FLOW SHEET

Addressograph: DATE: _____

DRUG: _____

DOSE: _____

	LABORATORY Initials Time	NURSING Initials Time
TROUGH		
MED STARTED		
MED FINISHED		
(NEW TUBING) Y/N		
PEAK		
RANDOM LEVEL		

NOTES/PROBLEMS:

tear here & insert bottom in medication cardex

Drug Level in progress:
Blood to be drawn _____ (peak/random)

FIGURE 20–3. Example of a corrective action. [Courtesy of Anita Sutherland, MT(ASCP), The Fauquier Hospital, Warrenton, VA.]

sealed sterile containers. Phlebotomists should not use puncture equipment if the seal has been broken. Visual inspection for nonpointed or barbed needles detects manufacturing defects.

Manufacturers of evacuated tubes must ensure that tubes, anticoagulants, and additives meet the standards established by the National Committee for Clinical Laboratory Standards. These standards specify the acceptable concentrations to provide quality specimens. Evacuated tubes produced at the same time are referred to as a **"lot"** and have a distinguishing lot number printed on the packages. There is also an expiration date printed on each package. This represents the last day the manufacturer guarantees the stability of the specified amount of vacuum in the tube and the reactivity of the anticoagulants and additives. The expiration date should be checked each time a new package of tubes is opened, and outdated tubes should not be used. Donate them to your local phlebotomy teaching program for use on artificial arms. For the most economical management of phlebotomy supplies, packages of tubes should be stored in groups by lot number, and lots with the shortest expiration dates should be placed in the front of the storage area.

Use of expired tubes may cause incompletely filled tubes (short draws), clotted anticoagulated specimens, improperly preserved specimens, and insecure gel barriers. Short draws in tubes containing anticoagulants and additives affect specimen quality because the amount of anticoagulant or additive present in the tube is based on the assumption that the tube will be completely filled. Errors that may occur include excessive dilution of the specimen by liquid anticoagulants and distortion of cellular structures by increased chemical concentrations.

Defects in the manufacturing of evacuated tubes are possible and, when present, frequently affect an entire lot of tubes. When a new lot of tubes is opened, the tubes should be checked for vacuum by measuring the amount of water drawn into the tube. They should also be checked for the presence of small clots in anticoagulated tubes, the visual appearance of additives, stability during centrifugation, and stopper integrity and ease of stopper removal. Results of these checks should be documented, and testing may need to be repeated if problems with tube integrity develop at a later date. Manufacturers must be notified when defects are discovered.

Patient Preparation

Numerous variables in patient preparation can affect specimen quality, and the phlebotomist cannot be expected to control and monitor all variables; however, phlebotomists should be aware of the most critical variables, such as fasting prior to glucose testing, and abstaining from aspirin prior to a bleeding time test. Any discrepancies should be reported to the nursing staff or a supervisor. Phlebotomists should also be alert for noticeable unusual circumstances and should note this information on the requisition form. Special patient preparation procedures must be included in the floor book.

Patient variables that may affect test results are summarized in Table 20-1 and include:

1 **FASTING** Test results will be most consistent with reference values when patients have been fasting for 8 to 12 hours prior to specimen collection. Increases in glucose and triglyceride levels are most noticeable in nonfasting patients. Prolonged fasting, longer than 48 hours, will increase bilirubin and triglyceride values and markedly decrease glucose levels.

2 **POSTURE** Change in posture from a supine to an erect position shifts the balance of water in the blood and interstitial fluid and affects the concentration of large molecules not filtered by the kidneys. Therefore, variations can be ex-

TABLE 20–1. **MAJOR TESTS AFFECTED BY PATIENT VARIABLES**

Variable	Increased Results	Decreased Results
Nonfasting	Glucose and triglycerides	
Prolonged fasting	Bilirubin, fatty acids, and triglycerides	Glucose
Posture	Albumin, bilirubin, calcium, enzymes, lipids, total protein, RBCs, and WBCs	
Short-term exercise	Creatinine, fatty acids, lactate, AST, CK, LD, and WBCs	
Long-term exercise	Aldolase, creatinine, sex hormones, AST, CK, and LD	
Stress	Adrenal hormones, fatty acids, lactate, and WBCs	
Alcohol	Lactate, triglycerides, uric acid, GGT, HDL, and MCV	
Tobacco	Catecholamines, cortisol, hemoglobin, MCV, and WBCs	
Diurnal variation (AM)	Cortisol	Serum iron and WBCs

pected between results obtained for a patient on an inpatient and outpatient basis.

3 **EXERCISE**   Transient strenuous exercise and prolonged exercise or weight training affect test results differently. Test results affected by transient exercise include primarily the enzymes associated with muscles and the WBC count associated with the release of cells attached to the venous walls into the circulation. The values usually return to normal within several hours of relaxation. Prolonged exercise also increases the muscle-related waste products and the sex hormones.

4 **STRESS**   Failure to calm a patient prior to specimen collection may increase levels of adrenal hormones and markedly affect ABG results. As described previously, WBC counts collected from children who are struggling or crying may be noticeably elevated.

5 **ALCOHOL**   In general, moderate consumption of alcohol does not affect test results. Glucose levels are transiently elevated in inebriated persons, and chronic alcohol consumption affects tests associated with the liver.

6 **SMOKING**   Immediate effects of tobacco include increases in plasma catecholamines and cortisol, with a resulting decrease in eosinophils and increase in neutrophils. Chronic smoking increases hemoglobin, WBC counts, and the MCV.

7 **DIURNAL VARIATION**   As discussed in Chapter 15, the concentration of some blood constituents, such as cortisol and iron, is affected by the time of day, so that specimens must be collected at specified times. Specific times for collection must be stated on the requisition form, and specimens must be collected in a timely manner by the phlebotomist.

8 MEDICATIONS Administration of medications prior to specimen collection may affect test results, either by changing a metabolic process within the patient or by producing interference with the testing procedure. Administration of materials such as radiographic dyes used in diagnostic procedures will also interfere with some laboratory tests. Understanding the affect of medications on laboratory test results is the responsibility of the physician and clinical laboratory scientists; however, phlebotomists should be aware of any therapy provided at the time they are performing the specimen collection and note this on the requisition form. Samples collected from patients while a transfusion is being administered may not be representative of the patient's true condition and this should be noted on the requisition form.

Monitoring and evaluation of quality assurance in patient preparation must be done jointly by the laboratory, nursing staff, and physicians.

Tourniquet Application

Application of the tourniquet for longer than 1 minute increases the concentration of large molecules such as bilirubin, lipids, protein, and enzymes, and may produce a slight hemolysis that affects potassium levels.

Site Selection

In general quality assurance is not affected by the choice of a puncture site, unless it is located in an area where contamination may occur or patient safety may be compromised.

Sites to be avoided because of the possibility of specimen contamination include:

1 Hematomas
2 Edematous areas
3 Arms adjacent to mastectomies
4 Arms receiving intravenous fluids

Sites to be avoided to prevent injury to the patient are:

1 Burned and scarred areas
2 Arms adjacent to mastectomies
3 Arms with fistulas and shunts
4 The back of the heel
5 Previous dermal puncture sites
6 Arteries for routine testing

Errors in site selection are detected by delta checks, test results that are markedly affected by intravenous fluids, and complaints from patients and nursing staff. Phlebotomists associated with poor choices in site selection may require counseling, retraining, or dismissal.

Cleansing the Site

Blood culture contamination is the most frequently encountered variable associated with improper cleansing of the puncture site. Records of contaminated blood cultures are maintained by the microbiology section and increases are investigated for possible errors in collection technique.

Failure to remove iodine from the patient's arm after specimen collection will produce patient complaints.

Use of iodine for dermal puncture collections will falsely elevate bilirubin, phosphorus, and uric acid levels.

Performing the Puncture

Variables in phlebotomy technique affect both specimen quality and patient safety. Errors affecting specimen quality include collection in the wrong tube, failure to adequately mix the specimen, failure to follow the correct order of draw or fill, and excessive dilution of dermal puncture specimens with tissue fluid.

The patient's impression of the laboratory quality is heavily influenced by phlebotomy technique. Painful probing, hematomas, unsuccessful attempts, repeat draws due to poor specimen quality, and excessive and inappropriately located heel punctures will cause complaints from patients, nursing staff, and physicians. Phlebotomists should remember how often patients tell them about previous bad experiences and strive to not become another bad memory on the part of the patient.

Documentation of poor technique affecting patients or specimen quality is frequently made in the form of an incident report generated by a nursing or laboratory supervisor. Incident reports describe the incident and the problem caused, document the corrective action taken, and become a part of an employee's permanent record. Errors in the identification and mislabeling of specimens are primary reasons for the generation of an incident report.

Disposal of Puncture Equipment

The availability of and the proper use of sharps containers is essential to quality performance by phlebotomists. Punctures with contaminated sharps must be immediately reported to a supervisor. A protocol that includes immediate and follow-up testing and counseling for the affected employee must be in place and followed. Documentation of excessive puncture injuries can lead to changes in the type of equipment used and its availability, or to disciplinary action against employees who are not following acceptable disposal procedures.

TRANSPORTATION OF SPECIMENS

Variables in the transportation of specimens include the method and timing of delivery to the laboratory and the use of special handling procedures discussed in previous chapters.

Specimen quality is most frequently compromised when red blood cells are hemolyzed as a result of excessive vibration during delivery of tubes to the laboratory. Tubes should be placed in an upright position in racks provided in the phlebotomy tray. This permits uniform clotting and prevents tubes from hitting against each other, thereby eliminating excessive vibration and the possibility of breakage.

Many hospitals have **pneumatic tube systems** running between the units and support areas. These systems increase the timeliness of specimen delivery to the laboratory; however, they must be carefully monitored to ensure that specimens are not hemolyzed or broken during transit. The most frequently affected tests are potassium, lactic dehydrogenase, plasma hemoglobin, and acid phosphatase. To transport laboratory specimens, the system should be designed to avoid sharp turns, provide a soft landing, and utilize containers that can be equipped with shock-absorbent lining materials. Records of unacceptable specimens must be maintained to verify satisfactory performance of the pneumatic tube system.

Phlebotomists' duties include timely delivery of specimens to the laboratory. This requires the ability to efficiently organize the work load and to adapt to emergency situations. Documentation of the time between the delivery of a requisition to the laboratory and the arrival of the specimen in the laboratory can be acquired by using a time-stamping machine (Fig. 20-4). This data can then be evaluated to determine the need for possible changes in phlebotomy staffing patterns.

SPECIMEN PROCESSING

Variables associated with specimen processing include the length of time between collection and processing or testing, centrifugation time and speed, contamination, evaporation, storage conditions, and labeling.

No more than 2 hours should elapse between specimen collection and separation of serum or plasma from the cells and less time is recommended for potassium, ammonia, ACTH, and cortisol determinations. When delays in separation are longer than 2 hours the most noticeable changes are decreased glucose, and increased potassium and lactic dehydrogenase concentrations. Serum or plasma does not have to be removed after centrifugation from tubes containing separator gel, providing a tight seal has been obtained.

Documentation of centrifuge calibration and maintenance is required for accreditation. Centrifuges are routinely calibrated every 3 months using a **tachometer** to confirm revolutions per minute at various settings. This information can then be converted into relative centrifugal force using nomograms provided by the centrifuge manufacturer. Marked changes in the calibration may indicate the need to replace the centrifuge brushes, or problems with the bearings. Procedure manuals should include specifications for centrifuge speed, type, and time, for each specimen. Failure to routinely perform centrifuge calibration or to follow the specifications stated in the procedure manual can affect specimen quality due to incomplete separation of liquid and formed elements, cellular damage caused by use of excessive speed or time, and deterioration of chemical elements if special requirements such as the use of a refrigerated centrifuge are needed.

Poor technique during specimen processing can seriously alter specimen com-

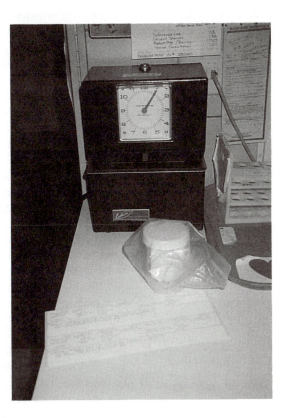

FIGURE 20–4. A time-stamping machine to document the time and date of specimen deliveries.

position by causing contamination or evaporation. All specimens left uncovered for extended periods of time are subject to external contamination and fluid evaporation. Small aliquots are particularly affected by evaporation, and specimens for blood gases, ammonia, and alcohol are severely affected if they are uncovered for even short periods of time. External contamination can be caused by air-borne materials, and also by the talc from powdered gloves, which contains calcium. Aliquots of serum or plasma may contain red blood cells if separation is not carefully performed. Very serious interference with test results will occur if specimens collected in different anticoagulants or additives are combined.

The temperatures of refrigerators and freezers used for specimen storage must be monitored, either continually with automatic temperature recorders or daily by recorded checks of thermometer readings. Self-defrosting freezers should not be used, as specimens may be thawed and refrozen during defrosting cycles.

When aliquoting specimens into different tubes, particular attention must be paid to labeling to ensure that specimen numbers are correctly transferred. Computer-generated labels often include additional labels for this purpose.

Errors in specimen processing are often difficult to detect immediately. They are usually discovered as a result of observing noticeable trends in test results, such as increased values due to specimen evaporation. Monitoring of temperature records, centrifuge calibration, and maintenance and observation of processing techniques must be assigned to a responsible supervisor.

TOTAL QUALITY MANAGEMENT

Laboratory quality assurance is part of the institutional **total quality management (TQM)** and **continuous quality improvement (CQI)** programs. Quality assurance is designed to monitor and control processes to provide a specified level of quality and is concerned only with maintaining the established level. In recent years the concepts of TQM and CQI have been incorporated into accreditation requirements, so as to expand the role of quality assurance from one of simply meeting prescribed standards of individual processes to one that also is continuously striving to improve the quality of all health care.

Total quality management is based on a team concept involving personnel at all levels working together to achieve a final outcome of customer satisfaction through implementation of policies and procedures identified by the CQI program. In the medical setting the patient is the ultimate consumer; however, the clinical laboratory has additional consumers, including the physicians and other personnel who provide patient treatment based on laboratory results. Areas of concern in medical TQM are the infrastructure, including physical, personnel, and management structure; support services, of which the clincial laboratory is a part; and direct patient care associated with physicians and the nursing service. Phlebotomists are involved in all of these areas, and their actions and suggestions are valuable to CQI.

Examples of infrastructure organization affecting the phlebotomist include the distance between patients and the laboratory, availability of safety and collection equipment, methods for transporting specimens, phlebotomy staffing patterns, and the volume of assigned duties. The role of phlebotomists in providing quality specimens for analysis affects the quality of the clinical laboratory as a support service and they should be alert for methods to improve this function.

As the laboratory member with the most direct patient contact, the phlebotomist plays a critical role in customer (patient) satisfaction. Unprofessional actions and appearance, and poor technique causing patient discomfort, all contribute to patient dissatisfaction. Phlebotomists should think about how often they hear people characterize a recent hospital stay by describing their experience with blood collection, and should strive to always make this a positive experience.

BIBLIOGRAPHY

Henry, JB: Clinical Diagnosis and Management by Laboratory Methods. WB Saunders, Philadelphia, 1991.

Joint Commission on Accreditation of Healthcare Organizations: Accreditation Manual for Hospitals. JCAHO, Oakbrook Terrace, IL, 1992.

National Committee for Clinical Laboratory Standards Approved Guideline H18-A: Procedures for the Handling and Processing of Blood Specimens. NCCLS, Villanova, PA, 1990.

Study Questions

1. State three reasons why actions of the phlebotomist are critical to laboratory quality assurance.

   a. _____

   b. _____

   c. _____

2. State a circumstance when the procedure manual must be used by the phlebotomist.

   _____

3. Give examples of two times when a phlebotomist might consult the procedure manual.

   a. _____

   b. _____

4. State the role of variables in the development of a quality assurance program.

   _____

   _____

   _____

5. Identify each of the following as a preanalytical, analytical, or postanalytical variable.

   a. _____ CBC on an elective surgery patient ordered STAT

   b. _____ Decimal point misplaced when results are entered into the computer

   c. _____ Hemolyzed specimen

   d. _____ Outdated reagents for chemistry analyzer

   e. _____ Increase in contaminated blood cultures

6. State advantages or disadvantages of the following times for phlebotomy sweeps.

   a. 0700 _____

   b. 0900 _____

   c. 1300 _____

   d. 1700 _____

7. Explain how a floor book improves the quality of patient testing.

   _____

   _____

   _____

8. State a corrective action to be taken for each of the following.

a. Excessive turn-around-times for ER tests

_____

_____

b. Increased STAT requests for CBCs from the OB unit

_____

_____

c. Increased rejection of specimens collected by personnel in pediatrics

_____

_____

d. Delays in the collection of timed tests

_____

_____

9. List three phlebotomy errors that may be detected by a delta check.

a. _____

b. _____

c. _____

10. State two ways to ensure the quality of venipuncture needles.

a. _____

b. _____

11. What is the purpose of an expiration date on evacuated tubes?

_____

_____

12. List two ways that a short draw may affect the quality of test results.

a. _____

b. _____

13. True or False. A package of lavender top tubes and a package of light-blue top tubes manufactured in the same plant on the same day will have the same lot number. Why?

_____

_____

14. List five procedures performed to check the quality of evacuated tubes.

    a. _____

    b. _____

    c. _____

    d. _____

    e. _____

15. Match the following patient variables with the possible effect on test results.

Effect	**Variable**
a. ____ Increased Hgb	1. Prolonged fasting
b. ____ Decreased glucose	2. Stress
c. ____ Increased adrenal hormones	3. Erect posture
	4. Long-term exercise
d. ____ Increased sex hormones	5. Tobacco
e. ____ Increased albumin	
f. ____ Increased CK	

16. Differentiate between the effects of short-term and long-term exercise on test results.

    _____

    _____

    _____

17. List two patient variables affecting bilirubin.

    a. _____

    b. _____

18. Why will stress and exercise increase WBCs?

    _____

    _____

19. How does prolonged tourniquet application affect test results?

    _____

    _____

20. In what two ways can puncture site selection affect the quality of patient care?

    a. _____

    b. _____

21. Unusually high bilirubin, phosphorus, and uric acid results on specimens collected in the nursery may be caused by

_____ .

22. Following the phlebotomist's rounds in the nursery, the nursing supervisor notices that four babies have an excessive number of punctures located at the back of the heel.

a. How could the supervisor formally document this problem?

_____

_____

b. What should the phlebotomy supervisor do?

_____

_____

c. What will happen to this documentation?

_____

_____

23. List four tests that may be affected by transport in a pneumatic tube system.

a. _____

b. _____

c. _____

d. _____

24. A specimen collected in a red top tube is centrifuged and stored unseparated in the refrigerator overnight. Will this affect any test results? If so, what tests and how will they be affected?

_____

_____

_____

25. Briefly describe the quality control of centrifuges, refrigerators, and freezers.

_____

_____

_____

_____

_____

26. True or False. It is acceptable to combine plasma collected in lavender and green top tubes, but not lavender and light-blue top tubes. Explain your answer.

_____

27. How could poor technique in specimen processing cause the following?

   a. Increased calcium _____

   b. Decreased alcohol levels _____

   c. Overall increased results
      in a general health profile _____

   d. Increased potassium _____

28. Identify the role of the phlebotomist in the TQM areas of infrastructure, support services, and direct patient care by stating a possible concern that might be associated with each area.

   a. Infrastructure _____

   b. Support services _____

   c. Direct patient care _____

Index

An "f" following a page number indicates a figure. A "t" following a page number indicates a table.

AABB. *See* American Association of Blood Banks (AABB)
Ab. *See* Antibody (Ab)
Abduction, definition of, 119
ABGs. *See* Arterial blood gases (ABGs)
ABO. *See* Blood group(s)
Abscess, definition of, 50
Accessioning, 333–334, 341–342
Accreditation, 3, 7, 30
   quality control and, 363–364
ACD. *See* Acid citrate dextrose (ACD)
Acetylcholine, definition of, 126
Acid, 67
Acid citrate dextrose (ACD), 182
Acid-base balance, 146
Acne, 85
Acquired immunodeficiency syndrome (AIDS), 103, 107
Acromegaly, 159
ACTH. *See* Adrenocorticotropic hormone (ACTH)
Activated partial thromboplastin time [APTT (PTT)], function of, 41t, 100
   clinical correlation, 103t
Adapter(s), needle, 176–177, 177f, 178
Addison's disease, 159
Additive(s)
   collection tubes and, 178–179, 182, 184, 265
   quality control and, 359, 364
Adduction, definition of, 119
ADH. *See* Antidiuretic hormone (ADH)
Adrenaline, 155, 159
Adrenocorticotropic hormone (ACTH), 155, 159, 252, 363
Aerobe, definition of, 50
Aerosol, 61–62, 343
Afferent neuron(s), 126–127, 128f
Ag. *See* Antigen (Ag)
Agglutination, definition of, 48
AIDS. *See* Acquired immunodeficiency syndrome (AIDS)
Air bubble(s), 271
Air contamination, 313
Albino, definition of, 83
Albumin, 42
   tests on, 45t
Alcohol level(s), 253, 360
Aldosterone, 156, 158
Alimentary tract, 142–143
Aliquoting, 333, 341–343, 363
ALS. *See* Amyotrophic lateral sclerosis (ALS)
Alveolar duct(s), 132f, 122
Alveoli, 132f, 133–135

Alzheimer's disease, 129
Amber-colored collection tube(s), 288
American Association of Blood Banks (AABB), 225, 337, 339
American Hospital Association Patient's Bill of Rights, 8–9
American Medical Technologists (AMT), 4, 8t
American Society for Clinical Laboratory Science (ASCLS), 4
American Society of Clinical Pathologists (ASCP), 4, 8t
Amino acids, 142–143
Ammonia measurement, 312, 363
Amniocentesis, definition of, 162
Amniotic fluid, 340–341
AMT. *See* American Medical Technologists (AMT)
Amyotrophic lateral sclerosis (ALS), 129
Anaerobe, definition of, 50
Anatomic pathology, definition of, 28
Anatomic position, 80
Ancillary blood glucose test, 296
   instrument for, 296f
Androgen, 156, 158
Anemia, 37–38, 102, 180
Aneurysm, 101
Antecubital fossa, 113, 203
Anterior, 78, 8, 81f
Antibody(ies) (Ab), 45–48
Anticoagulant(s), 37, 39–40, 337, 342
   arterial blood gases and,
   collection tubes and, 178–180, 180f, 181–182, 184, 251
      microcollection tubes, 265, 271
   patients receiving therapy with, 317, 319, 342
   quality control and, 359, 364
Antidiuretic hormone (ADH), 156, 159
Antigen(s) (Ag), 45–46
Antigen-antibody reactions, 49
Antiglycolytic agent(s), 173, 182
Antimicrobial, definition of, 50
Antimicrobial removal devices (ARDs), 251
Antiseptic, 173–174, 187
Antiserum, definition of, 45
Antithrombin III
   clinical correlation, 103t
   function of, 41t
Anuria, 149
Aorta, 91, 96–97
Apnea, 131
Appearance, 6. *See also* Professional image

Appendectomy, 142–143
Appendicitis, 143
Appendix, 143, 144f, 145
APTT (PTT). *See* Activated partial thromboplastin time [APTT (PTT)]
ARDs. *See* Antimicrobial removal devices (ARDs)
Arm
   bandaging of, 212, 212f
   veins in, 204, 204f
Arterial blood gases (ABGs), 133, 229, 252, 312
   collection of, 311–312
      complications of, 319–320
      equipment for, 313–314
         kit for, 314f
      Modified Allen Test, 316f
      procedure for, 314–318
      puncture procedure for, 317f
      technician performing determination, 313f
   effect of technical errors on results of, 319t, 360
Arterial puncture(s), 27, 187, 234
Arteriole(s), 90, 92, 97
Arteriosclerosis, 130
Arteriospasm, 311, 319
Artery(ies), 90–91, 96–97
   comparison to veins and capillaries, 92f, 95f
Arthritis, 113, 118t
Articulation, definition of, 113
Ascites, definition of, 142
ASCLS. *See* American Society for Clinical Laboratory Science (ASCLS)
ASCP. *See* American Society of Clinical Pathologists (ASCP)
Aseptic technique, 247, 250–251
Asphyxia, definition of, 131
Aspirin, 292, 359
Assault, definition of, 3, 10
Asthma, 133
Atherosclerosis, 101
Atrophy, 119
Autoimmunity, 48
Autologous transfusion, 47, 333, 338–339
Automated disposable incision device(s), 292
Automated hematology analyzer(s), 39, 40f
Automatic needle removal device(s), 176, 177f
Autonomic nervous system (involuntary), 126–127
Azotemia, 146

B lymphocyte(s), 103 – 105
Bacillus, definition of, 50
Bacteria, 50 – 51
Bacterial endocarditis, 102
Bacterial growth, inhibition of, 251
Bacterial inhibition test, 294, 295f
Bacteriology, definition of, 50
Bacteriostatic, 173, 187
Bandage(s), 212, 212f, 234, 272, 293, 318
Bar code(s), 344
Barrier gel(s), 343
Basal state, 247 – 248, 355
Basophil(s), 98, 100
Battery, definition of, 3, 10
BB. *See* Blood bank (BB)
Bedside blood glucose test, 296
    instrument for, 296f
Bell's palsy, 129
Benign, definition of, 83
Bevel(ed), 173, 175, 175f
Bilateral, definition of, 79
Bilirubin, neonatal, 288, 341
Biologic hazards, 61 – 66
    safety practices related to, 63f, 212
Black top(s), 180, 183t
Bladder, 146 – 147, 147f – 148f, 149
Blanch(es), 311, 315
Bleeding, puncture site and, 210 – 211,
    272, 292, 317, 319
Bleeding time (BT), 359
    clinical correlation, 103t
    dermal puncture and, 292 – 294
        template procedure for, 293f
        wicking of blood during, 294f
    function of, 41t, 100
Blood, 91 – 92, 97 – 100, 157, 176
    coagulation of, 100, 101f
    disorders associated with, 102
    pathway of through heart, 94 – 96, 96f
    transfer from syringe to evacuated tube,
        185f
Blood alcohol level(s), 182, 229
Blood bank (BB), 45 – 46, 47f, 211, 337
    specimen collection and handling in,
        47, 181 – 182
    tests in, 46f, 47, 48t
Blood cell(s), formation of, 114
Blood clot(s). *See* Clot(s)
Blood collection, 28 – 231
    possible reasons for failure of, 232f
    specimen processing, 341f
Blood culture(s), 52, 283, 287, 361
    collection systems for, 251f
    incubation of, 52f
    performed in microbiology section, 52t
    special venipuncture and, 250 – 252
    venipuncture complications and,
        228 – 229
Blood donor collection, 337 – 339
Blood gas determinations, 271, 312
Blood glucose test, 296
    instrument for, 296f
Blood groups (ABO), 45 – 46, 98, 98t
Blood level(s), medications and, 248
Blood pressure (BP), 96, 159
    cuffs for, 292 – 293
    tourniquets and, 186, 226

Blood smear(s), 266, 271
    preparation of, 288 – 290, 290f
        effect of technical errors on, 291t
        malaria and, 290 – 291
        slide positioning examples, 291f
Blood sugar, 159, 161
Blood test(s), 27, 39, 175
Blood transfusion. *See* Transfusion
Blood type, 47
    definition of, 45
Blood vessels, 90 – 93
    comparison of, 92f, 95f
    disorders associated with, 101
    major arteries, 93f
    veins used for arm venipuncture, 94f
Blood urea nitrogen (BUN), 181
Blood-borne pathogen(s), 65 – 66, 176
    donor collection and, 337 – 339
Board of Trustees, hospital's, 24
Body, 79 – 80
    cavities of, 81 – 82, 82f, 82t
    planes of, 81, 81f
Body fluid analysis, definition of, 39
Body language, 6
Bone(s), 114 – 115, 119
    contact with, 263, 267
    fractures of, 115 – 116
    major, 116f
Bone marrow, 97 – 100, 102, 107,
    113 – 114, 117
Bone marrow test, 39
    clinical correlation, 103t
Bowel, definition of, 142
BP. *See* Blood pressure (BP)
Brachial artery, arterial blood gases and,
    315, 320
Brain, 129
Bronchi, 132f, 133 – 134
Bronchitis, 134
Brown top(s), 182, 183t
Bruising. *See* Ecchymoses
BT. *See* Bleeding time (BT)
Buffer, definition of, 42
BUN. *See* Blood urea nitrogen (BUN)
Butterfly apparatus, 66, 173, 185, 186f, 204
    venipuncture complications and,
        229 – 230, 231f

C & S. *See* Culture and sensitivity (C & S)
Calcaneus area, 261, 268, 268f
Calcitonin, 156 – 157
Calibration of centrifuge, 363
Calluses, 269
Cannula, 223, 229
    arterial blood gases and, 315, 319
CAP. *See* College of American Pathologists
    (CAP)
Capillary(ies), 90, 92, 95, 97, 104
    comparison with arteries and veins, 92f,
        95f
Capillary blood, 262, 267
Capillary blood gases, 267, 314, 320
Capillary tubes, 264, 271 – 272, 288, 295
Caraway pipets, 265
Carbon dioxide (CO_2), 97, 312
    respiratory system and, 132 – 133, 135

Carcinoma, 165
Cardiac cycle, 96
Cardiac muscle, 120, 121f
Cardiovascular, definition of, 90
Carpal(s), 113, 115
Carpal tunnel syndrome (CTS), 121
Carrier, definition of, 50
Cartilage, 113, 115, 118
Cast, 52 – 53
Catheter(s), 224, 228. *See also* Central
    venous catheter(s)
Caudal, definition of, 79
Cavities of the body, 81, 82f
CBC. *See* Complete blood count (CBC)
CDC. *See* Centers for Disease Control
    (CDC)
Cell(s), 48, 80, 84
    metabolism of, 157, 161
Cell-mediated immunity, 99, 103 – 104, 107
Centers for Disease Control (CDC), 66
Central nervous system (CNS), 126, 129
Central neuron(s), 127
Central venous catheter(s) (CVCs),
    228 – 229
Centrifuge, 42, 44, 181
    microspecimens and, 264 – 265
    specimen handling with, 342, 342f, 343,
        363 – 364
Cerebellum, 126, 129
Cerebral palsy, 129
Cerebrovascular accident (CVA), 130
Cerebrospinal fluid (CSF), 126, 129
    handling specimens of, 340 – 341
Cerebrum, 126, 129
Certification, 3, 7 – 8, 8t
Certified laboratory phlebotomist
    (CLP1b), 4, 8t
Certified phlebotomy technician (CPT),
    4, 8t
CEU. *See* Continuing education unit (CEU)
Chain of infection, 62 – 63, 63f
Chemical hazards, 67, 68f, 69
Chemical Hygiene Plan, 67
Chemistry profile(s), 44
Chemistry section, 42 – 43, 129
    instrumentation in, 43f-44f
    specimen collection handling in, 44,
        340
    tests performed in, 44, 45t
CHF. *See* Congestive heart failure (CHF)
Chief of Staff, hospital's, 24
Children, 320, 337, 360
    dermal puncture in, 262 – 263,
        267 – 268, 272
Chilled specimens, 252
    blood gases, 314, 317 – 318, 320
Cholecystectomy, 142
Cholecystitis, 144
Cholesterol, 42
    tests on, 45t
Chronic obstructive pulmonary disease
    (COPD), 134, 312
Circulatory system, 89 – 102
    blood, 97 – 100
        ABO blood group system, 98t
        normal white cells, 99f
        blood vessels, 91 – 93

arm veins used for venipuncture, 94f
  comparison of, 92f, 95f
  major arteries, 93f
  coagulation, 100, 101f
  disorders associated with, 101 – 102
  heart, 93 – 97
    pathway of blood through, 96f
  laboratory tests associated with, 103,
    103t
Cirrhosis, 144
Civil law suit, definition of, 3, 10
Clavicle, definition of, 114
Clean-catch, 356
CLIA '88. *See* Clinical Laboratory
    Improvement Act of 1988 (CLIA
    '88)
Clinical chemistry instrumentation, 43f
Clinical laboratory department, 25, 32, 364
  blood bank section of, 45 – 47, 47f, 48t
  chemistry section of, 42 – 44, 45t
  hematology section of, 37 – 40, 41t
  hospital's, 27 – 28
  immunology section of, 48 – 49, 49t
  microbiology section of, 49 – 51,
    51f – 52f, 52t
  organization of, 28f
  personnel of, 28 – 29, 29f, 30
  regulation of, 30 – 31
  serology section of, 48 – 49, 49t
  urinalysis section of, 52 – 53, 53f, 54, 54t
Clinical Laboratory Improvement Act of
    1988 (CLIA '88), 31
Clinical laboratory scientist (CLS), 30
Clinical laboratory technician (CLT), 30
Clinical pathology, definition of, 28
Clot(s), 37, 39, 90, 100, 102
  activator(s) of, 180 – 181
Clotting time, 342, 362
CLP1b. *See* Certified laboratory
    phlebotomist (CLP1b)
CLS. *See* Clinical laboratory scientist (CLS)
CLT. *See* Clinical laboratory technician
    (CLT)
CNS. *See* Central nervous system (CNS)
CO_2. *See* Carbon dioxide (CO_2)
Coagulation, 100
  disorders associated with, 102, 234, 319
  studies of, 178, 180, 182, 184, 228, 252
Coagulation cascade, 101f, 179, 180f,
    181 – 182
Coagulation laboratory, 40
Coccus, definition of, 50
Cold agglutinins, 252
Colitis, 144
Collateral circulation, 311, 315, 319
Collection tray(s), 174, 174f
  dermal puncture equipment for, 262
Collection tube(s), 176, 178, 362
  color-coding principles, 179 – 182
  evacuated tube examples, 178f – 179f
  fill order of, 184f
  labeling of, 211, 211f, 233, 272, 338, 341,
    363
  serum separator tubes, 181f
College of American Pathologists (CAP),
    30 – 31
  accreditation certificate from, 31f

Colon, 143 – 144, 144f
Color-coding, 178, 265, 271
  principles of, 179 – 182
Communicable, definition of, 50
Communication skills, 6 – 7, 7f
Compassion, 5
Compatibility test(s), 45 – 46
Complete blood count (CBC), 38 – 39, 41t,
    179
  clinical correlation, 103t
  dermal puncture and, 271, 289
  hemolysis and, 233t
Computer(s), 355
  laboratories and, 343 – 344, 345f
Confidentiality, 3, 6, 9 – 10
Congestive heart failure (CHF), 101, 135
Consent form(s), 338
Contamination
  dermal punctures and, 289, 295 – 296
  quality control to prevent, 361,
    363 – 364
  specimens and, 234, 251, 270 – 271, 339,
    341 – 342
Continuing education, 8, 357
Continuing education unit (CEU), 4, 8
Continuous quality improvement (CQI),
    353 – 354, 364 – 365
Contraction(s), 119
COPD. *See* Chronic obstructive
    pulmonary disease (COPD)
Corpus luteum, definition of, 162
Corrective action(s), 355, 357, 358f, 363
Cortisol, 156, 158, 360
Costal, definition of, 114
Coumadin, 90, 100
CPT. *See* Certified phlebotomy technician
    (CPT)
CQI. *See* Continuous quality improvement
    (CQI)
Creatinine, 146, 149, 150t
Criminal law suit, definition of, 3, 10
Crohn's disease, 145
Crossmatch (X-match), 45 – 46
Cryoprecipitate, 46 – 47
CSF. *See* Cerebrospinal fluid (CSF)
CT. *See* Cytotechnologists (CT)
CTS. *See* Carpal tunnel syndrome (CTS)
Cubitus/cubital, definition of, 114
Culture(s), 50, 51f – 52f
Culture and sensitivity (C & S), 51, 52t
Culture media, 251
Cushing's disease, 159 – 160
CVA. *See* Cerebrovascular accident (CVA)
CVCs. *See* Central venous catheter(s)
    (CVCs)
Cyanosis, definition of, 131
Cystic fibrosis, 339
Cystitis, 149
Cystoscope, 146
Cytogenetics, 28, 341
Cytotechnologists (CT), 27 – 28

Dark-blue top(s), 182, 183t
Delta check, 353, 357, 361
Dendrite(s), 126 – 127, 128f, 129
Deoxyhemoglobin, 133

Dependability, 5
Dermal, definition of, 261
Dermal puncture, 5, 261 – 273, 361 – 362
  equipment for, 262 – 266
    microspecimen, 265f
    skin puncture devices, 263f
  finger puncture sites, 269f
  heel puncture posture, 270f
  heel puncture sites, 268f
  procedure for, 267 – 273
  special, 287 – 296
    bedside glucose testing instrument,
      296f
    blood smear preparation, 290f – 291f
    correct and incorrect blood
      collection with filter paper, 295f
    effect of technical errors on blood
      smears, 291t
    sample bacterial inhibition test, 295f
    template bleeding time procedure,
      293f
    wicking of blood during time
      procedure, 294f
  specimen collection from finger, 271f
  Unopette procedure, 266f
  vascular area of skin, 264f
Dermis, 83 – 84, 84f, 85
Diabetes insipidus, 160
Diabetes mellitus, 160, 249
Diagnostic related groups (DRGs), 32
Diarrhea, 142, 144 – 145
Diastole, 90, 96
Differential (Diff), function of, 41t, 98
Digestion, 142 – 143
Digestive system, 141 – 142, 144f
  disorders associated with, 143 – 145
  laboratory tests associated with, 145,
    145t
Dilution system(s), 265 – 266
Disciplinary action, 362
Disinfectant, 61, 66
Disposal systems, 176, 177f, 211, 211f
Disseminated intravascular coagulation,
    102
Distal, definition of, 79
Distal convoluted tubule, 148f, 149
Diurnal variation, 247 – 250, 360
DNA analysis, 253
Documentation, 353 – 355, 362 – 363
Dorsal, 80 – 81, 81f
Dorsal hand vein collection technique,
    295
Draw order, 182 – 184, 184f, 362
  dermal puncture, 271 – 272
Drawing station, 175f, 201, 262
DRGs. *See* Diagnostic related groups
    (DRGs)
Drug levels, 253
Duke method, 292
Duodenum, 142, 144f, 145
Dwarfism, 161
Dysentery, 142
Dysuria, 146

Earlobe(s), dermal punctures in, 267, 292
Ecchymoses, 261, 263

EDTA. *See* Ethylenediaminetetraacetic acid (EDTA)
Edema, 27, 224
Education, 7
Efferent neuron(s), 126 – 127, 128f
Effusion, definition of, 131
EIA. *See* Enzyme immunoassay (EIA)
Electrical hazards, 69
Electrocardiography, 23, 25
Electroencephalography, 23, 25
Electrolyte(s), 42, 181
    tests on, 45t
Electrophoresis, 42 – 43
Embolus, 90
Emesis, 142
Emphysema, 134
Endocardium, 90, 94
Endocrine, definition of, 156
Endocrine gland(s), 157 – 159
Endocrine system, 155 – 158, 158f, 159
    disorders associated with, 159 – 161
    hormones of the pituitary gland and their target organs, 160f
    laboratory tests associated with, 161, 161t
Endogenous, definition of, 42
Endometriosis, 165
Endometrium, 162, 165
Endothelium, 90 – 91
Enteric, definition of, 142
Enzyme, definition of, 42
Enzyme immunoassay (EIA), 43
Eosinophil(s), 98 – 99
Eosinophil count, 39
Epidermis, 83 – 84, 84f, 85
Epiglottis, 132f, 133
Epilepsy, 130
Epinephrine, 155, 159
Epithelium, 83 – 84
Equipment
    assembly of, 202, 202f, 226
    examination of, 207, 207f
    quality control of, 357, 359, 362
Erythema, 83, 85
Erythrocyte(s), 90, 97 – 98, 102
Erythrocyte sedimentation rate (ESR), 39
Esophagus, 133
ESR. *See* Erythrocyte sedimentation rate (ESR)
Estradiol, 162, 166t
Estrogen, 158 – 159, 162 – 163
Ethics, 3, 8, 10
Ethylenediaminetetraacetic acid (EDTA), 39
    collection tubes and, 179, 182 – 183, 183t, 184
    dermal punctures and, 289, 291
Evacuated collection systems, 175f, 176 – 178, 178f – 179f, 349. *See also* Vacutainer
    blood transfer to, 185, 185f
    specimen handling with, 340, 343
Evaporation, 364
Exchange transfusion, 288
Exercise, 360
Exogenous, definition of, 42
Expiration date, 359

Explosive hazards, 69
Extension, definition of, 119
External respiration, 132

Factor assays, function of, 41t
Fainting. *See* Syncope
Fallopian tubes, 162 – 164, 164f
Fasting specimens, 44, 247 – 249, 359
FDA. *See* Food and Drug Administration (FDA)
FDP. *See* Fibrin degradation products (FDP)
Feathered edge, 287, 289
Febrile, definition of, 50
Feces, 142 – 143
    specimen collection, 335f, 336
Femur, 114 – 115
Femoral, definition of, 114
Fertilization, 162 – 164
Fever of unknown origin (FUO), 250
Fibrin, 90, 100
Fibrin degradation products (FDP), 180
    clinical correlation, 103t
    function of, 41t
Fibrinogen, 39, 41t, 90, 100
Fibrinolysis, 100
Fibroids, 165
Filter paper, 292, 294 – 295
    correct and incorrect blood collection with, 295f
Finger puncture(s), 263, 267, 270 – 271
    sites for, 267, 269, 269f
Fire hazards, 69
    types of 70t
First morning specimen, 335
Fiscal services, hospital's, 25
Fist(s), 205, 205f, 338
Fistula, 224, 228
Flexion, 119, 120f
Floor book(s), 353, 355 – 357
Fluid balance, 146
Follicle-stimulating hormone (FSH), 156, 159
Food and Drug Administration (FDA), 337, 339
Forensic specimens, 247, 252 – 253
    sample chain-of-custody form for, 253f
Fracture(s) (Fxs), 115 – 116
Fresh frozen plasma, 46 – 47
Frontal plane, 79, 81
Frozen specimen(s), 343
Fungal culture(s), 51, 52t
Fungal infection(s), 85
FUO. *See* Fever of unknown origin (FUO)
Fxs. *See* Fracture(s) (Fxs)

Gallbladder (GB), 142 – 144, 144f
Gamete, 162 – 163
Gastroenteritis, 145
Gauge, 173, 175 – 176
Gauze pad(s), 187
GB. *See* Gallbladder (GB)
Genitalia, definition of, 162
Geriatric, 261 – 262
Gestation, definition of, 162

GH. *See* Growth hormone (GH)
Gigantism, 161
Glass slides, dermal punctures and, 266
Globulin, definition of, 42
Glomerulonephritis, 149
Glomerulus, 148f, 149
Gloves, 64, 66, 187, 289
    removal of, 65f, 212
    specimen handling and, 342 – 343, 364
Glucose, 42, 182
Glucose tolerance test (GTT), 249 – 250, 359
    sample test schedules, 249t
Glycosuria, 52
Gold top(s), 180, 183t
Gonads, 162 – 163
Gout, 116
Gowns, 64
Gram stain, 50 – 51, 51f, 52t
Gram-negative, definition of, 50
Gram-positive, definition of, 50
Granulocyte(s), 37, 98, 100
Graves' disease, 161
Gray matter, 127, 129
Gray top(s), 182, 183t, 184
Green top(s), 181, 183t, 184, 184f
Growth hormone (GH), 156, 159, 161
GTT. *See* Glucose tolerance test (GTT)

Hair, 83 – 84, 84f, 85
Hand, 204, 315
    position of during routine venipuncture, 207, 208f
Handling procedures, special collections and, 252 – 253
Handwashing, 63 – 64
Hardware, 333, 343
HBV. *See* Hepatitis B virus (HBV)
HCG. *See* Human chorionic gonadotropin (HCG)
Hct. *See* Hematocrit
HDN. *See* Hemolytic disease of the newborn (HDN)
Health Maintenance Organization(s) (HMOs), 31
Healthcare delivery system, 23 – 32
Healthcare settings, phlebotomist's role in, 31 – 32
Heart, 91 – 94
    pathways of blood through, 94 – 96, 96f
    disorders associated with, 102
Heart rate, 92, 96
Heel puncture(s), 263, 267, 279, 294, 362
    correct position for, 270f
    sites for, 268, 268f, 269
Heel warmer, 266
Hematocrit (Hct), 180, 264
    clinical correlation, 103t
    function of, 41t
Hematology section, 37, 129
    blood cell examination in, 38f
    coagulation area of, 40, 40t
    specimen collection and handling in, 38 – 39, 340 – 341
    tests performed in, 39 – 40, 41t

Hematoma, 177, 210, 227, 231, 233
  arterial blood gases and, 315, 318–319
  site selection and, 361–362
Hematopoiesis, 114
Hematuria, 52
Hemochromatosis, 339
Hemoconcentration, 197, 202, 205, 338
Hemoglobin (Hgb), 43, 97, 102, 248, 360
  function of, 41t, 133
Hemolysis, 37, 39, 44, 47, 202
  dermal punctures and, 262–263, 269,
    271, 288
  laboratory tests affected by, 233t
  specimens and, 232–234, 338, 342,
    361–362
  venipuncture causing, 175, 178, 185,
    206
Hemolytic disease of the newborn (HDN),
    288, 341
Hemophilia, 102
Hemorrhage(s), 319
Hemostasis, 37, 40, 100
Hemostats, 333, 338
Heparin, 90, 100, 228
  collection tubes and, 181–182
Heparin lock(s), 224, 228
Heparinized blood gas pipet(s), 320
Heparinized syringe(s), 313–314,
    316–317
Hepatitis, 145
Hepatitis B virus (HBV), 65–66
Hernia, 142
Hgb. See Hemoglobin
Histologists, 28
Histology section, 341
HIV. See Human immunodeficiency virus
    (HIV)
HMOs. See Health Maintenance
    Organization(s) (HMOs)
Hodgkin's disease, 107
Home glucose monitoring, 262, 269
Homeostasis, 79, 82, 157
Honesty, 6
Hormone(s), 156, 250
  function of, 157–159
Hospital(s), 51, 362
  identification numbers, 200, 211
  organization of, 24–25, 26f
Human chorionic gonadotropin (HCG),
    162–163, 166t
Human experimentation, 9
Human immunodeficiency virus (HIV),
    65, 107
Humoral immunity, 99, 103, 106
Hyperglycemia, 156, 160, 249
Hyperinsulinism, 161
Hypoglycemia, 161, 249
Hypothyroidism, 294
Hysterectomy, 162

Icteric, definition of, 42, 44
Identification (ID) band(s), 197, 200, 200f,
    201, 267
Ileum, 142
Iliac crest, 114
Immune, definition of, 103

Immune response, 48, 105
Immune system, 105, 105f, 106–107
Immunochemistry, 43
Immunoglobulin(s), 48
Immunohematology, 46
Immunology section, 48–49
  tests performed in, 49t
Impetigo, 85
In vitro tests, 27
In vivo tests, 27
Incident report(s), 362
Incision(s), dermal puncture and, 264, 292
Independent reference laboratories,
    phlebotomist's role in, 32
Indicator(s), 354–355
Indices, function of, 41t
Indwelling lines, 224, 228–229. See also
    Catheter(s)
Infant(s), 339, 341
  arterial blood gas collection in, 312,
    315, 320
  dermal puncture in, 262, 264, 267–268,
    272
  special dermal punctures in, 288, 292,
    294–295
Infant respiratory distress syndrome
    (IRDS), 134
Infarct, definition of, 90
Infection, 61
  risk of, 316, 319
  transmission of, 62–64
Infectious mononucleosis, 107
Inferior, definition of, 79
Informed consent, 3, 9
Inherited metabolic disorder(s), 294
Inservice education, 357
Insulin, 156, 159–161
Integumentary system, 83–85
  cross-section of, 84f
  disorders associated with, 85
  laboratory tests associated with, 86, 86t
Integrity, 6
Internal respiration, 132
Interneurons, 127
Interstitial fluid, 103–104
Intravenous fluid(s), 185, 228, 361
  veins for, 204–205
Invasion of privacy, definition of, 3, 10
Involuntary muscle(s), 120
Involuntary nervous system. See
    Autonomic nervous system
Iontophoresis, 333, 339
IRDS. See Infant respiratory distress
    syndrome (IRDS)
Isoenzyme, 42–43
Isolation, 50
  classification of, 64t
  procedures for, 64–65

Jaundice, 42
JCAHO. See Joint Commission on
    Accreditation of Healthcare
    Organizations (JCAHO)
Jejunum, 142
Joint(s), 114–115. See also Synovial
    joint(s)

Joint Commission on Accreditation of
    Healthcare Organizations
    (JCAHO), 30–31, 354

Keloid, 85
Keratin, 83, 85
Ketonuria, 52
Kidney, 146–147, 147f, 149–150
Kidney stone(s), 149

Labeling, 211, 211f, 233, 272, 338, 341, 363
  arterial blood gases and, 314, 317
  computers and, 343–344
  special collections, 250–251
Labile, 173, 180
Laboratory
  computers in, 343–344, 345f, 355
  management of, 28–29
  quality in, 353–365
  reference manuals in, 353, 355
  safety in. See also Chemical hazards
    equipment station for, 68f
    supplies and information manuals for,
      68f
Laboratory information management
    systems (LIMS), 344
Laboratory test(s), 9, 82, 212
  circulatory system and, 103, 103t
  digestive system and, 145, 145t
  endocrine system and, 161, 161t
  hemolysis effect on, 233t
  integumentary system and, 86, 86t
  lymphatic system and, 107, 107t
  muscular system and, 122, 122t
  nervous system and, 130, 130t
  normal values for, 248, 312
  requisition of, 250, 355–357, 336, 341,
    343–344
    arterial blood gases and, 314, 320
    complicated procedures, 224–225,
      228, 234
    dermal punctures and, 262, 267
    routine procedures, 198–199, 199f,
      200, 212
    sample requisition, 356f
  respiratory system and, 135, 135t
  skeletal system and, 118, 118t
  urinary system and, 150, 150t
  variables affecting, 360t
Lactic acid determinations(s), 226, 312
Lancet(s), 66, 270, 292
Laryngitis, 135
Larynx, 132f, 133, 135
Lateral, definition of, 79
Lavender top(s), 179, 183t, 184, 184f, 271
LE. See Lupus erythematosus (LE)
Lead determination(s), 182
Leg vein(s), use for venipuncture, 227
Legal issues, 10
Legal specimens, 252–253
  sample chain-of-custody form for, 253f
Length of stay, 32
Leukemia, 37–38, 102
Leukocyte(s), 90, 98–100, 102
  normal, 99f

Leukocytosis, 98
Leukopenia, 98
LH. *See* Luteinizing hormone (LH)
Ligament(s), 114, 118
Light, specimens sensitive to, 252, 288
Light-blue top(s), 179 – 180, 183, 183t, 184, 184f
LIMS. *See* Laboratory information management systems
Lipemic specimens, 44, 247 – 248
Listening skills, 6
Lithium, 42
    tests on, 45t
Lithotripsy, 149
Litigation, 4, 10
Liver, 143 – 144, 144f, 145
Loop of Henle, 148f, 149
Lot, 354, 359
Lower respiratory tract, 132
LP. *See* Lumbar puncture (LP)
Luer tip(s), 311, 313
Lumbar, definition of, 126
Lumbar puncture (LP), 129
Lumen, 90 – 91
Lung(s), 131, 132f, 133 – 135
Lupus erythematosus (LE) prep, definition of, 39
Luteinizing hormone (LH), 156, 159
Lyme disease, 117
Lymph, 103 – 104
Lymph node(s), 103 – 104, 107
Lymph vessel(s), 103 – 104
    relationship to cardiovascular system, 106f
Lymphatic system, 103 – 104, 105f, 227, 319
    disorders associated with, 107
    immune system, 105 – 107
    laboratory tests associated with, 107, 107t
    relationship to cardiovascular system, 106f
Lymphocyte(s), 98 – 99, 104, 107. *See also* B lymphocyte(s), T lymphocyte(s)
Lymphoma, 107
Lymphostasis, 224, 227

Magnetic resonance imaging (MRI), 27
Magnetized "flea," 311, 320
Malaria, blood smears for, 290 – 291
Malignant, 83, 85
Malpractice, 4, 10
Masks, 64, 66
Mastectomy, 227, 361
Material Safety Data Sheets (MSDS), 67
MCH. *See* Mean corpuscular hemoglobin (MCH)
MCHC. *See* Mean corpuscular hemoglobin concentration (MCHC)
MCV. *See* Mean corpuscular volume (MCV)
MD. *See* Muscular dystrophy (MD)
Mean corpuscular hemoglobin (MCH), function of, 41t
Mean corpuscular hemoglobin

concentration (MCHC), function of, 41t
Mean corpuscular volume (MCV), function of, 41t
Medial, definition of, 80
Medical laboratory technician(s) (MLT), 30
Medical technologist(s) (MT), 29 – 30
Medication(s), therapeutic monitoring of, 250, 360
Melanin, 83 – 84
Melanocyte-stimulating hormone (MSH), 156, 159
Melatonin, 159
Meninges, 126, 129 – 130
Meningitis, 130
Menopause, 162 – 163
Menstruation, 162 – 163, 166
Metacarpal(s), 113, 115
Metastasis, definition of, 162
Metatarsal(s), 114 – 115
MI. *See* Myocardial infarction (MI)
Microbiology, definition of, 50
Microbiology section, 49 – 50, 129
    specimen handling and collection in, 51, 51f – 52f, 340 – 341
    tests performed in, 51, 52t
Microcollection tube(s), 265, 271 – 272
Microhematocrit test, 264
Microorganism(s), 50 – 51
Micropipet(s), 265 – 266, 271
Microsample(s), 261, 267, 270, 272
    containers for, 264 – 265, 265f, 266
Midstream clean-catch, 54, 335
Mitosis, 84
MLT. *See* Medical laboratory technician(s) (MLT)
Mnemonics, 33, 344
Modem(s), 333, 343
Modified Allen Test, 315 – 316, 316f, 317 – 319
Monocyte(s), 98 – 99
Morphology, 37, 51
Motor neuron(s), 126 – 127, 128f
MRI. *See* Magnetic resonance imaging (MRI)
MS. *See* Multiple sclerosis (MS)
MSDS. *See* Material Safety Data Sheets (MSDS)
MSH. *See* Melanocyte-stimulating hormone (MSH)
MT. *See* Medical technologist(s) (MT)
Multiple myeloma, 107
Multiple sclerosis (MS), 130
Multiple specimens, 271
Multi-draw needle(s), 176 – 177
Muscular dystrophy (MD), 121
Muscular system, 118
    disorders associated with, 121
    laboratory tests associated with, 122, 122t
    movement in, 120f
    muscle types, 119 – 120, 121f
Myasthenia gravis, 121
Mycology, definition of, 50
Mycoplasma pneumoniae, 252
Mycosis, 50

Myelin sheath, 126 – 127, 128f, 130
Myocardial infarction (MI), 102
Myocarditis, 90
Myxedema, 161

Nail(s), 83, 85
Nasopharynx, 131
Natelson pipet(s), 265
National Certification Agency for Medical Laboratory Personnel (NCA), 4, 8t
National Committee for Clinical Laboratory Standards (NCCLS), 31, 359
National Fire Protection Association (NFPA), 69
National Phlebotomy Association (NPA), 4, 8t
Natremia, 156
Nausea, 142, 145
NCA. *See* National Certification Agency for Medical Laboratory Personnel (NCA)
NCCLS. *See* National Committee for Clinical Laboratory Standards (NCCLS)
Needle(s), 175 – 176, 178, 338, 357
    adapters for, 176 – 177, 177f
    disposal of, 66, 176, 177f, 211, 211f, 357, 362
    inspection of, 207, 207f – 208f, 210f
    removal of, 210, 233
    structure of, 175f
Negligence, 4, 10
Neonatal, definition of, 23
Neonatal bilirubin determination, 262, 288
Neonatal screening, 294
Nephron, 147, 149
    relationship to urinary system, 148f
Nerve damage, arterial blood gas collection and, 319 – 320
Nerve impulse(s), 127, 129 – 130
Nervous system, 125 – 127
    disorders associated with, 129 – 130
    laboratory tests associated with, 130, 130t
    sensory and motor neurons, 128f
Neuroglia, 126 – 127
Neuron, 126 – 127, 128f, 129
Neutrophil(s), 98 – 99
NFPA. *See* National Fire Protection Association (NFPA)
Nonverbal skills, 6
Noradrenalin, 156, 159
Norepinephrine, 156, 159
Normal values, 248, 312
    quality control and, 355 – 356, 364
Nose, 133
Nosocomial infection(s), 61, 63
NPA. *See* National Phlebotomy Association (NPA)
Nuclear medicine department, hospital's, 27
Nursery, dermal punctures in, 267, 272
Nursing services, hospital's, 25

O_2. See Oxygen (O_2)

O & P. See Ova and parasites (O & P)

Occlusion, 224, 227

Occult blood, 51, 52t, 336

Occupational Safety and Health
        Administration (OSHA), 66 – 67
    specimen processing regulations,
        341 – 342

Occupational therapy (OT) department,
        hospital's, 27

Oliguria, 149

Oncology, 23

Orange top(s), 181, 183t

Organ(s), 80 – 82, 82t

OSHA. See Occupational Safety and Health
        Administration (OSHA)

Osmotic fragility test, 39

Osteoblast(s), 115

Osteoclast(s), 115

Osteomalacia, 117

Osteomyelitis, 117, 267

Osteoporosis, 117

Osteosarcoma, 117

OT. See Occupational therapy

Outcome(s), 355, 364

Ova, 162 – 163

Ova and parasites (O & P), 51, 52t

Ovulation, 162, 164

Oxygen (O_2), 132 – 133, 135, 312,
        314 – 315

Oxyhemoglobin, 133

Oxytocin, 156, 159

Packed cells (RBCs), 46 – 47

Paget's disease, 117

Palmar area, 261, 268, 269, 271
    angle of, 269f
    specimen collection from, 271f

Palpation, 197, 205f, 206

Pancreas, 143, 144f, 145

Pancreatitis, 145

Panic value(s), 287, 96

Parasitology, 50

Parathyroid hormone, 156 – 157

Parental consent, 267

Parkinson's disease, 130

Partial pressure, 133, 311 – 312

Pathogen(s), 61, 65 – 66

Pathogenic, definition of, 50

Pathologist, 28 – 29

Pathology, 23

Patient(s), 234
    communication with, 6 – 7, 7f, 199, 200f,
        212, 224, 225, 234, 292, 315
    education of, 51, 334 – 336
        sample laboratory instructions for,
            336f
    identification of, 47, 200, 200f, 201, 225,
        267, 292, 315, 357
        legal specimens and, 253
    preparation and positioning of, 201,
        225 – 226, 267, 315
        major tests affected by, 360t
        quality control and, 359 – 361
    refusal of treatment by, 226
    safety of, 6, 62 – 64, 69, 250, 312

quality control and, 357, 361 – 362
    satisfaction of, 362, 364 – 365

Patient's Bill of Rights, 4, 8 – 9

PBT. See Phlebotomy technician (PBT)

Peak level, 247, 250

Pediatric, definition of, 23

Pelvic inflammatory disease (PID), 165

Pelvis, 114

Pericarditis, 102

Pericardium, 90, 94

Peripheral nervous system, 126 – 127, 129
    sensory and motor neurons of, 128f

Peristalsis, 142 – 143

Peritonitis, 145

Personal protective equipment (PPE),
        64 – 65

Petechiae, 197, 203

PF3. See Platelet factor 3 (PF3)

pH, 312 – 313

Pharmacology, definition of, 23

Pharmacy department, hospital's, 27

Pharyngitis, 135

Pharynx, 133, 135

Phenylaline, 287, 294

Phenylketonuria (PKU), 287, 294

Phlebotomist, 9 – 10, 23, 30, 197
    accidental needle sticks and, 176, 185,
        362
    blood donor collection, 337 – 339, 341
    certification of, 7 – 8, 8t
    computer use by, 343 – 344, 345f, 355
    duties of, 5, 47, 51, 54, 174, 267,
        333 – 345, 362
    errors by, 361 – 362
    failure by, 272
    hospitals and, 25, 364
    patient greeting by, 200f
    patient identification by, 200f
    patient instruction by, 334 – 336
        sample laboratory instructions for,
            336f
    personal characteristics of, 5 – 7
    preparation for arterial blood gases,
        314 – 315
    professionalism of, 8
    role of, 4 – 5
    specialized training for, 312, 320
    sweat electrolytes collection, 339 – 340,
        340f
    throat culture collection, 337f

Phlebotomy, 4
    collection tray for, 174f, 362
    drawing station for, 175f
    education and certification for, 7 – 8, 8t
    errors in, 357, 361 – 364
    ethical and legal aspects of, 8 – 10
    quality in, 353 – 365

Phlebotomy technician (PBT), 4, 8t

Physical hazards, 70

Physical therapy (PT) department, 27

Physician office laboratories (POLs),
        phlebotomist's role in, 31

PID. See Pelvic inflammatory disease (PID)

Pilocarpine, 334, 339

Pineal gland, 159

Pituitary gland, hormones of, 159, 160f

PKU. See Phenylketonuria (PKU)

Planes of the body, 81, 81f

Plantar area, 261, 267 – 269

Plasma, 39, 40, 40f, 44, 97, 107, 248, 250.
        See also Fresh frozen plasma
    chemistry tests of, 44
    in tests, 180 – 182
    microspecimens and, 264 – 265
    specimen processing of, 342 – 343,
        363 – 364

Plasma hemoglobin test, 39

Plasma separator tube(s) (PST), 181

plasmodium, 287, 290

Platelet(s) (Plts), 38, 40, 46, 90, 100, 102
    aggregation of, 41t, 103t
    counts of, 41t, 271

Platelet factor 3 (PF3), 100

Platelet plug, 287, 292 – 293

Pleura/pleural, 131, 132f, 135

Pleurisy, 135

Plts. See Platelet(s) (Plts)

PMS. See Premenstrual syndrome (PMS)

Pneumatic tube system(s), 354, 362

Pneumonia, 135

Poliomyelitis, 121

POLs. See Physician office laboratories
        (POLs)

Polycythemia, 102, 180, 339

Polydipsia, 146

Polyuria, 146

Posterior, 80 – 81, 81f

Posture, 226, 359

Potassium determination(s), 181, 361,
        363

PPD. See Purified protein derivative (PPD)

PPE. See Personal protective equipment
        (PPE)

Preanalytical variables, 355

Preferred provider organizations (PPOs),
        32

Prefixes, 15 – 16

Pregnancy, 68, 162 – 163, 165, 166t

Premenstrual syndrome (PMS), 166

Preservation requirement(s), 341

Primary hemostasis, 100, 102

Privacy, 3, 9

PRL. See Prolactin (PRL)

Procedure manual(s), 354 – 355, 363

Proficiency testing, 31

Professional image, 26

Professional service departments, 25
    hospital organization and, 26 – 28

Professionalism, 4, 8

Progesterone, 156 – 159, 162 – 163

Prolactin (PRL), 159

Prone, definition of, 80

Protective apparel, 342

Protective barriers, 64

Protein electrophoresis, 43

Proteinuria, 52

Prothrombin, 90, 100

Prothrombin time (PT)
    clinical correlation, 103t
    function of, 41t, 100

Proximal, definition of, 80

Proximal convoluted tubule, 148f, 149

Psoriasis, 85

PST. See Plasma separator tube(s) (PST)

PT. *See* Physical therapy; Prothrombin time (PT)
Pulmonary artery, 95, 97
Pulmonary circulation, 90–91
Pulmonary edema, 135
Pulmonary vein(s), 96–97
Pulse, 92, 96
Puncture depth, 263–264
Puncture-resistant container(s), 66–67, 67f
Purified protein derivative (PPD), 135t
Pyelonephritis, 149
Pyuria, 53

Quality assurance (QA), 354–357, 364
Quality control (QC), 353–365
    example of a corrective action, 358f
    major tests affected by patient variables, 360t
    sample laboratory collection schedule, 356f
    sample requisition with special instructions, 356f
    time-stamping machines for, 363f
Quality patient care, clinical laboratories and, 30

Radial, definition of, 114
Radial artery, arterial blood gases and, 315–316, 318
Radiation therapy department, hospital's, 27
Radioactive hazards, 68
Radioactivity, 61, 68
Radioimmunoassay (RIA), 43
Radioisotope(s), 61, 68
Radiologist, definition of, 23, 27
Radiology department, 27
Radius, definition of, 114
Random specimen(s), 335–336
Rapid immunologic Group A strep test, 337
RBCs. *See* Red blood cell(s) (RBCs)
RCF. *See* Relative centrifugal force (RCF)
RDS. *See* Respiratory distress syndrome (RDS)
RDW. *See* Red blood cell distribution width (RDW)
Reagent strip(s), 296, 336
Rectum, 142–143, 144f
Red blood cell(s) (RBCs), 38, 90, 97–98, 102
    counts of, 41t
    malaria and, 290–291
    specimen handling and, 362, 364
Red blood cell distribution width (RDW), function of, 41t
Red top(s), 181–182, 183t, 184, 184f
Red/gray top(s), 180–181, 183t, 184
Reference laboratories, 343
Reference ranges, 248, 359
Refractometer(s), 53
Refrigerated specimens, 343

Registered phlebotomy technician (RPT), 4, 8t
Relative centrifugal force (RCF), 342
Renal, definition of, 146
Renal artery, 147f–148f, 149
Renal calculi, 149
Renal dialysis, 146, 150, 228–229
Renal failure, 150
Reproductive system, 161–164
    disorders associated with, 165–166
    female, 164f
    laboratory tests associated with, 166, 166t
    male, 165f
Requisition(s), 336, 341, 343–344
    arterial blood gases and, 314, 320
    complicated procedures, 224–225, 228, 234
    dermal punctures and, 262, 267
    quality control of, 355, 357, 362
    routine procedures, 198–199, 199f, 200, 212
    special collections, 250
    sample of, 356f
Respiration rate, 311, 314
Respiratory distress syndrome (RDS), 312
Respiratory system, 131–132
    components of, 132f
    disorders associated with, 133–135
    laboratory tests associated with, 135, 135t
    pathway of, 134f
Respiratory therapy (RT) department, hospital's, 27
Restraint(s), 267
Reticulocyte(s), 90, 97
Reticulocyte (Retic) count, 39, 289
    clinical correlation, 103t
Rh, 46, 98
Rheumatic heart disease, 102
Rheumatoid arthritis, 118
Rhinitis, 135
RIA. *See* Radioimmunoassay (RIA)
Rolling vein(s), 207
RPT. *See* Registered phlebotomy technician (RPT)
RT. *See* Respiratory therapy

Safety, 61, 68–70
    biologic hazards, 62–66
        chain of infection and, 63f
    fire hazards, 70t
    laboratory equipment station, 68f
    laboratory supplies and information manuals, 68f
    sharp hazards, 66–67
    types of hazards, 62t
Sagittal plane, 80–81, 81f
Sarcoma, 114, 117
Scheduling, 212, 355
    routine specimen collection schedule, 356f
    sample glucose tolerance testing, 248–250
    staff and, 362, 364

Scoliosis, 118
Sebaceous gland, 83–84, 84f, 85
Secondary hemostasis, 100
Section supervisor, 29–30
Seizure(s), 130
Semen, 162, 164
    specimen collection, 336, 336f
Sensitivity, 50
Sensory neuron(s), 126–127, 128f
Separator gel, 265, 363
Sepsis, 50
Septicemia, 247, 250
Serology (Immunology) section, 48–49
    tests performed in, 49t
Serum, 39, 40f, 248, 250
    chemistry tests of, 43–44, 181–182
    microspecimens and, 264–265
    specimen processing of, 342–343, 363–364
Serum separator tube(s) (SST), 180–181, 181f, 184, 184f
Sexually transmitted diseases (STD), 166
Sharp hazards, 66–67, 362
Shingles, 130
Shock, 61, 69, 166, 312
Sickle cell test, 39
Site
    preparation of, 206, 315
        cleansing puncture site, 206f, 229, 251, 269, 361
    selection of, 203–206, 361
        arterial blood gases and, 315
        dermal punctures and, 267–269
        vein selection for, 205f
Skeletal muscle(s), 119, 121f
Skeletal system, 113–114
    disorders associated with, 115–118
    laboratory tests associated with, 118, 118t
    major bones in, 116f
    synovial joints, 117f
Skin, 83–85
    cross-section of, 84f
    vascular area of, 264f
Skin contamination, 251
Skin puncture devices, 263, 263f, 264
SLE. *See* Systemic lupus erythematosus (SLE)
Slide(s), positioning for blood smear preparation, 291f
Smoking, 360
Smooth muscle(s), 120, 121f
Sodium citrate, 40, 179–180
Sodium hypochlorite, 66
Sodium polyanetholesulfonate (SPS), 182, 251
Software, 334, 344
Somatotropin, 156, 159
Sore throat, 135
Special collections, 247–253
    blood culture collection systems, 251f
    handling procedures for, 252–253
    sample chain-of-custody form, 253f
    sample glucose tolerance test schedules, 249t
Special handling, 211–212
Special stains, 39

Specimen(s), 234, 362
  blood specimen processing, 341f
  collection and handling of, 198, 212, 253, 314, 341 - 343
    blood gases and, 314, 318, 320
    contamination of, 234, 270 - 271
    laboratory sections for, 39, 44, 47, 49, 51, 54
    receiving and transporting of, 340 - 341, 362
    serology section and, 49
    special collections, 252 - 253
  dermal puncture, 270 - 271
  finger and, 271f
  labeling of, 5, 211, 211f, 233
  quality control and, 355 - 357, 359, 361 - 363
Spermatozoa, 159, 162 - 164
Spina bifida, 118
Spinal cord, 129
Splenomegaly, 103 - 104, 107
Spreader slide(s), 289 - 290f
SPS. *See* Sodium polyanetholesulfonate (SPS)
SST. *See* Serum separator tube(s) (SST)
Standard System for the Identification of Fire Hazards of Materials, 69
STAT requests, quality control and, 357
STD. *See* Sexually transmitted diseases (STD)
Steady state, 311, 315
Stem cell(s), 97 - 98
Sterile, definition of, 50
Sterility, equipment and, 357, 359
Sternum, 114 - 115
Stomach, 144 - 145
Stool(s), 142, 144
Stop watch(es), bleeding time and, 292 - 293
Strep throat, 135, 337
Streptokinase, 311, 317
Stress, 360
Striated muscle(s), 119 - 120, 121f
Stroke, 130
Subclavian, definition of, 114
Subcutaneous, 83, 84f, 85
Superficial, definition of, 80
Superior, definition of, 80
Supine, definition of, 80
Support services, hospital's, 25
Surfactant, 134
Sweat electrolyte(s), collection of, 339 - 340, 340f
Sweat gland(s), 83 - 84, 84f, 85
Sweeps, 355
Synapse, 126 - 127, 129
Syncope, 224 - 226
Synovial joint(s), 115, 117f
Syringe(s), 176, 184 - 185, 207. *See also* Heparinized syringe(s)
  arterial blood gas collection and, 313 - 314
  blood transfer from, 185f
  needle structure of, 175f
  tube fill order in, 184f
  venipuncture complications and, 229, 229f, 230, 232 - 233

Systemic circulation, 90 - 91
Systemic lupus erythematosus (SLE), 118
Systole, 90, 96

T lymphocyte(s), 103 - 106
T3. *See* Triiodothyronine (T3)
T4. *See* Thyroxine (T4)
Tachometer(s), 354, 363
Tarsal(s), 114 - 115
TAT. *See* Turn-around-time (TAT)
TB. See Tuberculosis (TB)
TC. *See* Throat culture(s) (TC)
TDM. *See* Therapeutic drug monitoring (TDM)
Technical errors, 364
  effect on arterial blood gas results, 319t
  effect on blood smears, 291t
Telephone skills, 6 - 7
Template bleeding time procedure, 292, 293f
Tendon(s), 114, 118 - 119
Testosterone, 159, 162 - 164
Therapeutic drug monitoring (TDM), 43, 250
Therapeutic phlebotomy, 4, 102, 334, 339
Thixotropic gel, 173, 181, 181f
Thoracentesis, 131
Throat culture(s) (TC), 51
  collection of, 337, 337f
Thrombin, 90, 100
  collection tubes and, 181 - 182
Thrombin time (TT), function of, 41t
Thrombocyte(s), 90, 100
Thrombocytopenia, 102
Thrombolytic therapy, 311, 317, 319
Thrombus, 90, 227, 319
Thymosin, 159
Thymus gland, 104, 157, 159
Thyroid-stimulating hormone (TSH), 156, 159
Thyroxine (T4), 156 - 157, 159
Tibia, 114 - 115
Tibial, definition of, 114
Timed specimen(s), 27, 248 - 251
  sample glucose tolerance test schedules for, 249t
  special dermal puncture tests, 288, 291
  urine and fecal, 335 - 336
Time-stamping machine(s), 362, 363f
Tissue(s), specimen handling of, 340 - 341, 362
Tissue plasminogen activator (t-PA), 317
Tissue thromboplastin, 182, 184
Toe(s), dermal punctures in, 267 - 268
Tort, definition of, 4, 10
Total quality management (TQM), 354, 364 - 365
Tourniquet(s), 185 - 186, 186f, 233
  application of, 202 - 203, 203f, 205 - 206, 360
  venipuncture complications and, 226 - 227
Toxic shock syndrome (TSS), 166
Toxin, definition of, 50
t-PA. *See* Tissue plasminogen activator (t-PA)

TQM. *See* Total quality management (TQM)
Trachea, 132f, 133
Tracheotomy, 131
Transfusion, 46 - 47, 175, 225, 361
  blood donor collection for, 337 - 339
Transfusion reaction, 98
Transverse plane, 80 - 81, 81f
Triglycerides, 42
  tests on, 45t
Triiodothyronine (T3), 156 - 157, 159
Trough level, 250
TSH. *See* Thyroid-stimulating hormone (TSH)
TSS. *See* Toxic shock syndrome (TSS)
TT. *See* Thrombin time
Tuberculosis (TB), 135
Turn-around-time (TAT), 354, 357
Two-hour postprandial glucose, 249

UA. *See* Urinalysis (UA)
Ulcer, 145
Ulnar artery, 315
Unit(s) of blood, 46 - 47, 334, 337, 339
Universal precautions, 61, 65 - 66, 31
Unopette System, 265 - 266, 266f, 271
Upper respiratory infection (URI), 135
Upper respiratory tract, 132
Urea, 42
  tests on, 45t
Uremia, 146, 149
Ureter(s), 146 - 147, 147f - 148f
Urethra, 146 - 147, 147f - 148f, 149, 164
URI. *See* Upper respiratory infection (URI)
Uric acid, 42
  tests on, 45t
Urinalysis (UA), 335
  laboratory section for, 52 - 53, 53f, 54, 54t
Urinary, definition of, 146
Urinary system, 145 - 147, 148f
  disorders associated with, 149
  laboratory tests associated with, 150, 150t
  relationship of nephron to, 148f
Urinary tract infection, 150
Urine, 146, 149, 249
  specimen collection, 335, 335f
Urokinase, 311, 317
Urologist, definition of, 146

Vacutainer, 173, 176, 178, 185
Vacuum tube(s), 178, 179f, 181, 183, 185, 207
  summary of venipuncture technique with, 213
  venipuncture complications and, 226 - 227, 230, 232 - 233
Valve, 90, 92, 94 - 97
Variable factor(s)
  quality control and, 354 - 355
  specimen collection, handling, and, 357, 361 - 363
  major tests affected by, 360t
Varicella-zoster, 130

Varicose vein(s), 101
Vascular, 90
    skin area, 264f
Vasopressin, 156
Vector(s), 61 – 62
Vein(s), 90, 92 – 94, 97, 233, 262, 338
    comparison with arteries and
        capillaries, 92f, 95f
    selection of, 94f, 204, 204f, 205, 205f,
        206, 227
    small, needles and, 175 – 176, 178, 185
    tourniquet and, 186, 202
Venipuncture, 5, 92, 197 – 213, 362
    arm sites for, 94f, 204f
    complications of, 223 – 234
        possible reasons for failure, 232f
    equipment and for, 173 – 187, 202, 202f
        bandage on patient's arm, 212f
        butterfly apparatus, 230, 231f
        collection tubes, 178, 178f, 179, 179f,
            180 – 181, 181f, 182 – 183, 183t,
            184
        needles, 175, 175f, 176 – 177, 177f,
            207f, 211f
        phlebotomy collection tray, 174f
        phlebotomy drawing station, 175f

        syringes, 184f, 185, 185f, 229, 229f,
            230
        tourniquets, 185 – 186, 186f,
            202 – 203, 203f
        winged infusion sets, 185, 186f
    hand positioning during, 208f – 210f
    labeling the tube, 211f
    requisitions for, 198 – 199, 199f
    site selection for, 187, 203 – 206
        cleansing of, 206f
        complications with, 227 – 229
        locating the veins for, 205f
    special collections, 247 – 253
        blood culture collection systems,
            251f
        handling procedures for, 252 – 253
        sample chain-of-custody form, 253f
        sample glucose tolerance test
            schedules, 249t
Ventilation device(s), 311, 314
Ventral, 78, 81, 81f
Ventricle, 90, 94 – 97
Venule, 90, 92, 97
Verbal identification, 200, 267
Verbal skills, 6
Virology, definition of, 50

Volar surface, 287, 292
Voluntary muscle(s), 119
Voluntary nervous system, 127
Vomiting, 250

Warming, 262, 266 – 267, 320
Water and electrolyte balance, 149
Westergren sedimentation rate(s), 180
WBCs. See White blood cell(s) (WBCs)
White blood cell(s) (WBCs), 38, 90,
        98 – 100, 102, 360
    counts of, 41t
    normal, 99f
White matter, 127, 129
Whole blood, 38 – 39
Wicking of blood, bleeding time
        procedures and, 292, 294f
Winged infusion set(s), 185, 186f

X-match. See Crossmatch

Yellow top(s), 182, 183t
Yellow/gray top(s), 181 – 182, 183t